Endocrinology Research and Clinical Developments

nova
Medicine & Health
New York

Endocrinology Research and Clinical Developments

Management of Diabetes Mellitus Based on Natural Products
Yachana Mishra, PhD (Editor)
Vijay Mishra, PhD (Editor)
2023. ISBN: 979-8-88697-853-7 (Hardcover)
2023. ISBN: 979-8-88697-970-1 (eBook)

The Biochemical Guide to Hormones
David Aebisher, PhD, DSc (Editor)
2023. ISBN: 979-8-88697-492-8 (Hardcover)
2023. ISBN: 979-8-88697-534-5 (eBook)

Natural Products for Treatment of Metabolic Syndrome
Ajmer Singh Grewal, PhD (Editors)
Ashwani Kumar Dhingra, PhD (Editors)
2022. ISBN: 979-8-88697-152-1 (Hardcover)
2022. ISBN: 979-8-88697-233-7 (eBook)

A Clinical Guide to Thyroidectomies
Anand Mishra (Editor)
2022. ISBN: 978-1-68507-814-0 (Hardcover)
2022. ISBN: 979-8-88697-033-3 (eBook)

Polycystic Ovary Syndrome: Causes, Diagnosis and Management
Katherine Webb (Editor)
2021. ISBN: 978-1-53619-527-9 (Softcover)
2021. ISBN: 978-1-53619-586-6 (eBook)

More information about this series can be found at
https://novapublishers.com/product-category/series/endocrinology-research-and-clinical-developments/

Ajmer Singh Grewal
Geeta Deswal
Ashwani Kumar Dhingra
Priyanka Kriplani
Bhawna Chopra
and Shikha Baghel Chauhan
Editors

Naturally Occurring Chemicals for the Treatment and Management of Diabetes Mellitus and Related Disorders

nova
Medicine & Health
New York

DOI: https://doi.org/10.52305/WBBQ6236

NOTICE TO THE READER

Library of Congress Cataloging-in-Publication Data

Names: Grewal, Ajmer Singh, editor. | Deswal, Geeta, editor. | Dhingra, Ashwani K., editor. | Kriplani, Priyanka, editor. | Chopra, Bhawna, editor. | Chauhan, Shikha Baghel, editor.
Title: Naturally occurring chemicals for the treatment and management of diabetes mellitus and related disorders / editors Ajmer Singh Grewal (Associate Professor, Guru Gobind Singh College of Pharmacy, Yamuna Nagar, Haryana, India), Geeta Deswal, PhD (Professor, Guru Gobind Singh College of Pharmacy, Yamuna Nagar, Haryana, India), Ashwani Kumar Dhingra, PhD (Professor, Guru Gobind Singh College of Pharmacy, Yamuna Nagar, Haryana, India), Priyanka Kriplani, PhD (Professor, Guru Gobind Singh College of Pharmacy, Yamuna Nagar, Haryana, India), Bhawna Chopra, PhD (Professor, Guru Gobind Singh College of Pharmacy, Yamuna Nagar, Haryana, India), Shikha Baghel Chauhan, PhD (Associate Professor, Amity Institute of Pharmacy, Amity University, Noida, Uttar Pradesh, India).
Description: New York : Nova Science Publishers, [2024] | Series: Endocrinology research and clinical developments | Includes bibliographical references and index. |
Identifiers: LCCN 2024006358 (print) | LCCN 2024006359 (ebook) | ISBN 9798891134911 (hardcover) | ISBN 9798891136137 (adobe pdf)
Subjects: LCSH: Diabetes--Alternative treatment. | Herbs--Therapeutic use. | Materia medica, Vegetable.
Classification: LCC RC661.A47 N38 2024 (print) | LCC RC661.A47 (ebook) | DDC 616.4/62--dc23/eng/20240313
LC record available at https://lccn.loc.gov/2024006358
LC ebook record available at https://lccn.loc.gov/2024006359

Published by Nova Science Publishers, Inc. † New York

Contents

Preface

The field of diabetes mellitus and its management has witnessed remarkable advancements in recent years. As the prevalence of diabetes continues to rise globally, the need for effective treatments and interventions has become increasingly pressing. This book, "Naturally Occurring Chemicals for the Treatment and Management of Diabetes Mellitus and Related Disorders" is a comprehensive exploration of the potential of natural compounds derived from plants and marine sources in the management of diabetes and its associated complications. Diabetes, a complex metabolic disorder, poses significant health challenges for individuals and healthcare systems worldwide. This book aims to shed light on the multifaceted nature of diabetes mellitus, encompassing its diverse forms and the intricate interplay of factors contributing to its pathogenesis. It delves into the chronic hyperglycemia that characterizes diabetes, arising from deficiencies in insulin secretion, insulin action, or both, and how this condition manifests through symptoms such as increased thirst, urinary output, and the presence of ketone bodies in the blood or urine, signifying ketoacidosis. The chapters in this book are written by experts from various esteemed institutions, and they provide in-depth insights into the therapeutic potential of phytoconstituents for diabetes management. The research presented in these chapters spans a wide spectrum, covering herbal products, Thai traditional herbal plants, marine-based products, and the role of mushrooms, carbohydrates, glycosides, alkaloids, phenolic compounds, terpenoids, gingerols, organo-sulphur compounds, steroidal derivatives, saponins, catechins, allicin, arginine, berberine, charantin, curcumin, gallic acid, hesperidin, kaempferol, quercetin, resveratrol, rutin, and silymarin in managing diabetes mellitus. These natural compounds have garnered significant attention due to their potential to mitigate diabetes-related oxidative stress and inflammation, protect pancreatic β-cells, and enhance insulin sensitivity. Additionally, they exhibit minimal side effects, making them promising candidates for diabetes management. The chapters provide a wealth of knowledge on the biological properties, mechanisms of action, and clinical applications of these phytoconstituents, offering valuable insights for researchers, clinicians, and anyone interested in the field of diabetes mellitus.

As editors, we are honored to present this compilation of research and insights into the world of phytoconstituents and their role in diabetes management. We hope this book serves as a valuable resource in the ongoing quest to better understand, prevent, and treat diabetes mellitus and its complications. We extend our heartfelt gratitude to all the authors for their dedication and contribution to this book. We also thank the publishers for their support in bringing this important work to fruition.

We are extremely thankful to Prof. (Dr.) Kumar Guarve (Principal, Guru Gobind Singh of Pharmacy, Yamuna Nagar, Haryana, India) for his guidance, encouragement, and immense support during this assignment. We are also grateful to Ms. Nadya S. Gotsiridze-Columbus (President) and Mr. Thomas Mazzaferro of Nova Science Publishers, Inc., who took over the management of the production of this book and whose contribution is much appreciated. We sincerely hope that this book proves to be an informative and enlightening resource for all readers, ultimately contributing to improved diabetes care and the well-being of individuals affected by this global health challenge.

Dr. Ajmer Singh Grewal
Dr. Geeta Deswal
Dr. Ashwani Kumar Dhingra
Dr. Priyanka Kriplani
Dr. Bhawna Chopra
Dr. Shikha Baghel Chauhan
Editors

Chapter 1

Introduction to Diabetes Mellitus and Its Management

Sangya Dubey[1]
Janhavi Singh[1,*]
Manasvi Saini[1]
Chaitanay Vinayak Narayan[1]
Shallu Singh[2]
Shikha Baghel Chauhan[2]
Indu Singh[2]
Harsh Yadav[3]
and Sachin Gupta[3]
[1]I. T. S. College of Pharmacy, Muradnagar, Ghaziabad, Uttar Pradesh, India
[2]Amity Institute of Pharmacy, Amity University, Noida, Uttar Pradesh, India
[3]Department of Pharmacy, Indira Gandhi National Tribal University, Lal Pur, Amarkantak, Madhya Pradesh, India

Abstract

Diabetes mellitus is a rapidly progressing metabolic disorder characterized by increased insulin resistance, insufficient insulin production, or both, resulting in persistent hyperglycemia and impaired metabolism of proteins, carbohydrates, and fats. The financial burden of diabetes treatment affects all patients, regardless of their socioeconomic status. Diabetes is associated with an elevated risk of mortality due to

* Corresponding Author's Email: janhavisingh96@gmail.com.

In: Naturally Occurring Chemicals …
Editors: A. Singh Grewal, G. Deswal, A. Kumar Dhingra et al.
ISBN: 979-8-89113-491-1

complications such as pneumonia, kidney failure, cardiovascular disease, and influenza. These complications arise either due to inadequate insulin production, leading to elevated blood sugar levels, or the body's improper response to insulin. According to the World Health Organization (WHO), the number of adults with diabetes is expected to continue rising, with the majority of diabetic patients having type 2 diabetes mellitus, accounting for around 90-95% of cases. Effectively managing this disease requires a deep understanding of its underlying pathophysiology. In insulin-dependent diabetes mellitus, there is a severe deficiency in insulin production, necessitating the administration of insulin via intramuscular injection as the primary treatment option. Conversely, in non-insulin-dependent diabetes mellitus (NIDDM), the challenges are different. In NIDDM, cells in the body exhibit reduced sensitivity to insulin, or there is a decrease in insulin secretion from the pancreas. Therefore, the approach to treatment depends on the type and severity of diabetes in individual patients.

Keywords: diabetes mellitus, hyperglycemia, metabolism, NIDDM, pathophysiology, treatment

Abbreviations

AIDS	Acquired immune deficiency syndrome
DM	Diabetes mellitus
GDM	Gestational diabetes mellitus
HIV	Human immunodeficiency virus
IDDM	Insulin-dependent diabetes mellitus
NIDDM	Non-insulin-dependent diabetes mellitus
PPAR	Peroxisome proliferator-activated receptor
WHO	World health organization.

Introduction

Diabetes mellitus (DM) is a prevalent global public health concern affecting more than 400 million people worldwide (Khursheed et al., 2019). The term "diabetes" originates from the Greek word for "siphon," indicating the movement through a channel, and the Latin word "mellitus," meaning sweet. This metabolic disorder leads to chronic microvascular and neuropathic complications, as well as macrovascular issues. Effective treatment of diabetes depends on a thorough understanding of the underlying mechanisms responsible for these specific conditions (Simó and Hernández, 2002). The two most common types of diabetes are Type 1 diabetes mellitus (T1DM) and Type 2 diabetes mellitus (T2DM). In T1DM, the immune system targets and damages the beta cells within the islets of Langerhans in the pancreas, resulting in a complete lack of insulin production. Type 1B diabetes also involves insulin deficiency and a tendency toward ketosis but lacks the immunologic signature that signifies an autoimmune attack on β-cells. Genetic and metabolic factors often contribute to anomalies in insulin production and activity, leading to hyperglycemia. T1DM is a complex and multifaceted disease influenced by various non-HLA loci (Barroso et al., 1999). Despite affecting only 5 to 10% of all individuals with diabetes, an effective treatment for T1DM has not yet been discovered (Garg et al., 1988). According to the WHO and the American Diabetes Association, Type 1 diabetes has been categorized as autoimmune-based diabetes (Type 1A) and idiopathic diabetes associated with beta-cell dysfunction (Type 1B) (Jenkins et al., 1989). Management of this type of diabetes requires exogenous insulin to prevent diabetic ketoacidosis. T2DM, on the other hand, is considerably more common and can result from both insulin resistance and impaired insulin production, with either factor potentially occurring first. Individuals with T2DM often do not require exogenous insulin to regulate blood glucose levels but may need it if diet and oral hypoglycemic medications are insufficient. T2DM affects 90-95% of individuals with diabetes (Brenner et al., 1982). In cases where islet β-cell function is compromised, insulin secretion becomes inadequate, leading to increased glucose production by the liver and reduced glucose utilization by peripheral tissues (Hoewitz, 1990). Glucose homeostasis in the body is primarily regulated by two key hormones: insulin and glucagon. When blood glucose levels rise, beta cells release insulin, which works to reduce blood glucose through two main mechanisms. Firstly, it inhibits liver processes responsible for glucose production, namely gluconeogenesis and glycogenolysis. Secondly, it enhances the transport of glucose into cells, including muscle and adipose tissue. Conversely, when glucose levels drop, alpha cells in the pancreas secrete glucagon, which counteracts hypoglycemia by stimulating the liver to increase glucose release through glycogenolysis and gluconeogenesis. This intricate hormonal balance is essential for maintaining glucose levels within a narrow and healthy range (Okur et al., 2017; Galicia-Garcia et al., 2020).

Complications of DM

Cardiovascular Diseases

Atherosclerosis, a condition characterized by the buildup of plaque in the arteries due to chronic hyperglycemia and dyslipidemia, poses a significant risk of myocardial infarction (heart attack) and cerebral stroke, both of which can be fatal. In individuals with diabetes, cardiovascular diseases rank as the leading cause of death (Atkinson and Eisenbarth, 2001). It's worth noting that people with diabetes may not always experience the typical chest discomfort associated with heart issues, often referred to as silent ischemia. Therefore, a comprehensive cardiac assessment is advisable, especially for those undergoing significant surgical procedures. While there is evidence that better glycemic control can reduce microvascular complications in diabetes, its impact on macrovascular issues is less clear and may even exacerbate them. However, intensive treatment aimed at managing blood sugar levels may have a positive effect on lipid profiles, potentially reducing the risk of cardiovascular-related mortality. Additionally, individuals with diabetes are at a higher risk of cerebrovascular disease, such as strokes, in addition to coronary artery disease, further emphasizing the importance of managing these conditions (WHO, 1999).

Diabetic Nephropathy

Diabetes-related metabolic and hemodynamic changes can lead to glomerular sclerosis and fibrosis, both of which are characteristic of diabetic nephropathy. Diabetic nephropathy is associated with persistent albuminuria, high blood pressure, and can progress to end-stage renal failure. Notably, renal failure is observed in about 20-30% of individuals with type 2 diabetes, particularly those who have had the condition for an extended period, typically around 10 years. Microalbuminuria, an early sign of glomerular filtration dysfunction, is caused by alterations in the production and breakdown of various components of the glomerular basement membrane, including collagen and proteoglycans. These alterations lead to thickening of the glomerular basement membrane (Defronzo et al., 1997; Artasensi et al., 2020).

Diabetic Eye Diseases

Diabetic retinopathy is a condition that affects approximately three-quarters of individuals who have had diabetes for over 15 years. It progresses in severity, often leading to the development of new blood vessels in the retina. There are two primary types of diabetic retinopathy: non-proliferative and proliferative. The non-proliferative stage is characterized by retinal vascular microaneurysms, retinal hemorrhages, cotton-wool spots, loss of retinal pericytes, alterations in regional blood flow, increased retinal vascular permeability, and abnormal retinal microvasculature, all of which contribute to retinal ischemia. In the proliferative stage, new blood vessels may form near the optic nerve and/or macula, where they can be prone to ruptures, leading to fibrosis, retinal detachment, and vitreous hemorrhage (Lernmark and Ott, 1998). Diabetes can result in various visual problems, including diabetic retinopathy, cataracts, and glaucoma.

Diabetic Neuropathy

Diabetic neuropathy encompasses a spectrum of nerve disorders, ranging from polyneuropathy to mononeuropathy to autonomic neuropathy. Polyneuropathy can result in a loss of sensation in the extremities, and when combined with impaired microvascular and macrovascular function in the periphery, it can lead to chronic ulcers and, in severe cases, non-traumatic amputations. This condition involves changes such as microfilament reduction, axon thickening, and capillary narrowing in both small myelinated and non-myelinated C-fibers. These changes occur due to direct damage caused by the effects of hyperglycemia on nerve tissue and neuronal ischemia, leading to microvascular abnormalities. Mononeuropathy involves the dysfunction of individual cranial or peripheral nerves (Fajans et al., 2001). Diabetes affects nerve function, particularly in peripheral nerves and the autonomic nervous system, by impacting the small blood vessels that supply these nerves. Diabetic neuropathy can result in diabetic foot ulcers and lower limb amputations, as well as erectile dysfunction in males and diabetic gastropathy. Additionally, it can mask the symptoms of ischemic heart disease, potentially leading to clinically silent angina (Owen and Hattersley, 2001).

Infections

Infections tend to be both more frequent and more severe in individuals with DM. These increased infection risks can be attributed, in part, to incompletely understood abnormalities in cell-mediated immunity and phagocyte activity that are associated with hyperglycemia. The decreased vascularization that occurs as a result of long-term diabetes is another contributing factor. While many common infections are more severe and frequent in individuals with diabetes, there are also a few rare diseases that are almost exclusively observed in diabetics, such as rhinocerebral mucormycosis and malignant otitis externa. Urinary tract infections, pneumonia, and skin and soft tissue infections are the more common infections in the diabetic population (Taylor and Arioglu, 1999).

Treatments of DM

Non-Pharmacological Management

Diet

Calorific Value

Many individuals with T2DM (non-insulin-dependent diabetes mellitus (NIDDM)), are obese. Obesity is widely recognized as a significant factor contributing to insulin resistance, a hallmark of T2DM. Therefore, weight loss is a crucial component of managing NIDDM. In cases where rapid weight loss or extreme caloric restriction is necessary, an extremely low-calorie diet or a protein-sparing modified fast may be considered as part of the treatment plan. These interventions can help improve insulin sensitivity and glycemic control in overweight or obese individuals with T2DM.

Macronutrients

The ideal balance of carbohydrates, protein, and fat in the diet for patients with NIDDM is a topic of ongoing debate. Recent research has shown that a diet consisting of 60% carbohydrates, even if it doesn't include added sugars, can have an impact on the development of dyslipidemia (abnormal lipid levels in the blood). In the context of carbohydrates, it's advisable to focus on consuming complex carbohydrates that are high in soluble fiber and have low glycemic properties. However, moderate consumption of simple sugars like sucrose is generally considered to be harmless (Unger, 1971). Regarding protein intake, excessive consumption of high-protein diets can potentially have a negative effect on kidney function. Therefore, it's important for individuals with NIDDM not to exceed their daily protein requirements (Bin Rakhis et al., 2022; Unger, 1971). The optimal dietary balance for managing NIDDM may vary from person to person, and it's essential for individuals to work closely with healthcare professionals or registered dietitians to develop a personalized nutrition plan that suits their specific needs and health status.

Dietary Fibres

A recent study conducted by Hoewitz and published in Lancet in 1998 revealed that adding certain types of soluble fiber, particularly guar gum and pectin, to the diets of individuals with NIDDM can lead to significant reductions in postprandial (after-meal) glucose and insulin levels. Soluble fiber has been shown to have a beneficial impact on glycemic control by slowing down the absorption of glucose from the digestive tract and improving insulin sensitivity. These findings highlight the potential of dietary interventions, such as increasing soluble fiber intake, as a means to help manage blood glucose levels in individuals with NIDDM.

Fish Oils

Fish oils or fish-derived omega-3 fatty acids have been shown to reduce plasma triglyceride and lipoprotein levels, potentially aiding in the prevention of atherosclerotic vascular disease. However, studies have also indicated that in individuals with NIDDM, the reduction in plasma triglyceride levels is offset by negative effects on LDL cholesterol/ blood glucose (Groop, 1992).

Physical Activity

Current clinical studies have provided insight that exercise may aid in the management of high blood glucose levels. Additionally, strong evidence shows that daily exercise improves diagnosis in people with NIDDM/IDDM by influencing different cardiovascular disorders (Galloway et al., 1990). However, exercise may be detrimental to a tiny percentage of individuals and should not be advised. Regular exercise enhances insulin sensitivity, which can help with glucose tolerance. These benefits are a result of enzymatic adaptation in skeletal muscles, which is thought to increase maximum oxygen absorption, and also lead to a reduction in body weight. Such benefits are useful in diabetic patients because they improve the capacity to do work and quality of life, potentially lowering the need for insulin or oral hypoglycaemic medications (Stith et al., 1996).

Pharmacological Management of DM

Insufficient insulin release by an individual's β-cells leads to DM. Absolute insulin deficit occurs in patients with IDDM/NIDDM whose insulin activity is normal. Patients with insulin resistance often start with a relative shortage of insulin and develop absolute insulin deficiency over time. If patient education, dietary changes, and increased exercise have not helped a patient achieve their specific treatment objectives, drug therapy for NIDDM should be considered (Sharma et al., 2022). The most frequently used medications in NIDDM are listed in Table 1.

Table 1. Current treatments for type 2 diabetes and their molecular targets (Moller et al., 2001)

Drug class	Molecular target	Action site	Adverse events
Insulin	Insulin receptor	Liver, muscle, fat	Hypoglycemia, weight gain
Sulphonylureas (e.g., glibenclamide) plus nateglinide and repaglinide	SU receptor/K+ ATP channel	Pancreatic β cell	Hypoglycemia, weight gain
Metformin (biguanides)	Not disclose	Liver (muscle)	Gastrointestinal disturbance lactic acidosis
Acarbose	α-Glycosidase	Intestine	Gastrointestinal disturbances
Pioglitazone, rosiglitazone (thiazolidinediones)	PPAR-γ	Fat, muscle, liver	Weight gain, edema, anemia

Antidiabetic Drugs

Effective management of hyperglycemia is a crucial goal for type 2 diabetic patients to prevent macro- and microvascular complications (Lebovitz, 1997). The conventional approach begins with dietary modifications, exercise, and lifestyle recommendations aimed at helping obese individuals lose weight. However, more than four-fifths of currently diagnosed type 2 diabetes patients do not succeed with these interventions, and the progressive nature of the disease often necessitates pharmacological therapy for the majority of patients. Metformin, acarbose, and sulfonylureas are commonly used as monotherapies, and a new class of drugs called thiazolidinediones has recently been approved. If oral monotherapy fails to achieve adequate glycemic control, combinations of two different types of oral medications are often prescribed (Willson et al., 2000).

Treatment of NIDDM and Insulin Resistance

Insulin resistance is a prevalent feature of NIDDM and other components of this condition, although it is not commonly recognized as a clinical entity that requires its specific treatment. Using excessive amounts of insulin to amplify activation pathways or significantly reducing insulin levels to mitigate the effects of hyperinsulinemia are not straightforward strategies for addressing insulin resistance. Both approaches have their limitations. Increasing insulin levels can enhance the effects of insulin that are impeded by signal transduction bottlenecks. However, targeting the desired effect on a severely impaired insulin pathway (e.g., impaired glucose transport) may lead to an excess of other insulin effects. Insulin resistance can be exacerbated by excess insulin at both the receptor and post-receptor levels. Insulin therapy can, therefore, worsen the adverse consequences of hyperinsulinemia, with the added risk of excess insulin causing hypoglycemic episodes. Reducing insulin levels is a specific challenge in type 2 diabetes (Willson et al., 2000).

Conclusion

Recent research into the pathophysiology of diabetes has uncovered new pathways and factors that play a significant role in the onset and progression of the disease. The two main factors that contribute significantly to the development of diabetes are insulin resistance and beta cell dysfunction. In this chapter, we have discussed several factors that, while important, have not received enough attention in the etiology of T2DM. Multidrug combination therapy for diabetes may improve the health outcomes of T2DM patients but also present new challenges that require careful consideration. Multitargeting, which targets multiple pathways, is a promising approach for the treatment of T2DM. The primary challenge in treating T2DM is the inadequacy of single-target therapies.

References

Artasensi, A., Pedretti, A., Vistoli, G., Fumagalli, L. (2020). Type 2 diabetes mellitus: a review of multi-target drugs. *Molecules*, 25(8), 1987.

Atkinson, M. A., Eisenbarth, G. S. (2001). Type I diabetes: new prospective on disease pathogenesis and treatment. *Lancet*, 358(9277), 221-229.

Barroso, I., Gurnell, M., Crowley, V. E., Agostini, M., Schwabe, J. W., Soos, M. A., Maslen, G. L., Williams, T. D., Lewis, H., Schafer, A. J., Chatterjee, V. K., O'Rahilly, S. (1999). Dominant negative mutations in human PPARgamma associated with severe insulin resistance, diabetes mellitus and hypertension. *Nature*, 402(6764), 880-883.

Bin Rakhis, S., AlDuwayhis, N., Aleid, N., AlBarrak, A., Aloraini, A. (2022). Glycemic control for type 2 diabetes mellitus patients: a systematic review. *Cureus*, 14(6), e26180.

Brenner, B. M., Meyer, T. W., Hostetter, T. H. (1982) Dietary pattern and the progressive nature of kidney disease. *New England Journal of Medicine*, 307, 652-660.

Defronzo, R. A. (1997). Pathogenesis of type 2 diabetes: metabolic and molecular implication for identifying diabetes genes. *Diabetes Reviews*, 177-267.

Fajans, S. S., Bell, G. I., Polonsky, K. S. (2001). Molecular mechanisms and clinical pathophysiology of maternity-onset diabetes of the young. *New England Journal of Medicine*, 345, 971-980.

Galicia-Garcia, U., Benito-Vicente, A., Jebari, S., Larrea-Sebal, A., Siddiqi, H., Uribe, K. B., Ostolaza, H., Martín, C. (2020). Pathophysiology of type 2 diabetes mellitus. *International Journal of Molecular Sciences*, 21(17), 6275.

Galloway, J. A. (1990). Treatment of NIDDM with insulin agonists or substitute. *Diabetes Care*, 13, 1209-1239.

Garg, A., Bonanome, A., Grundy, S. M. (1999). Comparison of a high-carbohydrate diet with a high-monounsaturated-fat diet in patients with non-insulin-dependent diabetes mellitus. *New England Journal of Medicine*, 319, 829-834.

Groop, L. C. (1992). Sulfonylureas in NIDDM. *Diabetes Care*, 15, 737-754.

Hoewitz, D. L. (1990). Dietary adjuncts: Efficacy and inadequacy. In: Bailey et al. (eds.) *New Antidiabetic Drugs*. Smith-Gordon, London; pp. 53-63.

Jenkins, D. J. A., Jenkin, A. L., Volever, T. M. S. (1989). Aim of diet in diabetes management. In: Creutzfeldt, W., Lefebvre, P. (eds.) *Diabetes Mellitus: Pathophysiology and Therapy*. Springer Verlag, Berlin; pp. 299-308.

Khursheed, R., Singh, S., Wadhwa, S., Kapoor, B, Gulati, M., Kumar, R. (2019). Treatment strategies against diabetes: Success so far and challenges ahead. *European Journal of Pharmacology*, 862, 172625,

Lebovitz, H. E. (1997). alpha-Glucosidase inhibitors. *Endocrinology and Metabolism Clinics of North America*, 26(3), 539-551.

Lernmark, A., Ott, J. (1998). Sometimes it's hot, sometimes it's not. *Nature Genetics*, 1998, 213-214.

Moller, D. E. (2001). New drug targets for type 2 diabetes and the metabolic syndrome. *Nature*, 414, 821-827.

Okur, M., Karantas, I., Siafaka, P. (2017). Diabetes mellitus: a review on pathophysiology, current status of oral medications and future perspectives. *Acta Pharmaceutical Sciences*, 55, 61-82.

Owen, K, Hattersley, A. T. (2001). Maternity onset diabetes of the young: from clinical description to molecular genetics characterization. *Best Practice & Research Clinical Endocrinology & Metabolism*, 15, 309-323.

Sharma, P., Singh, S., Sharma, N., Singla, D., Guarve, K., Grewal, A. S. (2022). Targeting human glucokinase for the treatment of type 2 diabetes: an overview of allosteric glucokinase activators. *Journal of Diabetes and Metabolic Disorders*, 21(1), 1129-1137.

Sharma, P., Singh, S., Thakur, V., Sharma, N., Grewal, A. S. (2021). Novel and emerging therapeutic drug targets for management of type 2 diabetes mellitus. *Obesity Medicine*, 23, 100329.

Simó, R., Hernández, C. (2002). [Treatment of diabetes mellitus: general goals, and clinical practice management]. *Revista Española de Cardiología*, 55(8), 845-860.

Stith, B. J., Goalstone, M. L., Espinoza, R., Mossel, C., Roberts, D., Wiernsperge, N. (1996). The antidiabetic drug metformin elevates receptor tyrosine kinase and inositol 1,4,5-triphosphate mass in Xenopus oocytes. *Endocrinology*, 137, 2990-2999.

Taylor, S. I., Arioglu, E. (1999). Genetically defined forms of diabetes in children. *Journal of Clinical Endocrinology and Metabolism*, 84, 4390-4396.

UK Prospective Diabetes Study (UKPDS) Group. (1998). Intensive blood-glucose control with sulphonylureas or insulin compared with conventional treatment and risk of complications in patients with type 2 diabetes (UKPDS 33). *Lancet*, 352, 837-853.

Unger, R. H. (1971). Glucagon physiology and pathophysiology. *New England Journal of Medicine*, 285, 443-449.

Willson, T. M., Brown, P. J., Strenbach, D. D., Henke, B. R. (2000). The PPARs: from orphan receptors to drug discovery. *Journal of Medicinal Chemistry*, 43, 527-550.

World Health Organization (WHO). (1999). *Definition, Diagnosis and classification of diabetes mellitus and its complications. Part 1: Diagnosis and classifications of diabetes mellitus*. Department of Non-communicable Disease Surveillance, Geneva.

Chapter 2

Herbal Products for the Management of Diabetes Mellitus

Raj Kumari[1,*]
Meenakshi Sharma[1]
Sweta Pundir[1]
Kajal Chaudhary[2]
Anjali Rajora[3]
Anjali Nayak[4]
Paramita Das[4]
S. Lakshmi[4]
and Sakshi Bharadwaj[5]

[1]I. T. S. College of Pharmacy, Muradnagar, Ghaziabad, Uttar Pradesh, India
[2]Ram-Eesh Institute of Pharmacy, Knowledge Park-I, Greater Noida, Uttar Pradesh, India
[3]Lloyd School of Pharmacy, Knowledge Park-II, Greater Noida, Uttar Pradesh, India
[4]Krupanidhi College of Pharmacy, Chikka Bellandur, Carmelaram, Bengaluru, Karnataka, India
[5]Life Science Department, Altem Technologies, Bangalore, Karnataka, India

Abstract

Diabetes mellitus is a chronic non-communicable disease characterized by high blood sugar (glucose) levels. Challenges with conventional therapies have led to the exploration of alternative herbal treatments. Herbal medicinal products have been valued sources of medicine throughout human history. These products encompass natural remedies

* Corresponding Author's Email: rajkataria80@gmail.com.

In: Naturally Occurring Chemicals …
Editors: A. Singh Grewal, G. Deswal, A. Kumar Dhingra et al.
ISBN: 979-8-89113-491-1

that contain specific herbal medications or preparations composed of one or a combination of herbs. Medicinal plants, in addition to their natural therapeutic benefits for diabetes mellitus, have demonstrated antidiabetic properties due to the presence of compounds like phenolics, flavonoids, terpenoids, coumarins, and other components that can lower blood glucose levels. Herbal products are available in various forms, including powders, extracts, distillates, and juices, obtained by processing herbal substances for human use. *Galega officinalis*, for instance, is rich in hypoglycemic ingredients like guanidine. Many medicinal plants with known antidiabetic properties, such as *Withania somnifera, Tinospora cordifolia, Trigonella foenum graecum, Momordica charantia, Eugenia jambolana, Phyllanthus amarus, Pterocarpus marsupium,* and *Allium sativum*, offer additional health benefits alongside their potential in managing diabetes.

Keywords: diabetes mellitus, hypoglycaemic agents, herbal products, type I diabetes, type II diabetes

Abbreviations

LDL	Low-density lipoprotein
T1D	Type 1 diabetes
T2D	Type 2 diabetes
TCM	Traditional Chinese medicine.

Introduction

Millions of people worldwide suffer from chronic non-communicable conditions known as diabetes mellitus, which has been linked to the onset of various severe diseases, including microvascular (nephropathy, retinopathy, and neuropathy) and macrovascular (peripheral vascular disease and coronary heart disease) complications. Diabetes mellitus, commonly referred to as diabetes, was historically identified by the presence of "sweet urine" and muscle wasting. It is characterized by elevated blood sugar (glucose) levels due to the body's inability to efficiently produce or use insulin. Insulin, a pancreatic hormone, plays a critical role in the metabolism of carbohydrates, lipids, and proteins by promoting glucose uptake into cells. Diabetes mellitus is a non-communicable endocrine disorder that disrupts carbohydrate metabolism and results in hyperglycemia. Insulin, produced by the pancreas, regulates blood glucose levels. When blood glucose levels rise, the pancreas releases insulin to maintain glucose levels within a normal range. Among individuals with diabetes, inadequate insulin production leads to hyperglycemia. If not properly managed, diabetes can lead to serious complications, including cardiovascular diseases, kidney damage, neuropathy, and vision loss (Forouhi and Wareham, 2014). There are two main types of diabetes: Type 1 diabetes (T1D), characterized by an absolute lack of insulin due to autoimmune destruction of insulin-producing beta cells in the pancreas, and Type 2 diabetes (T2D), caused by a combination of insulin deficiency and insulin resistance (American Diabetes Association, 2020). T1D is also known as insulin-dependent diabetes mellitus because it results in a complete loss of functionality in all pancreatic islets of Langerhans cells. The aim of this chapter is to provide a comprehensive overview of herbal products used in the treatment of diabetes mellitus.

Conventional Treatment

The primary treatment for T1D involves the lifelong administration of exogenous insulin through injections or insulin pumps. This is necessary to replace the missing hormone and maintain blood sugar levels within a predefined range. To reduce the risk of complications, individuals with T1D must also regularly monitor their blood sugar levels, follow a healthy diet, and engage in regular physical activity (Chiang et al., 2015). T2D, on the other hand, accounts for 90-95% of all cases of diabetes, according to the American Diabetes Association (2020). Its defining characteristics are insulin resistance, where the body's cells do not respond to insulin as effectively as they should, and a gradual decline in pancreatic insulin production. T2D typically develops in individuals over the age of 40, but due to the increasing prevalence of obesity and sedentary lifestyles, it is now being diagnosed in younger populations as well. Risk factors for T2D include obesity, physical inactivity, a family history of diabetes, and belonging to specific ethnic groups (Forouhi and Wareham, 2014; Sharma et al., 2022). The management of T2D focuses on lifestyle measures, such as dietary changes and increased physical activity, to improve insulin sensitivity and lower blood sugar levels. If lifestyle modifications are not sufficient, oral hypoglycemic drugs like metformin or injectable medications like GLP-1 receptor agonists may be used to help regulate blood sugar. In advanced stages of T2D, when other treatments fail to maintain blood sugar levels within therapeutic ranges, insulin therapy may be necessary (Davies et al., 2018; Sharma et al., 2021).

Herbal Medicines

Herbal medicines have a long history of use in various civilizations, including Chinese, Indian, Egyptian, and Greek cultures, dating back to ancient times (Patwardhan et al., 2005). These traditional systems of medicine, such as Traditional Chinese Medicine (TCM), Ayurveda, and Unani, have relied heavily on the use of herbal remedies and continue to do so today (Ekor, 2014). In recent years, scientific research has shed light on the therapeutic potential of many medicinal plants, particularly in the treatment of diabetes and other chronic diseases. It's worth noting that numerous pharmaceutical drugs have their origins in plant sources. There is a growing demand for natural, safe, and cost-effective treatment options, which has further driven the interest in herbal products (Kooti et al., 2016). Medicinal plants contain a diverse array of active components, and their therapeutic effects are attributed to various compounds, including phenolic compounds, flavonoids, terpenoids, and coumarins. These components often work synergistically, providing antioxidant, anti-inflammatory, and anti-diabetic properties. This multifaceted nature of herbal medicines enhances their potential for treating diabetes and makes them attractive as complementary or alternative therapies to conventional treatments (Table 1).

Plants with Hypoglycaemic Activity

Ashwagandha (*Withania somnifera*)

Ashwagandha, also known as Indian ginseng, is a small woody shrub native to India, North Africa, and the Middle East. It has a history of use in Ayurvedic medicine spanning more than 3000 years and has been employed to address various health issues, including diabetes. The medicinal properties of Ashwagandha can be attributed to the rich array of bioactive compounds found in its roots and leaves, including withanolides, alkaloids, and steroidal lactones. One of the notable benefits of Ashwagandha is its ability to increase insulin sensitivity, making it valuable for individuals with insulin resistance who need to regulate their blood sugar levels. It achieves this by enhancing glucose uptake into skeletal muscle cells, contributing to its anti-diabetic effects. Research involving diabetic rats treated with Ashwagandha root extract demonstrated improved glycemic control and increased insulin production, which was attributed to the restoration of pancreatic islet structure and function. Additionally, Ashwagandha's anti-inflammatory and antioxidant properties help mitigate the chronic inflammation and oxidative stress often associated with diabetes. These protective effects can reduce the risk of diabetes-related complications such as nephropathy, neuropathy, and retinopathy. Furthermore, Ashwagandha has been found to have a positive impact on mental health. Studies have shown that Ashwagandha can help alleviate mental health issues (such as stress, anxiety, or depression), providing holistic support for individuals with diabetes (Choudhary et al., 2017; Chandrasekhar et al., 2012).

Guduchi (*Tinospora cordifolia*)

Guduchi, a perennial climbing shrub indigenous to India and other parts of South Asia, has a long history of traditional use for various health conditions, including diabetes, inflammation, and immune system disorders. Its antidiabetic properties are primarily attributed to the presence of bioactive compounds in different parts of the plant, including alkaloids, glycosides, and polysaccharides. Recent research has shed light on Guduchi's mechanisms of action in controlling diabetes. One significant way it benefits glycemic control is by stimulating the beta cells of the pancreas to secrete insulin. This effect helps in regulating blood sugar levels. Guduchi has also been found to enhance glucose uptake by skeletal muscle cells, further contributing to its antidiabetic effects. Another crucial aspect of Guduchi's antidiabetic benefits is its inhibition of α-glucosidase activity. α-glucosidase is an enzyme responsible for breaking down carbohydrates in the intestine.

Table 1. Medicinal plants and their specific constituents used for the management of diabetes mellitus (Pandey and Rizvi, 2009)

Plant name	Family	Plant part/ form used	Chemical constituents	Mode of action
Aegle marmelos (Bael)	Rutaceae	Leaves extracts	Aegle marmelosine	Improve the functional state of pancreatic β-cells
Allium cepa (Onion)	Lilliaceae	Dried powder	Dipropyl disulphide oxide	Stimulating the impact on glucose utilization and antioxidant enzyme
Allium sativum (Garlic)	Lilliaceae	Petroleum ether extract from bulbs	Allyproyl disulphide oxide, allicin	Improve plasma lipid metabolism and have antioxidant activity
Aloe barbadensis (Ghikanwar)	Asphodelaceae	Leaf pulp extract	β-Sitosterol, campesterol	Improvement in glucose tolerance
Andrographis paniculate (Kalmegh)	Acanthaceae	Whole plant	Kalmeghin	Increases utilization of glucose and decreases plasma glucose
Annona squamosa (Sharifa)	Annonaceae	Leaf extract	Liriodenin, moupinamide	A spike in glucose tolerance
Artemisia pallens (Dhavanam)	Asteraceae	Leaf and flowers extract	Germacranolide	Lower plasma level
Areca catechu (Areca nut)	Arecaceae	Seeds extract	Arecaine, Arecoline	Improve glucose tolerance
Azadirachta indica (Neem)	Meliaceae	Leaf Extract	Azadirachitin, nimbin	Epinephrine's glycogenolytic impact was inhibited
Bauhinia forficate (Kachnar)	Leguminosae	Leaves	Astragalin, kaempferitrin	Act by antiglycation activity
Beta vulgaris (Beet root)	Amaranthaceae	Root extract	Phenolics, betacyanins	Reduced insulin and blood sugar levels
Boerhavia diffusa (Punarnava)	Nyctaginaceae	Whole plant	Punarnavine and ursolic acid	Reduced insulin and blood sugar levels
Brassica juncea (Mustard)	Brassicaceae	Aqueous extract	Sulforaphane	Increased glycogen synthetase activity
Cajanus cajan (Arhar)	Fabaceae	Seeds	2'-Methyl cajanone, isoflavones, cajanin, cahanones	Decrease in blood sugar that is significant
Carica papaya (Papaya)	Caricaceae	Aqueous seed extract	Papain, chymopapin	Reduced triglyceride, and values of fasting blood sugar and total cholesterol
Carum carvi (Caraway)	Apiaceae	Aqueous seed extract	Furfurol, carvone	Significant lowering high blood sugar

Plant name	Family	Plant part/ form used	Chemical constituents	Mode of action
Cassia auriculata (Tanner's cassia)	Leguminosae	Aqueous seed extract	Limonene, terpinol	Increase hepatic activity, hexohinase, phosphor fruictokinase
Catharanthus roseus (vinca)	Apocyanaceae	Decoction of leaves	Vincristine, vinblastine Catharanthaine	Lowering of blood sugar
Coccinia indica (Baby water melon)	Cucurbitaceae	Whole plant ethanolic extract	Glutamic acid, asparagine	Reduced glucose production results in decreased amounts of blood sugar
Coriandrum sativum (Coriander)	Apiaceae	Seed extract	p-Cymene, linalool	Decreases serum glucose and increases β-cells
Cinnamomum cassia (Cinnamon)	Lauraceae	Bark	Cinnamaldehyde, eugenol	Increases insulin levels receptor's sensitivity
Cinnamomum tamala (Tejpat)	Lauraceae	Leaf extract	Linalool, β-caryophyllene	Insulin is released from pancreatic β - cells.
Curcuma longa (Turmeric)	Zingiberaceae	Powdered form	α -Phellantrene, tripinolene	Reduces blood sugar and boosts glucose metabolism
Elephantopus scaber (Gobhi)	Asteraceae	Whole plant	Terpenoid and 2,6,23-trienolide	Reducing the elevated blood sugar level and re-establishing insulin levels
Eugenia jambolana (Jamun)	Myrataceae	Pulp of fruit	Oleanolic acid, ellagic acid	The liver's insulinase activity was obstructed
Ficus bengalensis (Bargad)	Moraceae	Stem bark extract	Leucodelphinidin	Increased synthesis of insulin from β-cells.
Ficus hispida (Daduri)	Moraceae	Alcoholic leaf extract	Ficustriol, O-methyltylophorinidine	A drop in blood glucose and an increase in serum insulin
Gymnena sylvestre (Gudmar)	Asclepidaceae	Dried leaves	Dihydroxy gymnemic triacetate	Increase the serum G peptide level which monitor the release of enogenous insulin
Gynandropsis gynandra (Safed hulhul)	Capparidaceae	Root extract	N, N-Diethyltoluamide	Increase sensitivity to insulin and subsequently lower the amount of blood sugar
Mangifera indica (Mango)	Anacardiaceae	Leaves extract	β-Carotene, α-carotene	Decrease in the glucose absorption by the gut
Lantana camara (Raimuniya)	Verbenaceae	Leaf extract	Lantanoside, lantanone	Glucose lowering activity
Liriope spicata (Border grass)	Liliaceae	Root extract	β-Sitosterol, stigmasterol	Activation of P13K and insulin induce glycogen synthesis

Table 1. (Continued)

Plant name	Family	Plant part/ form used	Chemical constituents	Mode of action
Momordica charantia (Bitter gourd)	Curcubitaceae	Fresh green leaves	Charantin, sterol	Lower plasma apo β-100 and activates PPARs in mice given a high-fat diet
Musa paradisiacal (Banana)	Musaceae	Flower	β-Sitosterol, leucocyanidin, syringin	Rise in total haemoglobin while lowering glucose levels and glycosylated haemoglobin levels
Ocimum sanctum (Tulsi)	Labiateae	Whole herbs	Eugenol	Boost insulin production
Panex ginseng (Ginseng)	Araliaceae	Root extract	Ginsenosides, pro-topanaxadiol	Reduces intake of glucose and inhibits α-glycosidase
Parinari excelsa (Guinea plum)	Chrysobalanaceae	Bark decoction	Myricetin, quercertin	Induced insulin secretion
Phyllanthus emblica (Amla)	Euphorbiaceae	Leaf methanolic extract	Phyllanthin	Lower blood sugar levels
Prunus amygdalus (Almond)	Rosaceae	Seed extract	Amygdalin	Reduce the amount of blood glucose
Pterocarpus marsupium (Bigasal)	Leguminosae	Whole plant	Kenotannic acid, pyrocatechin	Decrease the elevated α-TNF and high blood sugar
Punica grantum (Pomegranate)	Puniaceae	Methanolic seed extract	Punicalagin, punicalin	The reduction of blood sugar
Ricinus communis (Arandi)	Euphorbiaceae	Root extract	Ricinolic acid	Decreasing blood sugar levels
Salacia oblonga wall (Arhar)	Celastraceae	Root bark	Salacinol	The inhibition of metabolic enzymes, which prevents postprandial hyperglycemia
Sarcopoterium spinosum (Spiny burnet)	Rosaceae	Plant root	Catechin and epicatechin	It induced insulin secretion
Smallanthus sonchifolius (Yacon)	Asteraceae	Fresh and dried leaves	Sonchifolin, uvedalin, enhydrin, fluctuanin	Lower the blood glucose level
Swertia chirata (Chirata)	Gentinaceae	Whole herbs	Methyl swertianin	Lower amount of blood glucose
Terminelia arjuna (Arjuna)	Combertaceae	Stem bark	Arjunic acid, arjunolic acid	Lower levels of blood sugar and G6P activity

Plant name	Family	Plant part/ form used	Chemical constituents	Mode of action
Terminelia cattappa (Almond)	Combertaceae	Fruit extract in petroleum ether	Omega-9 fatty acid	Lower amount of blood sugar
Tinospora cardifolia (Geloy)	Menispermaceae	Root's aqueous extract	Tinosporone, tinosporic acid	Decrease in brain lipids and blood sugar
Trigonella foenum Graecum (Methi)	Fabaceae	Ethanolic leaf extract	4-Hydroxy-isoleucine	Increase insulin production, reduce insulin resistance and decrease sugar levels
Vernonia anthelmintica	Asteraceae	Seed	Epoxy acid or vernolic acid	Lowers amount of blood sugar
Zingiber officinalis (Sunth)	Zingiberaceae	Rhizome	Gingerol, shogaol	Rise insulin levels

By blocking this enzyme, Guduchi slows down carbohydrate digestion, preventing rapid spikes in blood sugar levels after meals. Additionally, Guduchi exhibits antioxidant and anti-inflammatory properties. These qualities play a vital role in reducing inflammation and lowering the risk of diabetes-related complications such as cardiovascular disease, nephropathy, and neuropathy. In diabetic rats, Guduchi has been shown to reduce elevated levels of total cholesterol, triglycerides, and LDL cholesterol, further contributing to its potential in managing diabetes and associated conditions (Rajalakshmi et al., 2013; Sannegowda et al., 2015).

Methi (*Trigonella foenum graecum*)

Fenugreek, commonly known as Methi, has been recognized for its antidiabetic properties, which include enhancing insulin sensitivity and improving glucose tolerance. It is native to regions like Western Asia, Southern Europe, and the Mediterranean area and has a long history of use in traditional medicinal systems such as Ayurveda, Unani, and Chinese medicine for various health conditions, including diabetes, digestive disorders, and inflammatory diseases. Fenugreek's seeds and leaves are the primary parts of the plant used for their therapeutic effects. These parts contain several bioactive compounds, including alkaloids, flavonoids, and saponins, contributing to their medicinal properties. One of fenugreek's key mechanisms in managing diabetes is its ability to modulate glucose metabolism. This action is primarily attributed to galactomannan, a soluble fiber abundant in fenugreek seeds. Galactomannan slows down the absorption of glucose in the intestine, which can help regulate blood sugar levels. Moreover, the fiber content in fenugreek promotes a feeling of fullness, potentially assisting individuals with diabetes in managing their weight. Another valuable component in fenugreek is 4-hydroxyisoleucine, an amino acid. This compound has been found to enhance insulin sensitivity in peripheral tissues and stimulate insulin production in pancreatic beta cells, further aiding in glycemic control. Beyond its direct antidiabetic effects, fenugreek also possesses anti-inflammatory and antioxidant properties. These additional qualities can be beneficial for individuals with diabetes by reducing oxidative stress and inflammation often associated with the condition. Moreover, there have been reports suggesting that fenugreek can lower lipid levels, including total cholesterol. This effect may contribute to the prevention and treatment of cardiovascular complications in individuals with diabetes, further highlighting the potential benefits of fenugreek in diabetes management (Kaviarasan et al., 2006; Alam et al., 2011).

Karela (*Momordica charantia*)

Karela, also known as bitter melon, belongs to the Cucurbitaceae family and has a history of use in traditional medicinal systems such as Ayurveda and African traditional medicine to treat various ailments, including diabetes, inflammation, and infections. Karela's notable antidiabetic properties are primarily attributed to its ability to lower blood glucose levels and improve glucose tolerance (Joseph and Jini, 2013). These effects are associated with several bioactive compounds found in the bitter melon, including charantin, vicine, and polypeptide-p. Charantin, a cucurbitane-type triterpenoid present in Karela's fruit, leaves, and seeds, exhibits insulin-like actions. It encourages glucose uptake in peripheral tissues and helps prevent the liver from producing glucose through gluconeogenesis. This dual mechanism contributes to its antidiabetic effects (Ahmed et al., 2001). In addition to its direct antidiabetic effects, Karela is linked to anti-inflammatory and antioxidant properties. These qualities can be beneficial for individuals with diabetes as they may help reduce inflammation and oxidative stress, which are often associated with the condition (Chen et al., 2003).

Jamun (*Eugenia jambolana*)

Jamun or Indian blackberry, is an evergreen tropical tree native to the Indian subcontinent. In traditional medical systems like Ayurveda and Unani, jamun has been used to treat various illnesses, including diabetes, diarrhea, and digestive issues. Jamun's antidiabetic properties are attributed to the presence of bioactive compounds found in its fruit, seeds, and bark. These compounds include jambosine, ellagic acid, and anthocyanins (Mandal et al., 2007). Jambosine has been shown to have hypoglycemic effects by inhibiting the digestion and absorption of carbohydrates in the gastrointestinal tract. It also promotes the production of insulin in the pancreas, contributing to better glycemic control. Ellagic acid, a polyphenolic molecule found in jamun, possesses antioxidant and anti-inflammatory properties. This compound may help prevent and alleviate diabetes-related complications, such as cardiovascular disease and neuropathy. Anthocyanins, the water-soluble pigments responsible for jamun's deep purple color, have demonstrated the ability to enhance insulin sensitivity and reduce insulin resistance in animal studies. This effect can be beneficial for individuals with diabetes. Jamun is also believed to have antibacterial, anti-inflammatory, and analgesic qualities in addition to its antidiabetic effects (Chattopadhyay, 2006; Pari and Satheesh, 2002; Basha and Sankaranarayanan, 2014).

Bhumyamalaki (*Phyllanthus amarus*)

Bhumyamalaki, commonly known as stonebreaker, is a widespread herbaceous plant found in tropical climates. It has demonstrated anti-diabetic effects by improving insulin sensitivity and facilitating glucose uptake in cells (Ilangkovan et al., 2016). In Ayurvedic and folk medicine, bhumyamalaki has been traditionally used to treat various ailments, including diabetes, liver diseases, and urinary tract infections. The antidiabetic properties of bhumyamalaki are attributed to the presence of bioactive compounds found in its leaves, stems, and roots. These compounds include flavonoids, alkaloids, and phenolic acids (Chatterjee et al., 2012). Phenolic acids such as gallic acid and ellagic acid found in bhumyamalaki have been shown to possess anti-inflammatory and antioxidant effects. These effects can be beneficial in preventing and managing diabetes-related complications like neuropathy and nephropathy. Additionally, bhumyamalaki has been found to have lipid-lowering properties. Studies in both animals and individuals with diabetes have indicated that bhumyamalaki extract can reduce levels of total cholesterol. This effect may contribute to the control and prevention of cardiovascular problems in individuals with diabetes (Saxena et al., 2013).

Indian Kino (*Pterocarpus marsupium*)

Indian kino, an indigenous deciduous tree of India, has been found to possess anti-diabetic characteristics by improving glucose utilization and stimulating insulin production (Grover et al., 2005). In Ayurvedic medicine, it has a long history of use in treating various ailments, including diabetes, diarrhea, and skin conditions. It contains bioactive compounds such as pterostilbene and epicatechin, which are believed to contribute to its antidiabetic potential.

Pterostilbene exhibits hypoglycemic effects by inhibiting the alpha-glucosidase and alpha-amylase enzymes responsible for breaking down carbohydrates in the gut (Singh et al., 2011). This action can slow the rate at which glucose enters the bloodstream, reducing post-meal blood sugar levels. Epicatechin has demonstrated anti-inflammatory and antioxidant effects. These effects may help prevent and manage diabetes-related complications like retinopathy and nephropathy (Sultan et al., 2014). Additionally, this plant has been associated with anti-inflammatory, analgesic, and wound-healing properties, in addition to its antidiabetic benefits.

Garlic (*Allium sativum*)

Garlic has demonstrated anti-diabetic properties by improving glucose tolerance and reducing blood glucose levels. It has been used for centuries in both culinary and medicinal contexts. While it is renowned for its cardiovascular benefits, it has also been found to possess antidiabetic properties. The primary active ingredients in garlic responsible for its medicinal benefits include organosulfur compounds, flavonoids, and arginine. Taking garlic powder supplements for 12 weeks significantly decreased fasting blood glucose levels and HbA1c in a randomized controlled trial involving 60 individuals with T2D. Additionally, garlic has cholesterol-lowering effects, which may assist diabetics in preventing and managing cardiovascular issues (Ashraf et al., 2005). Garlic also possesses antioxidant, antibacterial, and anti-inflammatory properties that contribute to its antidiabetic effects. These actions can help reduce infections, inflammation, and oxidative stress associated with diabetes-related complications, thereby improving the overall health of individuals with diabetes. It's important to note that while garlic is generally considered safe, individuals taking blood-thinning medications should exercise caution, as garlic may potentiate the effects of these medications (Ashraf et al., 2018).

Conclusion

Research on herbal products must continue in order to gain a better understanding of their effectiveness, safety, and optimal application in the treatment of diabetes. This research can help integrate herbal therapy with conventional medicine and provide individuals with diabetes with more treatment options. In conclusion, both traditional medicine and scientific studies have shown positive outcomes when using herbal medications for diabetes management. By understanding the various herbal products, their potential benefits, and addressing challenges and limitations, more effective and safe treatment solutions can be developed.

References

Ahmed, I., Adeghate, E., Cummings, E., Sharma, A. K. (2001). Beneficial effects and mechanism of action of Momordica charantia juice in the treatment of streptozotocin-induced diabetes mellitus in rat. *Molecular and Cellular Biochemistry*, 224(1-2), 45-51.

Alam, M. A., Sernia, C., Brown, L. (2011). Ferulic acid improves cardiovascular and kidney structure and function in hypertensive rats. *Journal of Cardiovascular Pharmacology*, 57(2), 177-183.

American Diabetes Association. (2020). Classification and diagnosis of diabetes: Standards of medical care in diabetes 2020. *Diabetes Care*, 43(Suppl 1), S14-S31.

Ashraf, R., Aamir, K., Shaikh, A. R., Ahmed, T. (2018). Effects of Allium sativum (garlic) on glycemic control in diabetic patients: A randomized controlled clinical trial. *Journal of Diabetes*, 10(1), 18-23.

Ashraf, R., Khan, R. A., Ashraf, I. (2005). Garlic (Allium sativum) supplementation with standard antidiabetic agent provides better diabetic control in type 2 diabetes patients. *Pakistan Journal of Pharmaceutical Sciences*, 23(4), 408-413.

Basha, S. K., Sankaranarayanan, C. (2014). Anthocyanins in Eugenia jambolana and their role in diabetes management: A comprehensive review. *Journal of Traditional and Complementary Medicine*, 4(3), 143-150.

Chandrasekhar, K., Kapoor, J., Anishetty, S. (2012). A prospective, randomized double-blind, placebo-controlled study of safety and efficacy of a high-concentration full-spectrum extract of Ashwagandha root in reducing stress and anxiety in adults. *Indian Journal of Psychological Medicine*, 34(3), 255-262.

Chang, C. L., Lin, Y. (2015). Herbal medicine for the management of diabetes mellitus: An evidence-based review. *Journal of Diabetes, Metabolic Disorders & Control*, 2(3), 00045.

Chatterjee, S. J., Mondal, S., De, R. K., Bhattacharya, S. K., Mandal, B. P. (2012). Study of antidiabetic activity of leaf extract of Phyllanthus amarus Schum. & Thonn. on alloxan induced diabetic rats. *Journal of Pharmacy Research*, 5(2), 1002-1005.

Chattopadhyay, R. R. (2006). Possible mechanism of antihyperglycemic effect of Eugenia jambolana seed extract. *Indian Journal of Biochemistry and Biophysics*, 43(1), 25-31.

Chen, Q., Chan, L. L. Y., Li, E. T. S. (2003). Bitter melon (Momordica charantia) reduces adiposity, lowers serum insulin and normalizes glucose tolerance in rats fed a high fat diet. *Journal of Nutrition*, 133(4), 1088-1093.

Chiang, J. L., Kirkman, M. S., Laffel, L. M., Peters, A. L. (2014). Type 1 diabetes through the life span: A position statement of the American Diabetes Association. *Diabetes Care*, 37(7), 2034-2054.

Choudhary, D., Bhattacharyya, S., Bose, S. (2017). Efficacy and safety of Ashwagandha (Withania somnifera (L.) Dunal) root extract in improving memory and cognitive functions. *Journal of Dietary Supplements*, 14(6), 599-612.

Davies, M. J., D'Alessio, D. A., Fradkin, J., Kernan, W. N., Mathieu, C., Mingrone, G., American Diabetes Association. (2018). Management of hyperglycemia in type 2 diabetes, A consensus report by the American Diabetes Association (ADA) and the European Association for the Study of Diabetes (EASD). *Diabetes Care*, 41(12), 2669-2701.

Ekor, M. (2014). The growing use of herbal medicines: issues relating to adverse reactions and challenges in monitoring safety. *Frontiers in Pharmacology*, 4, 177.

Forouhi, N. G., Wareham, N. J. (2014). Epidemiology of diabetes. *Medicine*, 42(12), 698-702.

Grover, J. K., Vats, V., Rathi, S. S. (2005). Anti-hyperglycemic effect of Eugenia jambolana and Tinospora cordifolia in experimental diabetes and their effects on key metabolic enzymes involved in carbohydrate metabolism. *Journal of Ethnopharmacology*, 73(3), 461-470.

Ilangkovan, M., Jantan, I., Mesaik, M. A. (2016). Immunosuppressive effects of the standardized extract of Phyllanthus amarus on cellular immune responses in Wistar-Kyoto rats. *Drug Design, Development and Therapy*, 10, 2779-2789.

Joseph, B., Jini, D. (2013). Antidiabetic effects of Momordica charantia (bitter melon) and its medicinal potency. *Asian Pacific Journal of Tropical Disease*, 3(2), 93-102.

Kaviarasan, S., Naik, G. H., Gangabhagirathi, R., Anuradha, C. V., Priyadarsini, K. I. (2006). In vitro studies on antiradical and antioxidant activities of fenugreek (Trigonella foenum graecum) seeds. *Food Chemistry*, 103(1), 31-37.

Kooti, W., Farokhipour, M., Asadzadeh, Z., Ashtary-Larky, D., Asadi-Samani, M. (2016). The role of medicinal plants in the treatment of diabetes: a systematic review. *Electronic Physician*, 8(1), 1832-1842.

Mandal, S. C., Mukherjee, P. K., Saha, K., Pal, M., Saha, B. P. (2007). Studies on the hypoglycaemic activity of Eugenia jambolana fruit juice in streptozotocin-induced diabetic rats. *Phytotherapy Research*, 11(4), 306-308.

Pandey, K. B., Rizvi, S. I. (2009). Plant polyphenols as dietary antioxidants in human health and disease. *Oxidative Medicine and Cellular Longevity*, 2(5), 270-278.

Pari, L., Satheesh, M. A. (2002). Antidiabetic activity of ellagic acid in streptozotocin-induced diabetic rats. *Journal of Medicinal Food*, 5(1), 19-23.

Patwardhan, B., Warude, D., Pushpangadan, P., Bhatt, N. (2005). Ayurveda and traditional Chinese medicine: a comparative overview. *Evidence-Based Complementary and Alternative Medicine*, 2(4), 465-473.

Rajalakshmi, M., Eliza, J., Priya, C. E., Nirmala, A., Daisy, P. (2013). Antihyperglycemic effect of Tinospora cordifolia leaf extracts on alloxan-induced diabetic rats. *African Journal of Traditional, Complementary and Alternative Medicines*, 10(1), 46-49.

Sannegowda, K. M., Venkatesha, S. H., Moudgil, K. D., Shaila, H. (2015). Tinospora cordifolia (Guduchi) ameliorates the oxidative stress and complications of streptozotocin-induced diabetes in rats. *Journal of Pharmacopuncture*, 18(3), 12-20.

Saxena, A., Vikram, N. K., Sharma, B. (2013). Hypoglycemic activity of methanolic extract of Phyllanthus amarus Schum. & Thonn. in alloxan induced diabetic rats. *Journal of Ethnopharmacology,* 150(2), 533-537.

Sharma, P., Singh, S., Sharma, N., Singla, D., Guarve, K., Grewal, A. S. (2022). Targeting human glucokinase for the treatment of type 2 diabetes: an overview of allosteric glucokinase activators. *Journal of Diabetes and Metabolic Disorders*, 21(1), 1129-1137.

Sharma, P., Singh, S., Thakur, V., Sharma, N., Grewal, A. S. (2021). Novel and emerging therapeutic drug targets for management of type 2 diabetes mellitus. *Obesity Medicine*, 23, 100329.

Singh, A. K., Rai, N. P., Mishra, S. K., Srivastava, S., Maurya, R. (2011). Pterocarpus marsupium extract (Vijayasar) prevented the alteration in metabolic patterns induced in the normal rat by feeding an adequate diet containing fructose as sole carbohydrate. *ISRN Pharmacology*, 2011, 823439.

Singh, J., Upadhyay, A. K., Prasad, K. (2012). Antioxidant and anti-inflammatory potential of bitter melon (Momordica charantia) fruits. *International Journal of Food Sciences and Nutrition*, 63(2), 178-184.

Sultan, S., Zafar, M., Saeed, S. A., Khan, M. R. (2014). Protective effects of Pterocarpus marsupium extract against diabetic nephropathy in streptozotocin-induced diabetic rats. *Asian Pacific Journal of Tropical Medicine*, 7(Suppl 1) S154-S159.

Chapter 3

Thai Traditional Herbal Plants for the Management of Diabetes Mellitus

Jiradej Manosroi[1,2]
Aranya Manosroi[1,2]
Charinya Chankhampan[1,2]
Worapong Kitdamrongtham[1,2]
Shikha Baghel Chauhan[3,*]
and Charu Gupta[4]

[1]North-Chiang Mai University, Chiang Mai, Thailand
[2]Manose Health and Beauty Research Centre, Chiang Mai, Thailand
[3]Amity Institute of Pharmacy, Amity University, Noida, Uttar Pradesh, India
[4]Amity Institute of Herbal Research & Studies, Amity University, Noida, Uttar Pradesh, India

Abstract

The global prevalence of diabetes mellitus presents a grave and intricate health challenge, marked by its substantial morbidity and mortality rates. Initially, North Africa and North America reported the highest incidence of diabetes cases; however, this malady has rapidly disseminated worldwide, encompassing nations like India, China, and Thailand. Characterized by elevated blood glucose levels, diabetes leads to disruptions in protein, lipid, and carbohydrate metabolism, intensifying its metabolic impact. Traditional diabetes treatments utilizing various plant species found in Thailand have gained prominence among rural Thai communities and ethnic minorities

* Corresponding Author's Email: shikha.pharma@gmail.com.

In: Naturally Occurring Chemicals …
Editors: A. Singh Grewal, G. Deswal, A. Kumar Dhingra et al.
ISBN: 979-8-89113-491-1

residing in rural enclaves. These botanical resources hold substantial promise as economic therapeutic avenues for an ailment that disproportionately affects the Thai populace. A multitude of indigenous Thai herbs warrants investigation for their potential ethnopharmacological properties in diabetes management. This chapter undertakes the task of enumerating medicinal plants utilized historically in Thailand for diabetes treatment, offering detailed insights into their attributes and applications. This chapter offers comprehensive insights into the medicinal plants indigenous to Thailand, which have a historical precedent for effectively addressing diabetes mellitus.

Keywords: medicinal plants, traditional medicines, thai herbal plants, traditional Thai knowledge, diabetes

Abbreviations

AA	Anogeissus acuminata
AD	Alzheimer's disease
DM	Diabetes mellitus
DPPH	1,1-Diphenyl-2-picrylhydrazyl
GK	Goto-Kakizaki
MO	Moringa oleifera
NLEM	National List of Essential Medicines
STZ	Streptozotocin
TTM	Thai traditional medicine.

Introduction

Thailand, a nation rich in its diversity of medicinal plant species, has long embraced traditional knowledge that has been utilized across rural Thai communities since ancient times. As technology advances, there has arisen a necessity to catalog and preserve this age-old wisdom in the form of a comprehensive database. This repository offers intricate insights into the diverse array of Thai medicinal plants, their manifold uses, and the formulations they have been incorporated into for addressing specific ailments. The creation of such databases serves a dual purpose: not only do they ensure the perpetuation of local traditional knowledge, but they also facilitate the fusion of this wisdom with scientific methodologies and substantiating evidence. Embedded within the fabric of Thai culture, these medicinal plants are emblematic of the symbiotic relationship between traditional practices and well-being. They have historically been wellsprings of health, contributing to the maintenance of a robust lifestyle. The abundance of locally available herbal medicinal plants has kindled a strong propensity for their employment, drawing on the wealth of traditional wisdom. This synergy has provided invaluable assistance in tackling a spectrum of diseases. In conjunction with modern medical approaches, these herbal medicinal resources offer a promising avenue for alternative treatments. This chapter undertakes the task of meticulously documenting and collating information pertaining to the prominent Thai medicinal plants that have been extensively harnessed in the management and treatment of diabetes mellitus. The focal point of this endeavor is the "MANOSROI IV" Thai medicinal plant formulations database, encompassing a compendium of formulations derived from Thai herbal plants (Manosroi et al., 2006). The meticulous process of collecting, interpreting, and systematically organizing recipes from every corner of Thailand has been expertly carried out for the development of this database. As of now, the "MANOSROI IV" database stands as a repository containing an impressive 200,000 recipes, although only 90,000 of these have undergone interpretation thus far. This comprehensive compilation encompasses a remarkable assortment of over 8,300 medicinal plant species and encompasses treatment for 3,900 distinct ailments and symptoms, including diabetes. Thai medicinal plant formulations have an illustrious tradition spanning more than seven centuries, proving to be a stalwart approach for addressing a wide spectrum of diseases and symptoms, diabetes included. Notably, empirical evidence has highlighted the value of employing multiple plants within a single recipe. This approach capitalizes on the diverse bioactive compounds sourced from various plants, each contributing to distinct mechanisms that synergistically enhance efficacy. Such an approach also holds the potential for reducing adverse side effects (Ruan et al., 2006). The symptoms of diabetes including frequent urination, thirst, blurred vision, fatigue and dry mouth were used as the keywords for searching the recipes for diabetes from the "MANOSROI IV" database. Some plants, such as *Zingiber cassumunar* Roxb, *Alpinia galanga* (L.) Willd., *Croton Stellatopilosus* Ohba, *Croton poilanei* Gagnep. and *Piper nigrum* L. usually appeared in Thai medicinal plant formulations for diabetes as shown in Table 1. The list of Thai hypoglycaemic plants for the management of Diabetes mellitus is presented in Table 2.

Table 1. Thai herbal plant formulations for diabetes were chosen from a library of Thai medicinal plant recipes "MANOSROI IV"

Sr. No.	Medicinal plants	
	Scientific name	Family name
1	*Zingiber cassumunar* Roxb.	Zingiberaceae
2	*Alpinia galanga* (L.) Willd.	Zingiberaceae
3	*Croton Stellatopilosus* Ohba	Euphorbiaceae
4	*Croton poilanei* Gagnep.	Euphorbiaceae
5	*Piper nigrum* L.	Piperaceae
6	*Zingiber offcinale* Roscoe	Zingiberaceae
7	*Plumbago indica* L.	Plumbaginaceae
8	*Plumbago zeylanica* L.	Plumbaginaceae
9	*Cassis fistula* L.	Leguminosae-Caesalpinoideae

Table 2. Thai hypoglycemic medicinal plants

Sr. No.	Scientific name	Family
1	*Anogeissus acuminata* (Roxb. ex DC.) Guill. & Perr. var lanceolata	Combretaceae
2	*Catunaregam tormentosa* (Blume ex DC.) Tirveng.	Rubiaceae
3	*Dendropthoe pentandra* (L.) Miq.	Loranthaceae
4	*Mimosa pudica* L.	Leguminosae-Mimosoideae
5	*Moringa oleifera* Lam.	Moringaceae
6	*Acanthus ilicifolius* L.	Acanthaceae
7	*Cyperus rotundus* L.	Cyperaceae
8	*Rhinacanthus nasutus* (L.) Kurz	Acanthaceae
9	*Curcuma zedoria* (Berg) Roscoe	Zingiberaceae
10	*Syzygium aromaticum* (L.) Merr. & L. M. Perry	Myrtaceae
11	*Piper chaba* Hunt	Piperaceae
12	*Myristica fragans* Houtt.	Myristicaceae
13	*Rauwolfia serpentina* (L.) Benth. ex Kurz	Apocynaceae

Zingiber cassumunar Roxb.

This plant, along with other herbs, has been incorporated into the National List of Essential Medicines (NLEM) for its therapeutic benefits in addressing conditions such as heartburn, menstrual disorders, stomach pain, and various other applications (Han et al., 2021). The extract fraction derived from *Z. cassumunar* Roxb. underwent in vitro testing. The plant extract was obtained through the maceration method using methanol as the solvent. The inhibitory activity of the *Z. cassumunar* extract against glucosidase was evaluated through a dedicated assay. The results of the DPPH radical scavenging assay indicated that the chloroform fraction exhibited the highest levels of antioxidant activity. This study underscores the potential of *Z. cassumunar* Roxb. as both an antioxidant and a potential therapy for diabetes (Deng et al., 2011).

Alpinia galanga (L.) Willd.

Alpinia galanga is an herb characterized by its subterranean rhizomes and small adventitious roots, capable of attaining a height of up to 3.5 centimeters. The external surface of the rhizomes displays a reddish-brown hue, while the internal sections are a combination of brown and orange tones. The flowers are intricate, measuring 3 to 4 centimeters in length, exuding a fragrant aroma, and featuring white buds with green flower crowns at their base. The fruit, elliptical and capsule-shaped, reaches a diameter of 1.5 centimeters and showcases hues ranging from orange to crimson (Kaushik, 2011). This can be used for the treatment of back pain, rheumatism, asthma, diabetes, heart disease, liver disorders, kidney diseases, and appetite enhancement (Verma et al., 2011). Preparations derived from galangal rhizomes have exhibited hypoglycemic effects (Akhtar et al., 2002). Galangal rhizome powder, along with methanolic and water extracts, was employed in the treatment. The outcomes revealed a notable reduction in blood sugar levels in healthy rabbits, accompanied by an enhancement in the lipid profile (Verma et al., 2015). An extract derived from galangal rhizome likewise hindered the glycosylation of hemoglobin. Additionally, galangal rhizome contributed to a reduction in blood sugar levels (Shettar et al., 2017).

Croton Stellatopilosus Ohba

Croton stellatopilosus, a diminutive tree or shrub, has the potential to attain a height of up to 5 meters. Its bole, characterized by branching near the base, boasts a diameter of approximately 8 centimeters. This plant holds a special place in Thailand, where it is often harvested from the wild and deliberately cultivated for its medicinal applications. Renowned as a popular traditional remedy, efforts have been made to cultivate the plant to ensure that the pharmaceutical sector can reliably access this vital ingredient (*Croton stellatopilosus - Useful Tropical Plants*, n.d.).

Croton poilanei Gagnep.

A member of the Euphorbiaceae family, Croton poilanei Gagnep. is a plant with its nomenclature derived from Pierre Poilane, the French botanist who acquired the type specimen in Laos back in 1928. This plant boasts petite flowers and fruits while flaunting expansive leaves. Within Thai traditional medicine, the plant's purported anti-inflammatory properties are harnessed. While scant information exists concerning Croton poilanei Gagnep.'s potential anti-diabetic attributes, certain studies have delved into its role in diabetes management. A study conducted in 2015 delved into the diabetic potential of Croton poilanei leaf extracts in rats. This research, published in the Journal of Ethnopharmacology, showcased how the extract effectively lowered blood sugar levels in diabetic rats. The researchers postulated that the presence of flavonoids and other phytochemicals within the plant instigated and contributed to the observed decrease in blood glucose levels (Salatino et al., 2007).

Piper nigrum L.

Plant sources have been utilized in traditional medical practices and everyday activities such as cooking and cosmetics since the dawn of humanity. Black pepper, owing to its primary pharmacological component, piperine, stands as a widely employed species. In animal models, phenols have demonstrated effectiveness in preventing diabetes. Black pepper oil possesses antioxidant and ferric-reducing properties, enabling it to effectively scavenge free radicals (Nabi et al., 2013). Oxidative stress primarily contributes to the onset of diabetes, and a multitude of studies have demonstrated piperine's antioxidant capabilities. In their study, Vijayakumar et al. revealed that the consumption of black pepper in rats led to a reduction in blood sugar levels (Vijayakumar et al., 2004). Rats induced with diabetes using alloxan, blood glucose levels were effectively controlled following four weeks of treatment with P. nigrum and V. rosea. Furthermore, the treatment had an impact on lipid levels and antioxidant capacity.

Zingiber officinal Roscoe

Zingiber officinale, commonly known as ginger, stands as one of the most popular herbs and food flavorings. This versatile herb boasts a range of medicinal attributes and proves efficacious in addressing various ailments (Kumar et al., 2011). In traditional medicine, Z. officinale is harnessed for the management of diabetes. A multitude of in vivo scientific studies employing animal models have been conducted to evaluate the anti-diabetic potential of Z. officinale. In rats induced with diabetes, Z. officinale was found to lower blood glucose levels (Al-Amin et al., 2006). Conversely, it's worth noting that Z. officinale's fresh juice exhibits hyperglycemic properties, as reported. In mice induced with diabetes through streptozotocin, the fresh extract of Z. officinale displayed antidiabetic effects (Asha et al., 2011).

Plumbago indica L.

Plumbago indica, a flowering plant species belonging to the Plumbaginaceae family, is indigenous to Southeast Asia, Indonesia, the Philippines, and the Yunnan region in southern China. Numerous studies have pointed towards the anti-diabetic properties of *Plumbago indica*. In rats induced with diabetes through streptozotocin, noteworthy observations were made. Hepatic hexokinase activity exhibited a substantial increase, while lactic dehydrogenase levels and hepatic glucose concentrations exhibited significant decreases (Shukla et al., 2021). Administration of Plumbago indica to diabetic rats resulted in a significant reduction in their blood glucose levels (Sunil et al., 2012).

Plumbago zeylanica L.

The shrub Plumbago zeylanica L., a member of the Plumbaginaceae family, is extensively distributed across India, Australia, Bangladesh, and Nepal. Numerous studies and investigations have revealed that Plumbago zeylanica L. exhibits a property of lowering blood glucose levels. It has been demonstrated that the extract derived from Plumbago zeylanica L. has the capacity to effectively reduce blood glucose levels and enhance hepatic hexokinase activity (Shukla et al., 2021).

Cassis fistula L.

Belonging to the Caesalpiniaceae family, Cassia fistula Linn is extensively recognized for its medicinal virtues. One of its primary advantages is its suitability as a gentle laxative that is considered safe for both children and pregnant women. The antidiabetic potential of Cassia fistula's bark was explored through the study of its complete alcoholic extract and the ethyl acetate fraction in alloxan-induced diabetic rats. The ethyl acetate extract displayed a reduction in blood glucose levels (Malpani et al., 2010). Additionally, the hydroalcoholic extract of Cassia fistula Linn showcased documented hypoglycemic and anti-diabetic effects in rat models. Furthermore, the ethanolic extract of Cassia fistula Linn stem bark was investigated for its antihyperglycemic properties (Ashraf Ali et al., 2012).

Thai Hypoglycemic Medicinal Plants

Anogeissus acuminata (Roxb. ex-DC.) Guill. & Perr. var lanceolata

The plant *Anogeissus acuminata* (AA) is encompassed within the Combretaceae family. This plant is commonly employed by locals as a remedy for various conditions, including diabetes mellitus (DM), in different parts of the world. Notably, AA is rich in phenolics, which hold the potential for diverse pharmacological impacts. Numerous studies have indicated that extracts of AA exhibit anti-inflammatory, antioxidant, analgesic, neuroprotective, and HIV reverse transcriptase inhibitor properties. Moreover, it has demonstrated hypoglycemic effects in mice afflicted with DM induced by alloxan. Given its multifaceted activities and constituent compounds, it has been hypothesized that AA could potentially serve as an effective antidiabetic agent, aiding in the prevention of long-term diabetic complications (Shaikh & Somani, 2010).

Catunaregam tormentosa (Blume ex DC.) Tirveng.

The plant species Catunaregam tormentosa has a longstanding history of medicinal usage across Southeast Asia and Africa, among other regions. An assessment of the blood-glucose-lowering potential of Catunaregam tormentosa leaf extract in diabetic rats was detailed in a 2012 publication in the Journal of Ethnopharmacology. The study's outcomes revealed that the extract notably reduced blood glucose levels and improved glucose tolerance. It's important to note that traditional remedies should not be substituted for established medical practices without proper guidance from a medical professional (Kaennakam et al., 2018).

Dendropthoe pentandra **(L.) Miq.**

The antidiabetic effectiveness of DPLME was evaluated using a previously documented procedure (Kumar et al., 2011). The experiment employed both diabetic and non-diabetic rats, with six rats allocated to each of the four primary groups comprising normal and alloxan-induced diabetic rats. Following the conclusion of the trial, all remaining animals underwent an overnight fasting period. Over the course of five consecutive days, blood samples were collected from the tail veins at intervals of 0, 30, 60, and 120 minutes subsequent to glucose administration. The determination of glucose levels was carried out using a conventional glucose oxidase assay (Hasan et al., 2018).

Mimosa pudica **L.**

Mimosa pudica has a longstanding history in the treatment of diabetes, with numerous trials validating its effectiveness (Ahmad et al., 2012). The initial evaluation of M. pudica's impact on diabetes was based on an herbal recipe named Ilogen-Excel (Babu & Prince, 2010). This formulation was administered to diabetic rats induced with streptozotocin (STZ), revealing significant antidiabetic properties and an elevation in plasma insulin levels (Babu & Prince, 2010). Sutar et al. conducted a comparative study utilizing *M. pudica* extracts from ethanolic and petroleum ether sources, comparing them with metformin, a conventional medication, on Wistar rats induced with alloxan. The ethanolic extract displayed a noteworthy reduction in blood glucose levels when compared to the common medication Metformin. In a Thai study centred on the Lanna people of Northern Thailand, five crucial herbal plants were evaluated for their antidiabetic potential, one of which was Catunaregam tormentosa (Bl. ex-DC.). Among these, Mimosa pudica exhibited notable anti-diabetic properties (Manosroi et al., 2011).

Moringa oleifera Lam.

Extensive research has been conducted on the potential of numerous medicinal plants to prevent, control, and manage diabetes, with the Moringa Oleifera (MO) plant playing a significant role. Studies have demonstrated the remarkable efficacy of MO leaves in reducing blood sugar levels in wistar diabetes models and Goto-Kakizaki (GK) rats (Ndong et al., 2007a). The presence of potent polyphenols like rutin, quercetin-3-glucoside, and kaempferol glycosides in MO is believed to explain its ability to lower glucose levels (S et al., n.d.). Aqueous extracts of MO leaves have been shown to possess robust hypoglycemic and anti-diabetic properties (Jaiswal et al., 2009). Notably, the combined extracts of MO and VA (Vernonia amygdalina) have displayed hepatoprotective properties, potentially lessening liver damage associated with diabetes. Recent research by Iwara et al. demonstrated that using VA in conjunction with MO leaf extract on STZ-induced diabetic rats proved beneficial in reducing renal damage. This combination seemed to mitigate the nephrotoxic effects caused by diabetes mellitus. This suggests that it's challenging to pinpoint which plant extract holds the most potent active ingredient for diabetes treatment, warranting further comprehensive research. The findings from studies suggest that MO has a beneficial effect on glucose intolerance, potentially mediated by compounds such as quercetin-3-glucoside and fiber content within MO leaf powder (Ndong et al., 2007). The research on MO indicates that it is a highly effective medicinal plant with minimal adverse effects, making it a promising candidate for diabetes management and treatment. This effect could stem from MO's potential to stimulate the islets of Langerhans' β-cells or its compounds that mimic insulin activity.

***Acanthus ilicifolius* L.**

An ethanolic extract of *A. ilicifolius* demonstrated noteworthy anti-diabetic effects in Wistar rats (G. Venkataiah et al., 2013). Notably, the extract exhibited antidiabetic properties when compared to glibenclamide. Moreover, it facilitated the regeneration of pancreatic beta cells, suggesting its potential usefulness in diabetes treatment. HBOA and its derivatives have been reported to effectively treat diabetes (Liu et al., 2013).

Cyperus rotundus L.

Oral administration of the extract in alloxan-induced diabetic rats led to a significant reduction in blood sugar concentrations (Raut & Gaikwad, 2006). The effective in vitro DPPH antioxidant properties exhibited by *C. rotundus* led researchers to suggest that its antihyperglycemic effect could be attributed to its antioxidant characteristics (Ardestani & Yazdanparast, 2007). Given the link between non-enzymatic glycation and the severity of diabetes mellitus and its complications, researchers concluded that *C. rotundus* could serve as a promising option for diabetes treatment (Singh et al., 2012).

Rhinacanthus nasutus (L.) Kurz

The methanolic extract of *R. nasutus* significantly elevates overall glucose concentrations in diabetic rats, akin to the effects of glibenclamide. Glibenclamide is a commonly used medication for treating diabetes mellitus due to its ability to enhance the production of insulin by pancreatic beta-cells. The key mechanism of glibenclamide involves inhibiting plasma membrane ATP-sensitive K+ (KATP) channels. This inhibition leads to membrane depolarization, activation of voltage-gated Ca2+ channels, and subsequent influx of Ca2+, resulting in elevated cytosolic calcium levels and consequently increased insulin release. Glibenclamide is widely employed as a reference medication to assess the antidiabetic properties of various compounds in diabetic models, evaluating their potential effects (Rajasekaran et al., 2005). The liver, a vital organ, plays a pivotal role in both glycolysis and gluconeogenesis. It serves as the primary site for endogenous glucose synthesis (Roden & Bernroider, 2003), achieved through processes like gluconeogenesis or glycogenolysis. In diabetes, there is an elevation in endogenous glucose production, contributing to hyperglycemia. This can arise from compromised pancreatic function or reduced glucose clearance (Schillinger et al., 2002; Wang et al., 2003). Insulin governs the uptake and utilization of glucose within these tissues. This regulation involves the control of various metabolic enzyme activities. A deficiency in insulin levels, whether partial or complete, will disrupt carbohydrate metabolism and subsequently diminish the activity of several pivotal enzymes. The study aimed to explore the effects of treatment using an extract of *R. nasutus* on hepatic carbohydrate concentrations in rats that had developed diabetes due to STZ induction (Grover et al., 2000).

Curcuma zedoria (Berg) Roscoe

Blood sugar levels can be effectively reduced by using a methanol extract obtained from *Curcuma zedoaria* rhizomes and *Sonneratia caseolaris* fruits, both of which are utilized in the traditional treatment of diabetes in Bangladeshi medicine. When subjected to a glucose load, mice treated with the methanolic extract of the rhizomes exhibited a significant and dose-dependent reduction in blood glycemia levels (Sahebrao Kharat & Deepak Lad, 2020).

Syzygiumaromaticum (L.) Merr. & L. M. Perry

Hyperinsulinemia and insulin resistance are interconnected with type 2 diabetes. Additionally, individuals with Alzheimer's disease (AD) often exhibit insulin resistance, which disrupts brain glucose metabolism and contributes to neurodegeneration (Ramesh & Govindaraju, 2022). Both hyperinsulinemia and insulin resistance accelerate the accumulation of Aβ and tau phosphorylation. Herbal plants that can enhance insulin secretion could be beneficial for both AD and diabetic patients due to their similar symptoms (Baliga et al., 2013). The anti-diabetic potential of eight *Syzygium* species was comprehensively investigated by Zulcafli et al. and noted that the extract from *S. cumini* stimulates insulin production in pancreatic β-cells in diabetic rats (S. B. Sharma et al., 2011). Furthermore, the ethanolic extract of *S. cumini* leaves demonstrates the ability to lower blood sugar levels and improve insulin resistance (Sanches et al., 2016). Moreover, administering *S. cumini* seed powder to 30 recently diagnosed type 2 diabetic patients led to a reduction in insulin resistance (Sahana et al., 2010). The aqueous seed extract also displayed a reduction in other diabetic indicators and blood glucose levels (Sharma et al., 2012). In a study conducted by Shen et al., using TNF-treated FL83B cells, a clear link between insulin resistance and inflammation was established. Treatment with *S. samarangense* fruit extract inhibited JNK activity, thereby preventing an inflammatory response. This intervention resulted in a decrease in insulin resistance triggered by TNF-α (Sharma et al., 2012). In a separate investigation, rats with hyperglycemia induced by a high-fructose diet exhibited improved outcomes with vescalagin isolated from *S. samarangense*. Through the stimulation of the insulin signaling pathway, vescalagin enhanced lipid deposition and glucose absorption. Similarly, myricitrin, a compound derived from *S. malaccense* leaf extract, demonstrated insulin-like actions by promoting lipid deposition and glucose absorption (Arumugam et al., 2019). Additionally, homoeopathic treatments using *Syzygium jambolanum* resulted in the reversal of insulin receptor (IR) mRNA levels in diabetic rats, restoring them to normal levels. This reversal indicated an enhancement in insulin secretion (Sharma et al., 2012).

Piper chaba **Hunt**

Researchers investigated the antihyperglycemic and anti-lipid peroxidative properties of ethanolic extracts from dried fruits of *Piper longum* and *Piper chaba* in rats that had developed diabetes due to alloxan-induced damage. They utilized precise colorimetric methods to assess parameters such as blood glucose levels, carbohydrate-digesting enzyme activity, antioxidant status, and lipid peroxidation. The study revealed that the dried fruits, when administered orally to diabetic rats, exhibited equivalent hypoglycemic, antioxidant, and anti-lipid peroxidative effects as those observed with the standard treatment (Manoharan et al., 2007).

Myristica fragans **Houtt**

In healthy rats as well as those with alloxan-induced diabetes, the extract of M. fragrans exhibited a capacity to lower sugar levels. The hypoglycemic effect might be attributed to an enhancement in insulin release from beta-cells. Furthermore, when the extract was orally administered, it effectively mitigated the rise in glucose levels triggered by glucose overload. This outcome could potentially arise from mechanisms such as the modulation of pancreatic secretions, a potential increase in intestinal glucose absorption, or an augmentation of glucose uptake. Notably, the extract also contributed to increased body weight in diabetic animals, potentially due to improved glycemic control and heightened insulin secretion Somani & Singhai, 2008). Similarly, the ethanolic extract of M. fragrans fruit led to a minor reduction in sugar levels when administered to diabetic mice (Ahmad et al., 2008).

Rauwolfia serpentina (L.) Benth. ex Kurz

An initial investigation into the effects of Rauwolfia serpentina's root extract on alloxan-induced mice was conducted, analyzing the outcomes of a single dose of methanolic extract. The study extended its exploration by evaluating immediate toxic effects and establishing the maximum lethal dose (LD50) of the same extract. The research delved into the phytochemistry of Rauwolfia serpentina and its influence on male Wistar mouse models with diabetes induced by alloxan. The methanolic root extract (MREt) exhibited a substantial quantity of total phenols through quantitative analysis, alongside qualitative assessments that indicated the presence of alkaloids, saponins, and flavonoids within the root powder (Qureshi et al., 2009). Methanolic root extract (MREt) demonstrated advantageous effects in various aspects. It contributed to the reduction of body weights, insulin and blood sugar levels, the insulin/glucose ratio, glycosylated and total hemoglobin levels, as well as blood pressure, when compared to the control group. Additionally, the test groups exhibited significantly lower levels of triglycerides, LDL, VLDL, and total cholesterol. Furthermore, ALT levels were maintained within acceptable limits, below permissible thresholds (Hafsa Azra, 2020).

Conclusion

Despite the availability of current treatment options, the quest for novel anti-diabetic medications remains a priority due to diabetes persisting as a significant modern metabolic ailment. The resurgence of Thai Traditional Medicine (TTM) has emerged as a prominent focus, with substantial efforts being directed towards expediting research on active constituents sourced from herbs and their potential incorporation into healthcare facilities across the nation. Moreover, in rural regions particularly, TTM practitioners frequently advocate herbal formulations for managing diabetes and its associated symptoms. In conclusion, Thai plants have a historical track record of being used to address a range of ailments, including diabetes. Numerous Thai herbal plants have been the subject of research studies, indicating their anti-diabetic properties and ability to aid in blood sugar level regulation. These plants encompass bioactive compounds like flavonoids, alkaloids, and triterpenoids that support insulin secretion, glucose absorption, and lipid metabolism. While additional clinical research is warranted to validate therapeutic efficacy and address potential toxicity concerns, integrating these herbal sources into a balanced diet and lifestyle could prove beneficial for individuals with diabetes mellitus. As such, Thai plants hold the potential to serve as a valuable complementary approach for managing diabetes mellitus.

References

Ahmad, H., Sehgal, S., Mishra, A., Gupta, R. (2012). Mimosa pudica L. (Laajvanti): an overview. *Pharmacognosy Reviews*, 6(12), 115.

Ahmad, R., Srivastava, S. P., Maurya, R., Rajendran, S. M., Arya, K. R., Srivastava, A. K. (2008). Mild antihyperglycaemic activity in Eclipta alba, Berberis aristata, Betula utilis, Cedrus deodara, Myristica fragrans and Terminalia chebula. *Indian Journal of Science and Technology*, 1(5), 1-6.

Akhtar, M. S., Khan, M. A., Malik, M. T. (2002). Hypoglycaemic activity of Alpinia galanga rhizome and its extracts in rabbits. *Fitoterapia*, 73(7-8), 623-628.

Al-Amin, Z. M., Thomson, M., Al-Qattan, K. K., Peltonen-Shalaby, R., Ali, M. (2006). Anti-diabetic and hypolipidaemic properties of ginger (Zingiber officinale) in streptozotocin-induced diabetic rats. *British Journal of Nutrition*, 96(4), 660-666.

Ali, M. A., Sagar, H. A., Khatun, M. C. S., Azad, A. K., Begum, K., Wahed, M. I. I. (2012). Antihyperglycemic and analgesic activities of ethanolic extract of Cassia fistula (L.) stem bark. *International Journal of Pharmaceutical Sciences and Research*, 3(2), 416.

Ardestani, A., Yazdanparast, R. (2007). Cyperus rotundus suppresses AGE formation and protein oxidation in a model of fructose-mediated protein glycoxidation. *International Journal of Biological Macromolecules*, 41(5), 572-578.

Arumugam, B., Palanisamy, U. D., Chua, K. H., Kuppusamy, U. R. (2019). Protective effect of myricetin derivatives from syzygium malaccense against hydrogen peroxide-induced stress in ARPE-19 cells. *Molecular Vision*, 25, 47–59.

Asha, B., Krishnamurthy, K. H., Devaru, S. (2011). Evaluation of anti hyperglycaemic activity of Zingiber officinale (Ginger) in albino rats. *Journal of Chemical and Pharmaceutical Research*, 3(1), 452-456.

Babu, P. S., Prince, P. S. M. (2010). Antihyperglycaemic and antioxidant effect of hyponidd, an ayurvedic herbomineral formulation in streptozotocin-induced diabetic rats. *Journal of Pharmacy and Pharmacology*, 56(11), 1435-1442.

Baliga, M. S., Fernandes, S., Thilakchand, K. R., D'Souza, P., Rao, S. (2013). Scientific validation of the antidiabetic effects of syzygium jambolanum dc (black plum), a traditional medicinal plant of India. *Journal of Alternative and Complementary Medicine*, 19(3), 191–197.

Bhakuni, D. S., Goel, A. K., Jain, S., Mehrotra, B. N., Srimal, R. C. (1990). Screening of Indian plants for biological activity: Part XIV. *Indian Journal of Experimental Biology*, 28(7), 619-637.

Deng, J., Cheng, W., Yang, G. (2011). A novel antioxidant activity index (AAU) for natural products using the DPPH assay. *Food Chemistry*, 125(4), 1430-1435.

Grover, J. K., Vats, V., Rathi, S. S. (2000). Anti-hyperglycemic effect of Eugenia jambolana and Tinospora cordifolia in experimental diabetes and their effects on key metabolic enzymes involved in carbohydrate metabolism. *Journal of Ethnopharmacology*, 73(3), 461–470.

Hafsa Azra, B. (2020). A Comprehensive Review and Evaluation of in Vitro Antifungal Potential of Rauvolfia Serpentina. *International Journal for Research in Applied Science & Engineering Technology*, 8, 2321-9653.

Han, A. R., Kim, H., Piao, D., Jung, C. H., Seo, E. K. (2021). Phytochemicals and bioactivities of Zingiber cassumunar Roxb. *Molecules*, 26(8), 2377.

Hasan, M., Ali, M. T., Khan, R., Palit, P., Islam, A., Seidel, V., Akter, R., Nahar, L. (2018). Hepatoprotective, antihyperglycemic and antidiabetic effects of Dendrophthoe pentandra leaf extract in rats. *Clinical Phytoscience*, 4(1), 1-7.

Jaiswal, D., Kumar Rai, P., Kumar, A., Mehta, S., Watal, G. (2009). Effect of Moringa oleifera Lam. leaves aqueous extract therapy on hyperglycemic rats. *Journal of Ethnopharmacology*, 123(3), 392–396.

Kaennakam, S., Rassamee, K., Siripong, P., Tip-Pyang, S. (2018). Catomentosaponin, a new triterpene saponin from the roots of Catunaregam tomentosa. *Natural Product Research*, 32(13), 1499-1505.

Kaushik, D., Yadav, J., Kaushik, P., Sacher, D., Rani, R. (2011). Current pharmacological and phytochemical studies of the plant Alpinia galanga. *Zhong Xi Yi Jie He Xue Bao*, 9(10), 1061-1065.

Kharat, R. S., Lad, M. D. (2020). A pharmacological review of karchoor (curcuma zedoaria): a potent herb mentioned in ayurved. *World Journal of Pharmaceutical Research*, 9, 2322.

Kumar, D., Kumar, S., Kohli, S., Arya, R., Gupta, J. (2011). Antidiabetic activity of methanolic bark extract of Albizia odoratissima Benth. in alloxan induced diabetic albino mice. *Asian Pacific Journal of Tropical Medicine*, 4(11), 900-903.

Kumar, G., Karthik, L., Rao, K. B. (2011). A review on pharmacological and phytochemical properties of Zingiber officinale Roscoe (Zingiberaceae). *Journal of Pharmacy Research*, 4(9), 2963-2966.

Liu, L., Fan, H., Qi, P., Mei, Y., Zhou, L., Cai, L., Lin, X., Lin, J. (2013). Synthesis and hepatoprotective properties of Acanthus ilicifolius alkaloid A and its derivatives. *Experimental and Therapeutic Medicine*, 6(3), 796–802.

Mahmoud, M. F., Abdelaal, S., Mohammed, H. O., El-Shazly, A. M., Daoud, R., El Raey, M. A., Sobeh, M. (2021). Syzygium jambos extract mitigates pancreatic oxidative stress, inflammation and apoptosis and modulates hepatic IRS-2/AKT/GLUT4 signaling pathway in streptozotocin-induced diabetic rats. *Biomedicine & Pharmacotherapy*, 142, 112085.

Malpani, S. N., Manjunath, K. P., Sholapur, H., Savadi, R. V., Akki, K. S., Darade, S. S. (2010). Antidiabetic activity of Cassia fistula Linn. bark in alloxan induced diabetic rats. *International Journal of Pharmaceutical Sciences and Research*, 2, 382-385.

Manohar, V. S., Jayasree, T., Kishore, K. K., Rupa, L. M., Rohit, D., Chandrasekhar, N. (2012). Evaluation of hypoglycemic and antihyperglycemic effect of freshly prepared aqueous extract of Moringa oleifera leaves in normal and diabetic rabbits. *Journal of Chemical and Pharmaceutical Research*, 4(1), 249-253.

Manoharan, S., Silvan, S., Vasudevan, K., Balakrishnan, S. (2007). Antihyperglycemic and antilipidperoxidative effects of Piper longum (Linn.) dried fruits in alloxan induced diabetic rat. *Journal of Biological Sciences*, 6(1), 161-168.

Manosroi, J., Moses, Z. Z., Manosroi, W., Manosroi, A. (2011). Hypoglycemic activity of Thai medicinal plants selected from the Thai/Lanna Medicinal Recipe Database MANOSROI II. *Journal of Ethnopharmacology*, 138(1), 92-98.

Nabi, S. A., Kasetti, R. B., Sirasanagandla, S., Tilak, T. K., Kumar, M. V. J., Rao, C. A. (2013). Antidiabetic and antihyperlipidemic activity of Piper longum root aqueous extract in STZ induced diabetic rats. *BMC Complementary and Alternative Medicine*, 13, 1-9.

Ndong, M., Uehara, M., Katsumata, S. I., Suzuki, K. (2007). Effects of oral administration of Moringa oleifera Lam on glucose tolerance in Goto-Kakizaki and Wistar rats. *Journal of Clinical Biochemistry and Nutrition*, 40(3), 229-233.

Ndong, M., Uehara, M., Katsumata, S. I., Suzuki, K. (2007). Effects of oral administration of Moringa oleifera Lam on glucose tolerance in Goto-Kakizaki and Wistar rats. *Journal of Clinical Biochemistry and Nutrition*, 40(3), 229-233.

Qureshi, S. A., Nawaz, A., Udani, S. K., Azmi, B. (2009). Hypoglycaemic and hypolipidemic activities of Rauwolfia serpentina in alloxan-induced diabetic rats. *International Journal of Pharmacology*, 5(5), 323-326.

Rajasekaran, S., Sivagnanam, K., Subramanian, S. (2005). Antioxidant effect of Aloe vera gel extract in streptozotocin-induced diabetes in rats. *Pharmacology Reports*, 57(1), 90-96.

Ramesh, M., Govindaraju, T. (2022). Multipronged diagnostic and therapeutic strategies for Alzheimer's disease. *Chemical Science*, 13(46), 13657-13689.

Raut, N. A., Gaikwad, N. J. (2006). Antidiabetic activity of hydro-ethanolic extract of Cyperus rotundus in alloxan induced diabetes in rats. *Fitoterapia*, 77(7-8), 585-588.

Roden, M., Bernroider, E. (2003). Hepatic glucose metabolism in humans—its role in health and disease. *Best Practice & Research Clinical Endocrinology & Metabolism*, 17(3), 365-383.

Sahana, D. A., Shivaprakash, G., Baliga, R., MR, A. P., Ganesh, J., Pai, M. R. S. M. (2010). Effect of Eugenia jambolana on plasma glucose, insulin sensitivity and HDL-C levels: Preliminary results of a randomized clinical trial. *Journal of Pharmacy Research*, 3(6), 1268-1270.

Salatino, A., Salatino, M. L. F., Negri, G. (2007). Traditional uses, chemistry and pharmacology of Croton species (Euphorbiaceae). *Journal of the Brazilian Chemical Society*, 18, 11-33.

Sanches, J. R., Franca, L. M., Chagas, V. T., Gaspar, R. S., Dos Santos, K. A., Goncalves, L. M., Sloboda, D. M., Holloway, A. C., Dutra, R. P., Carneiro, E. M., Cappelli, A. P. G., Paes, A. M. D. A. (2016). Polyphenol-rich extract of Syzygium cumini leaf dually improves peripheral insulin sensitivity and pancreatic islet function in monosodium L-glutamate-induced obese rats. *Frontiers in Pharmacology*, 7, 48.

Schillinger, D., Grumbach, K., Piette, J., Wang, F., Osmond, D., Daher, C., Palacios, J., Sullivan, G. D., Bindman, A. B. (2002). Association of Health Literacy with Diabetes Outcomes. *JAMA*, 288(4), 475-482.

Shaikh, A. S., Somani, R. S. (2010). Animal models and biomarkers of neuropathy in diabetic rodents. *Indian Journal of Pharmacology*, 42(3), 129.

Sharma, A. K., Bharti, S., Kumar, R., Krishnamurthy, B., Bhatia, J., Kumari, S., Arya, D. S. (2012). Syzygium cumini ameliorates insulin resistance and β-cell dysfunction via modulation of PPAR, dyslipidemia, oxidative stress, and TNF-α in type 2 diabetic rats. *Journal of Pharmacological Sciences*, 119(3), 203-213.

Sharma, S. B., Rajpoot, R., Nasir, A., Prabhu, K. M., Murthy, P. S. (2011). Ameliorative Effect of Active Principle Isolated from Seeds of Eugenia jambolana on Carbohydrate Metabolism in Experimental Diabetes. *Evidence-Based Complementary and Alternative Medicine*, 2011, 789871-789871.

Shettar, A. K., Sateesh, M. K., Kaliwal, B. B., Vedamurthy, A. B. (2017). In vitro antidiabetic activities and GC-MS phytochemical analysis of Ximenia americana extracts. *South African Journal of Botany*, 111, 202-211.

Shukla, B., Saxena, S., Usmani, S., Kushwaha, P. (2021). Phytochemistry and pharmacological studies of Plumbago zeylanica L.: a medicinal plant review. *Clinical Phytoscience*, 7, 1-11.

Singh, N., Pandey, B. R., Verma, P., Bhalla, M., Gilca, M. (2012). Phyto-pharmacotherapeutics of Cyperus rotundus Linn. (Motha): an overview. *Indian Journal of Natural Products and Resources*, 3(4), 467–476.

Somani, R. S., Singhai, A. K. (2008). Hypoglycaemic and antidiabetic activities of seeds of Myristica fragrans in normoglycaemic and alloxan-induced diabetic rats. *Asian Journal of Experimental Sciences*, 22(1), 95-102.

Sunil, C., Duraipandiyan, V., Agastian, P., Ignacimuthu, S. (2012). Antidiabetic effect of plumbagin isolated from Plumbago zeylanica L. root and its effect on GLUT4 translocation in streptozotocin-induced diabetic rats. *Food and Chemical Toxicology*, 50(12), 4356-4363.

Venkataiah, G., Ahmed, M. I., Reddy, D. S., Rejeena, M. (2013). Anti-diabetic activity of Acanthus ilicifolius root extract in alloxan induced diabetic rats. *Indo American Journal of Pharmaceutical Research*, 3(11), 9007-9012.

Verma, R. K., Garima, M., Pradeep, S., Jha, K. K., Khosa, R. L. (2011). Alpinia galanga-an important medicinal plant: a review. *Der Pharmacia Sinica*, 2(1), 142-154.

Verma, R. K., Mishra, G., Singh, P., Jha, K. K., Khosa, R. L. (2015). Anti-diabetic activity of methanolic extract of Alpinia galanga Linn. aerial parts in streptozotocin induced diabetic rats. *Ayu*, 36(1), 91.

Vijayakumar, R., Surya, D., Nalini, N. (2004). Antioxidant efficacy of black pepper (Piper nigrum L.) and piperine in rats with high fat diet induced oxidative stress. *Redox Report*, 9(2), 105-110.

Wang, F., Herrington, M., Larsson, J., Permert, J. (2003). The relationship between diabetes and pancreatic cancer. *Molecular Cancer*, 2(1), 1-5.

Chapter 4

Marine-Based Product for the Management of Diabetes Mellitus

Megha Sharma[1]
Chaitanay Vinayak Narayan[2,*]
Avinash Bajpai[2]
Neelam Singh[2]
and Janhavi Singh[2]
[1]Metro College of Health Sciences and Research, Greater Noida, Uttar Pradesh, India
[2]I. T. S. College of Pharmacy, Muradnagar, Ghaziabad, Uttar Pradesh, India

Abstract

In the past few decades, there has been a significant increase in the prevalence of diabetes, which is now recognized as a major global health concern. Due to the inconvenience, high costs, and adverse effects of synthetic drugs, many individuals with diabetes are seeking alternative therapies, and marine products have emerged as promising options. As a result, this chapter focuses on marine bioactive substances with antioxidant properties that can help mitigate diabetes and its related complications. The marine environment offers a diverse array of underutilized biologically active compounds. Exploring marine resources has the potential to yield valuable molecules with both commercial and practical significance. The primary motivation for investigating marine resources as medicinal sources and nutritional supplements lies in the relative safety of pharmaceuticals derived from natural origins. Various aquatic organisms, including bacteria, macro-

* Corresponding Author's Email: chaitanayvinayak@gmail.com.

In: Naturally Occurring Chemicals …
Editors: A. Singh Grewal, G. Deswal, A. Kumar Dhingra et al.
ISBN: 979-8-89113-491-1

algae, micro-algae, seagrasses, corals, sea anemones, sponges, fish, shark-derived proteins, and even components like salmon skin and fish/shellfish waste, have been studied to assess their potential anti-diabetic properties. Screening for anti-hyperglycemic and anti-diabetic properties of marine species has been conducted through both in vitro and in vivo studies. This chapter provides a summary of current findings regarding the anti-diabetic actions of numerous marine organisms, including marine waste products, and suggests potential research directions in this field for the future.

Keywords: marine organism, antidiabetic mechanism, metabolic disorder, bioactive compound

Abbreviations

AMPK	AMP-activated protein kinase
DM	Diabetes mellitus
GSK-3	Glycogen synthase kinase-3
IDDM	Insulin-dependent diabetes mellitus
NIDDM	Non-insulin dependent diabetes mellitus
NKT	Natural killer cell
PTP-1B	Protein tyrosine phosphatase-1B
SOD	Superoxide dismutase
TNF	Tumour necrotic factor.

Introduction

Carbohydrate metabolism disorders disrupt the normal metabolic processes of living organisms and are primarily responsible for prevalent pathological conditions, notably diabetes (Kaur et al., 2014). In 2013, diabetes accounted for 1.6 million reported fatalities according to government agencies, and an estimated 382 million individuals worldwide were projected to be affected by this disease (Zaccardi et al., 2016). Notably, the Western Pacific region (with 132 million cases) and South Asia (with 71.4 million cases) documented the highest prevalence of diabetes cases (Panunti et al., 2014). Projections indicate that by 2030, diabetes will rank as the 7th leading cause of death, and this number could potentially escalate to reach as high as 500 million cases (Barde et al., 2015). Diabetes mellitus (DM) is recognized as a significant and chronic metabolic disorder (En-Qin et al., 2017), typically stemming from a combination of natural and genetic factors. This condition is characterized by hyperglycemia, which leads to disruptions in the metabolism of carbohydrates, proteins, and fats due to insufficient insulin secretion (both relatively and absolutely) (Liu et al., 2014). Insulin, a peptide hormone consisting of amino acids, is synthesized within the β-cells of the pancreatic islets of Langerhans (Barde et al., 2015). Its role is two-fold: firstly, it facilitates the synthesis of lipids and the uptake of glucose; secondly, it inhibits the breakdown of proteins, glycogen, lipids, and the gluconeogenesis pathway (Joshi et al., 2007; Newsholmeet al., 2014; Sonksenet al., 2000). Numerous complications arise in individuals with diabetes, including ketoacidosis, nephropathy, retinopathy, neuropathy, diabetic foot conditions, and an elevated risk of hypertension and cardiovascular diseases (Liu et al., 2014). Many people with diabetes will eventually develop these complications. Notably, the progressive deterioration of microstructures—specifically neurons, retinal cells, and nephrons—affects the nerves, eyes, and kidneys, resulting in severe conditions related to diabetes. Furthermore, abnormal diabetes conditions are also linked to various cardiovascular and other health issues (Goldenberg et al., 2013; Groop et al., 2014). For the body's millions of cells to sustain their physiological functions, they require energy derived from food, primarily in the form of sugar. Two processes regulate the passage of sugar through cell membranes: a receptor that acts like a door, and insulin, which serves to open these receptors. Two primary classes of diabetes are IDDM (Type 1 DM) and NIDDM (Type 2 DM) (Figure 1). In Type 1 diabetes (T1DM), insulin generation is absent due to the destruction of β-cells caused by an autoimmune reaction (D'Orazio et al., 2012). Because individuals with T1DM require lifelong insulin injections, it's often referred to as insulin-dependent diabetes. On the other hand, in Type 2 diabetes (T2DM), the islets of Langerhans either fail to produce sufficient insulin for proper functioning, or the body's cells don't respond adequately to insulin (insulin resistance). This leads to reduced utilization of insulin by peripheral tissues, contributing to obesity and hyperglycemia (Heendeniya et al., 2020). In this context, patients can manage the condition through a healthy diet and exercise, or they might require regular insulin injections or oral medications. Globally, Type 1 diabetes affects over 20 million individuals, with its prevalence increasing by 2-5% annually in many countries (Groop et al., 2014). Type 2 diabetes, which is more prevalent, accounts for 90%–95% of all cases (Reimann et al., 2009). Moreover, this syndrome is closely linked to numerous cardiovascular diseases and related complications (Goldenberg et al., 2013; Groop et al., 2014).

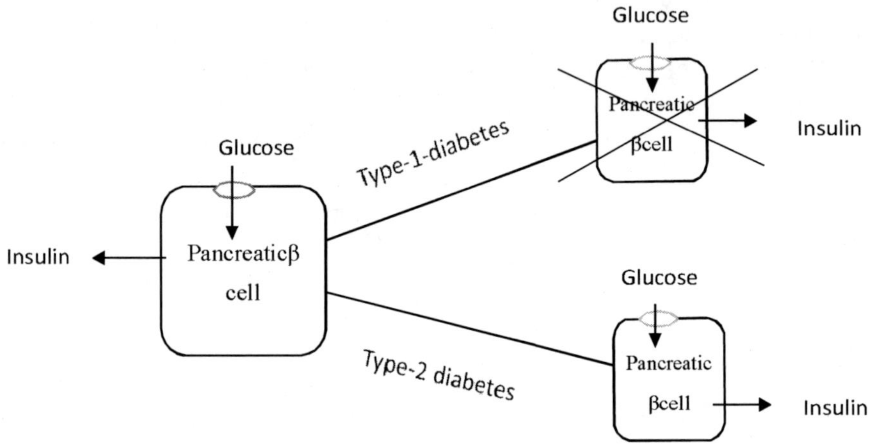

Figure 1. Diagrammatical representation of type1 & type 2 diabetes.

The precise pathophysiological mechanisms underlying diabetes are still not completely understood. Nevertheless, compelling evidence suggests that oxidative stress and inflammatory processes play a significant role in initiating or exacerbating the disease (Popov et al., 2013). Consequently, anti-inflammatory and antioxidant assessments are incorporated into screening protocols for potential anti-diabetic compounds. These assessments involve evaluating the activation of proteins and enzymes responsible for neutralizing free radicals, such as glutathione and superoxide dismutase (SOD), as well as the inhibition of certain inflammatory mediators like tumor necrosis factor (TNF) and interleukins 6 (IL6) (Liu et al., 2014; Zhang et al., 2011; Zhu et al., 2010). Selecting appropriate preventive measures is crucial to mitigate both the financial and health burdens associated with this condition. Although there are numerous synthetic pharmaceuticals available in the market for treating diabetes mellitus, none of them are entirely efficacious or cost-effective. Furthermore, prolonged usage of these medications may lead to undesirable side effects (Tabatabaei-Malazy et al., 2013). Preventing chronic and severe complications in individuals with Type 2 diabetes requires the identification of effective treatment strategies for managing blood serum glucose levels. The administration of daily insulin injections can be uncomfortable, and for those with Type 1 diabetes, reliance on exogenous insulin injections is necessary for maintaining a normal life. Type 2 diabetes can be managed through lifestyle modifications, oral antidiabetic drugs, and insulin therapy. Given the limited availability of anti-diabetic medications compared to the number of individuals with diabetes, various approaches are employed. These include antioxidant therapy, immunological interventions, islet therapy, α-glucosidase inhibitors, and a range of oral antidiabetic medications. These strategies constitute the primary therapies for Type 2 diabetes (Hinnen et al., 2018; Qaid et al., 2016; Hinnen et al., 2015). Due to their limited efficacy and significant side effects, these existing anti-diabetic medications impose a burden on the nation's economy and public health. Therefore, it is imperative to develop new and effective preventive therapies that can preserve the structure of β-cells and delay the onset of diabetes, thereby minimizing these adverse outcomes. Despite the considerable focus on herbal remedies in research, none of them has provided comprehensive relief for individuals with Type 2 diabetes (Sudasinghe et al., 2018). Given that marine seaweeds are a rich source of potentially bioactive compounds derived from their physiological and biochemical processes, their importance deserves particular attention. Marine bio-resources have been shown to yield a wide range of new molecular frameworks, often characterized by unconventional structural motifs (Thomas et al., 2010; Fountain et al., 2020). Numerous marine compounds have been introduced for the treatment of various human conditions. Trabectedin, an alkylating agent marketed as Yondelis®, is derived from the tunicate Ecteinascidia turbinate and is employed in the treatment of ovarian cancer and tissue sarcomas (Ustündağ et al., 2000; Singh et al., 2014; Khalid et al., 2018). Additionally, the pyrimidine nucleoside analog Cytosar-U® (Ara-C, DepoCyt®), sourced from the Caribbean sponge Tethya crypta, is used to treat non-lymphatic cancer and acute myelocytic leukemia (Khalid et al., 2018). The macrocyclic ketone Halaven®, originating from the sponge *Halichondria okadai* (Rengasamy et al., 2020), is employed in the treatment of advanced liposarcoma and metastatic breast cancer. Ziconotide (Prialt®), extracted from the Conus magus clam, is a notable seawater amalgam utilized to treat chronic pain (Gunathilaka et al., 2020). Purine nucleoside and beta-D-arabinoside (Ara-A), isolated from the sponge Tethya crypta, find application in the treatment of infections caused by the herpes simplex virus (Wijesekara et al., 2011). Additionally, dysidine, sourced from the sponge *Dysidea villosa*, is currently in pre-clinical trials for diabetes management. The smajority of marine seaweeds are able to thrive in extremely hostile settings, which offers tremendous potential for producing complex bioactive chemicals to tolerate harsh environments.

Therapeutic Targets for Type-II Diabetes Mellitus

Effective treatment of type 2 diabetes is essential to manage diabetic complications and hyperglycemia, as this condition is progressive in nature. A disruption in glucose homeostasis leads to hyperglycemia due to insulin resistance and diminished beta-cell functionality, ultimately resulting in the loss of control over postprandial glucose levels. Maintaining postprandial blood glucose control is vital for addressing the hyperglycemic state and associated issues in individuals with type 2 diabetes (Hinnen et al., 2018). Postprandial hyperglycemia in Type 2 diabetes patients can be controlled by targeting key anabolic and catabolic enzymes. These include alpha-amylase, dipeptidyl peptidase-IV (DPP-IV), and α-glucosidase inhibitors, as well as regulatory hormones like glucagon-like peptide-1 (GLP-1) and gut-derived peptide hormones known as incretins. Additionally, enzymes such as aldose reductase, angiotensin-converting enzyme, glucose-dependent insulinotropic peptide hormones, and protein tyrosine phosphatase enzyme IB contribute to the development of diabetic complications. Managing these factors is crucial for effective control of postprandial hyperglycemia and associated issues in Type 2 diabetes (Qaid et al., 2016). As a result, these enzyme inhibitors work by slowing down the absorption of glucose, leading to reduced postprandial blood glucose levels (Hinnen et al., 2015). Another significant enzyme, dipeptidyl peptidase-IV, functions as a protease responsible for breaking down incretins, a group of metabolic hormones that stimulate the insulin-producing ß cells in the Langerhans' islets. Following nutrient consumption, incretins are released, leading to the delay of stomach emptying and glucagon secretion, while also promoting insulin secretion (Gerich et al., 2013). Conversely, once a patient achieves euglycemia (normal blood sugar levels), the influence of incretins on insulin secretion gradually diminishes (Makrilakis et al., 2019). To mitigate the degradation of incretins and thus sustain hyperglycemic conditions in Type 2 diabetes, inhibitors of the dipeptidyl peptidase IV enzyme have proven effective as treatment methods. Similarly, the aldose reductase enzyme is integral to the polyol pathway and acts as a rate-limiting factor. Functioning in a NADP/H-dependent mechanism, it catalyzes the conversion of glucose to sorbitol. When hexokinase is saturated, aldose reductase, characterized by broad substrate specificity, attaches to reducing sugars and converts them into sorbitol, thereby elevating blood glucose levels. The accumulation of sorbitol within cells creates an ion gradient, leading to the development of diabetic neuropathy and cataracts (Tang et al., 2012; Thomas et al., 2010). Aldose reductase inhibitors play a crucial role in preventing the development of secondary complications associated with diabetes. Another set of enzymes, angiotensin-converting enzymes, play a vital role in modulating the angiotensin-aldosterone system, which maintains the body's physiological acid-base balance and blood pressure. These enzymes convert angiotensin I to angiotensin II, a potent vasoconstrictor that stimulates the narrowing of arterioles. This, in turn, triggers the release of aldosterone from the renal cortex, enhancing sodium reabsorption in the kidneys. Consequently, angiotensin-converting enzyme inhibitors mitigate prolonged microvascular and macrovascular complications by reducing peripheral resistance and cardiac output in the arteries (Fountain et al., 2020). A study has indicated that the activity of angiotensin-converting enzyme is elevated in diabetic patients compared to individuals without diabetes (Ustundag et al., 2000; Vieira et al., 2017). Additionally, regulators of protein tyrosine phosphatase IB (PTP IB) activity decrease serum glucose levels by enhancing insulin sensitivity, as evidenced by low to high directions (Singh et al., 2014). Therefore, identifying natural molecules that impede the formation of highly advanced glycation end products (AGEs) could serve as a promising therapeutic target. Such molecules could effectively mitigate the severity of diabetes associated with glycated products.

Marine Pharmacology

Natural resources serve as the cornerstone for a significant portion of disease treatments, and many of their constituents, including components utilized in modern pharmaceuticals, rely on these resources (Mayer et al., 2010). Marine sources, in particular, have yielded a diverse array of physiologically active compounds such as phycocolloids, phlorotannins, pigments, and fucoidans. These compounds find effective applications in industries ranging from cosmetics and fine chemicals to therapeutic agents and nutritional supplements. These natural sources have proven to be highly fruitful in producing various therapeutically effective compounds, including antiviral and anticancer agents, which are now being utilized in clinical settings (Yasuhara-Bell et al., 2010). In the quest for new alternative therapeutics and hypoglycemic medications for diabetes, researchers are increasingly focusing on marine sources as potential reservoirs of bioactive molecules. The pelagic sources primarily encompass trawl byproducts, salts, seaweed, and marine pathogens (Lee et al., 2013). Secondary metabolites found in marine organisms offer a rich source of bioactive compounds with significant potential for the development of new pharmacological drugs (Gamal et al., 2010). The nutritional bioactives required by the pharmaceutical industry, encompassing enzymes, receptors, and regulatory factors, are strikingly similar to those present in marine resources. These substances contribute to cellular homeostasis, a process often disrupted during disease progression, thereby exerting positive effects on health (Gamal et al., 2010; Freitas et al., 2012). These bioactive compounds are commonly utilized as dietary supplements. A range of marine bioactive substances has demonstrated efficacy against infections such as herpes simplex virus and tuberculosis (Vo et al., 2011; Bansemir et al., 2016). Seaweeds from the west coast of India were when extracted using methanol, exhibits anti-plasmodial activity. Furthermore, several marine bioactive compounds hold potential as antitumor agents (Namvar et al., 2012; Gul et al., 2005; Ravikumar et al., 2011). Ascophyllum nodosum, brown seaweed from the northeastern coast of the United States, contains phenol-containing compounds that exhibit both rutin-like activity and inhibition of the enzymes α-amylase and glucosidase (Apostolidis et al., 2011). The remarkable diversity of the marine environment is responsible for the wide distribution of numerous bioactive substances, including pigments, sterols, rutin, fatty acids with multiple double bonds, and sugars with various homo- and heterosaccharide units. Species from marine environments thrive within intricate ecosystems and endure harsh environmental conditions, resulting in the production of diverse biologically active compounds not found in other organisms. The fish oil component n-3PUFAs (omega-3 polyunsaturated fatty acids) possesses lipid-lowering properties that aid in the prevention of atherosclerosis and hypertension (Lordan et al., 2011).

Marine Seaweeds Contain Bio-Active Compounds

Marine seaweeds are categorized into three algal classes based on their natural colors: green (Chlorophyceae), red (Rhodophyceae), and brown algae (Phaeophyceae). Phaeophycean algae contain the brown pigment fucoxanthin, Rhodophyceae possess the red pigments phycoerythrin and phycocyanin, while Chlorophyceae are rich in chlorophyll, the green pigment. The majority of these marine algae types are considered "edible" and suitable for human consumption. Recent discoveries have revealed that marine seaweeds are abundant sources of bioactive compounds with positive impacts on the human biological environment. Specifically, marine seaweeds are prolific in the synthesis of various bioactive compounds, including flavonoids, polyphenols, sterols, basic amino compounds, tannins, proteins, amino acid derivatives, essential fatty acid esters, vitamins, enzymes, and pigments. These substances exhibit notable chemical and biological properties, showcasing activities such as anti-diabetic, rutin-like, cytotoxic, anti-fungal, anti-microbial, anti-coagulant, anti-inflammatory, and anti-proliferative effects (Khalid et al., 2018; Rengasamy et al., 2020). Abundant in marine seaweeds, sulfated polysaccharides have demonstrated beneficial effects on human health. Brown seaweeds, in particular, contain a variety of sulfated saccharides including fucoidan, alginates, and laminarins. These compounds have been associated with anti-diabetic, antioxidant, and anti-inflammatory effects (Gunathilaka et al., 2020). Red seaweeds typically contain carrageenans and agarans, which are sulfated sugar units. Similarly, green seaweeds contain sulfated polysugars known as ulvan (Wijesekara et al., 2011). These sulfated polysaccharides are recognized for their properties such as antiviral, antitumor, and anticoagulant effects (Udayangani et al., 2020). Sea water scums contain a variety of polyphenolic molecules, including flavonoids, bromophenols, phlorotannins, amino acids resembling mycosprine, and phenolic terpenoids. Amino acids resembling mycosprine are small molecules with hydroxyl groups in aromatic rings. Phlorotannins are a type of polyphenolic compound found in brown seaweeds, and they can be classified into six subgroups based on the linkage of their phloroglucinol units and hydroxyl groups: fuhalols, phloro-ethols, fucophloro-ethols, phucols, eckols, and carmalols. Flavonoids, phenolic terpenoids, phenolic acids, bromophenols, and mycosporine-like compounds are known to possess various beneficial properties including anti-diabetic, anticancer, anti-inflammatory, antioxidant, and anti-allergic effects (Ganesan et al., 2019; Cotas et al., 2020).

Antidiabetics from Marine Sources

Table 1 lists several marine-based bio-active anti-diabetic substances, their sources, and major modes of action.

Table 1. List of several marine bio-active anti-diabetic substances, their sources, and major modes of action

Bioactive Agents	Pelagic Sources	Mechanism of action	References
Bacteria	Marine sponge *Aka coralliphaga*	Blockage of β-glucosidase	Pandey et al., 2013
Polyphenols (Phlorotannins)	Brown Algae	Enhanced glucose uptake by skeletal muscles through the inhibition of α-glucosidase and α-amylase, increased insulin sensitivity is achieved by inhibiting the PTP 1B enzyme	Lee et al., 2013
Oligo-peptides	Salmon skin (*Oncorhynchus kerm*)	Lower anxiety	Zhu et al., 2010
Enrich phenol extract	Macroalgae *Palmaria, Ascophyllum, Alaria*	Amylase and glucose-6-phosphatase inhibitor	Nwosu et al., 2011
Alcohol methane extract	Tanned colored algae *Ecklonia cava*	Increase in AMP-activated protein kinase phosphorylation, radical scavenging ability	Kang et al., 2010
Eury-spongins A, B &C	Sea water sponge *Euryspongia* sp.	PTP1B (protein tyrosine phosphatase 1B) inhibition	Yamazaki et al., 2013
HPN analogues	Red agae Rhodomela confervoides	Hampering of PTP-1B	Shi et al., 2013; Shi et al., 2012
α-Galactosylceramide (α-GalCer)	Sea water sponge *Agelas mauritianus*	Switch on natural killer cells (NKT)	Van Kaer et al., 2001
Sesquiterpene Palinurin (Axel 2013)	Sponge *Ircinia dendroides*	GSK-3β (glucogen synthase kinase-3β) inhibition	Bidon-Chanal et al., 2013
Docosahexaenoic acid (DHA), Eicosapentaenoic acid (EPA)	Microalgae *Palmaria, Ascophyllum, Alaria*	maitains glucose and lipid metabolism	Nuno et al., 2013

Palinurin

The enzyme glycogen synthase kinase-3 (GSK-3) plays a significant role in various disorders, including diabetes, neurodegenerative conditions, tumors, and neurological abnormalities. Due to this involvement, GSK-3 has been recognized as a potential therapeutic target for treating diverse disorders. Laboratory experiments using isopropanol extracts from Ircinia dendroides exhibited strong inhibitory activity against human recombinant GSK-3. This inhibitory effect is attributed to the sesquiterpene compound palinurin. Palinurin achieves its inhibitory action by binding to a distinct site on the N-terminal lobe of the enzyme. This interaction alters the conformation of the glycine-rich loop, thereby affecting the accessibility of the ATP γ-phosphate. Notably, palinurin demonstrates selectivity for GSK-3β. This specific binding mechanism of palinurin to GSK-3 suggests its potential for treating GSK-3β-mediated disorders (Bidon-Chanal et al., 2013).

3,4-Dibromo-5-(2-bromo-3,4-dihydroxy-6-isopropoxymethyl benzyl)benzene-1,2-diol Analogues

A compound named 3,4-Dibromo-5-(2-bromo-3,4-dihydroxy-6-isopropoxymethyl benzyl)benzene-1,2-diol (HPN) has emerged as a promising and innovative candidate for diabetes treatment, acting as an artificial analog of bromo-containing phenols found in red algae from seawater. This compound was extensively studied in the red alga Rhodomela confervoides, known for its potent inhibition of the enzyme PTP1B. Research on HPN revealed that it exhibits a PTP1B inhibitory effect similar to that of BPN. Notably, HPN demonstrated even stronger inhibitory activity against PTP1B compared to BPN. In experimental settings, treatment with HPN resulted in a substantial and dose-dependent reduction in serum lipid levels, particularly triglycerides and total cholesterol, alongside glucose levels. Although insulin levels were reduced at higher doses, HbA1c levels saw noticeable reductions at both medium and high doses of HPN. The antihyperglycemic effects of HPN were comparable to those of the anti-diabetic medication rosiglitazone. Therefore, HPN holds significant promise as an advanced therapeutic option for managing type 2 diabetes (Shi et al., 2013; Shi et al., 2012).

Euryspongins A, B and C

The sea sponge species Euryspongia is responsible for the synthesis of three distinctive and newly discovered sesquiterpenes known as euryspongins A-C, as reported by Hiroyuki et al. in 2013. These euryspongins were identified on Iriomote Island in Okinawa, Japan, and have exhibited remarkable potential for diabetes treatment. Notably, the euryspongins A, B, and C effectively inhibit a crucial target enzyme for diabetes therapy, known as protein tyrosine phosphatase 1B (PTP1B) (Yamazaki et al., 2013).

Ecklonia Cava

The anti-diabetic potential of the brown algae Ecklonia cava was investigated using streptozotocin-induced type 1 diabetes mellitus rats and C2C12 myoblasts. In rats with type 1 diabetes mellitus, methane-mixed alcoholic extracts of Ecklonia cava significantly reduced plasma glucose levels and increased insulin levels. The antidiabetic effects of Ecklonia cava may be attributed to numerous polyphenolic compounds present in the algae. These polyphenols likely operate through various mechanisms, including AMP-activated protein kinase (AMPK), acting in a manner similar to insulin. AMPK, a key regulator in many cells, controls intracellular fatty acid metabolism and synthesis. The methane-alcoholic extract of Ecklonia cava was observed to enhance AMPK phosphorylation in C2C12 cells in a dose-dependent manner (Kang et al., 2010).

α-Galacto-sylcer-amide (α-GalCer)

The glycolipid α-GalCer has been identified as effective in the management of type 1 diabetes. Its dose-dependent anti-diabetic potential was observed in experiments conducted on nude mice. This glycoprotein, derived from the marine sponge-Alga mauritianus, initially underwent testing for its potential antimetastatic properties. The immune system plays a crucial role in the mechanism of action of α-GalCer's anti-diabetic effects. α-GalCer enhances natural cell-mediated immunity, selectively suppressing pathogenic T cells responsible for the destruction of insulin-producing pancreatic cells. Moreover, α-GalCer has the capability to modify immune responses by promoting cellular reactions that primarily work to suppress autoimmune reactions. Clinical studies involving α-GalCer revealed no adverse side effects, suggesting its potential as a viable option for diabetes prevention (Van Kaer et al., 2001).

Eicosapentaenoic Acid (EPA) and Docosahexaenoic Acid (DHA)

Isochrysis galbana and nannochloropsis oculate are two marine micro-algae that serve as abundant sources of protein, soluble and insoluble polysaccharides, and polyunsaturated essential fatty acids. While Nannochloropsis oculate is rich in EPA (eicosapentaenoic acid), Isochrysis galbana contains a high proportion of DHA (docosahexaenoic acid). In studies conducted by Nuno et al., in 2013, these biochemical components were found to regulate lipid and glucose metabolism in rats with high levels of sugars. They also positively influenced the upper layer of the intestine and epithelium, managing lipid-proteins and nitrogenous compounds. These biologically active constituents present in microalgae have the potential to be utilized in the development of nutraceuticals and functional foods. Treatment with Isochrysis galbana resulted in decreased blood glucose, triglyceride, and cholesterol levels. Interestingly, both microalgae elevated levels of both "bad" and "good" cholesterol in both healthy and diabetic rat groups, indicating a notable impact on lipid metabolism (Nuno et al., 2013).

Phenolic contents of Palmaria, Alaria and Ascophyllum

Nwosu et al., (2011) conducted a study exploring the anti-glucose properties of phenol-containing extracts from marine macro-algae commonly found in the UK. Phenolic extracts from Palmaria, Alaria, and Ascophyllum were found to inhibit α-amylase activity. Additionally, Ascophyllum extract exhibited inhibitory effects on α-glucosidase. Both of these enzymes play a significant role in the regulation of blood sugar levels and the digestion of starch (Nwosu et al., 2011).

Salmon Skin Oligopeptides

The anti-diabetic potential of oligo-peptides extracted from salmon skin was investigated by Zhu et al. in 2010. Rats were utilized to examine the effectiveness of oligo-peptides obtained from the skin of wild Oncorhynchus keta, found in the Eastern China Sea, in treating diabetes. Rats exhibiting diabetic symptoms and treated with these oligo-peptides showed reduced fasting blood sugar levels and a decrease in pancreatic islet cell necrosis. Additionally, the levels of malondialdehyde, interferon-gamma, and serum tumor necrosis factor-alpha were lower. Notably, in diabetic rats receiving oligo-peptide treatment, the levels of serum superoxide dismutase and glutathione increased significantly (Zhu et al., 2010).

Marine Bacteria

The glycosidic linkages within sugar moieties are formed through the catalytic activity of the enzyme glucosidase. Specifically, β-glucosidase plays a crucial role in the processing of glycoproteins, glycolipids, and the breakdown of polysaccharides. As a result, β-glucosidases have significant physiological implications in various diseases, including diabetes, obesity, and cancer. A study conducted by Pandey et al. (2013) revealed that numerous marine microorganisms produce metabolites with the potential to act as β-glucosidase inhibitors. One such microorganism, in conjunction with the marine sponge Aka coralliphaga, yielded a variety of alpha-glucosidase inhibitors. These inhibitors demonstrated strong inhibitory activity when assessed using a β-glucosidase inhibition assay. Phylogenetic analysis of these bacterial strains indicated that glucosidase inhibitors are produced by the phyla Firmicutes, Actinobacteria, Proteobacteria, and Bacteroidetes. The inhibition of β-glucosidase from marine sources holds promise for the treatment of diabetes and its associated complications (Pandey et al., 2013).

Polyphenols (Phlorotannin's) Obtained from Brown Algae

Phloroglucinol units undergo polymerization to give rise to polyphenols, which are abundantly produced by brown algae. These marine-derived polyphenols, commonly referred to as phlorotannins, are synthesized through the polyketide pathway within brown algae. Phlorotannins exhibit a diverse range of activities, including antineoplastic, anti-inflammatory, and rutin-like effects. These polyphloroglucinols exhibit their antidiabetic effects through a multitude of mechanisms. Their modes of action encompass inhibiting α-glucosidase and α-amylase enzymes, promoting increased glucose uptake by skeletal muscles, impeding the function of the protein tyrosine phosphatase 1B (PTP 1B) enzyme, and enhancing insulin sensitivity. This multifaceted approach contributes to the potential antidiabetic effects of phlorotannins derived from marine sources (Lee et al., 2013).

Conclusion

While various approaches rooted in plant-based and synthetic compounds have demonstrated success in diabetes treatment, a definitive pharmaceutical solution to effectively combat diabetes and its associated complications remains elusive. The complexity of diabetes management poses a significant challenge, and addressing this complexity requires innovative solutions. The marine environment offers a promising avenue for addressing these challenges, as it is an underutilized resource rich in potential bioactive molecules. The objective of the present chapter is to underscore the potential of diverse marine bioactive compounds in the context of diabetes management. The vast marine ecosystem, including sources such as trawl, seaweed, sponges, fungi, microorganisms, and seagrasses, provides an array of bioactive substances with potential anti-diabetic properties. These marine resources hold the promise of serving as a novel reservoir for the development of innovative and potent medications for diabetes.

References

Apostolidis, E., Karayannakidis, P. D., Kwon, Y. I., Lee, C. M., Seeram, N. P. (2011). Seasonal variation of phenolic antioxidant-mediated α-glucosidase inhibition of Ascophyllum nodosum. *Plant Foods for Human Nutrition*, 66(4), 313-319.

Bansemir, A., Blume, M., Schröder, S., Lindequist, U. (2006). Screening of cultivated seaweeds for antibacterial activity against fish pathogenic bacteria. *Aquaculture*, 252(1), 79-84.

Barde, S. R., Sakhare, R. S., Kanthale, S. B., Chandak, P. G., Jamkhande, P. G. (2015). Marine bioactive agents: A short review on new marine antidiabetic compounds. *Asian Pacific Journal of Tropical Disease*, 2020, S209-S213.

Bidon-Chanal, A., Fuertes, A., Alonso, D., Pérez, D. I., Martínez, A., Luque, F. J., Medina, M. (2013). Evidence for a new binding mode to GSK-3: allosteric regulation by the marine compound palinurin. *European Journal of Medicinal Chemistry*, 60, 479-89.

Cotas, J., Leandro, A., Monteiro, P., Pacheco, D., Figueirinha, A., Gonçalves, A. M. M., da Silva, G. J., Pereira, L. (2020). Seaweed phenolics: from extraction to applications. *Marine Drugs*, 18, 384.

D'Orazio, N., Gammone, M. A., Gemello, E., De Girolamo, M., Cusenza, S., Riccioni, G. (2012). Marine bioactives: pharmacological properties and potential applications against inflammatory diseases. *Marine Drugs*, 10, 812-833.

Xia, E. Q., Zhu, S. S., He, M. J., Luo, F., Fu, C. Z., Zou, T. B. (2017). Marine peptides as potential agents for the management of type 2 diabetes mellitus-a prospect. *Marine drugs*, 15(4), 88.

Fountain, J. H., Lappin, S. L. (2020). *Physiology, Renin Angiotensin System*; StatPearls Publishing: Treasure Island, Florida, 2020.

Freitas, A. C., Rodrigues, D., Rocha-Santos, T. A., Gomes, A. M., Duarte, A. C. (2012). Marine biotechnology advances towards applications in new functional foods. *Biotechnology Advances*, 30(6), 1506-1515.

Gamal, A. A. E. (2010). Biological importance of marine algae. *Saudi Pharmaceutical Journal*, 18(1), 1-25.

Ganesan, A. R., Tiwari, U., Rajauria, G. (2019). Seaweed nutraceuticals and their therapeutic role in disease prevention. *Food Science and Human Wellness*, 8, 252-263.

Gerich, J. (2013). Pathogenesis and management of postprandial hyperglycemia: role of incretin-based therapies. *International Journal of General Medicine*, 6, 877-895.

Goldenberg, R., Punthakee, Z. (2013). Canadian Diabetes Association Clinical Practice Guidelines Expert Committee, Definition, classification and diagnosis of diabetes, prediabetes and metabolic syndrome. *Canadian Journal of Diabetes*, 37(Suppl 1), S8-S11.

Groop, L., Pociot, F. (2014). Genetics of diabetes - are we missing the genes or the disease? *Molecular & Cellular Endocrinology*, 382(1), 726-739.

Gul, W., Hamann, M. T. (2005). Indole alkaloid marine natural products: an established source of cancer drug leads with considerable promise for the control of parasitic, neurological and other diseases. *Life Sciences*, 78(5), 442-453.

Gunathilaka, T. L., Samarakoon, K., Ranasinghe, P., Peiris, L. D. C. (2020). Antidiabetic potential of marine brown algae—a mini review. *Journal of Diabetes Research*, 2020, 1230218.

Heendeniya, S. N., Keerthirathna, L. R., Manawadu, C. K., Dissanayake, I. H., Ali, R., Mashhour, A., Alzahrani, H., Godakumbura, P., Boudjelal, M., Peiris, D. C. (2020). Therapeutic Efficacy of Nyctanthes arbor-tristis flowers to inhibit proliferation of acute and chronic primary human leukemia cells, with adipocyte differentiation and in silico analysis of interactions between survivin protein and selected secondary meta. *Biomolecules*, 10, 165.

Hinnen, D., Strong, J. (2018). A New Once-Daily Fixed-Ratio Combination of Basal Insulin Glargine and Lixisenatide for the Management of Type 2 Diabetes. *Diabetes Spectrum*, 31, 145-154.

Hinnen, D. A. (2015). Therapeutic options for the management of postprandial glucose in patients with type 2 diabetes on basal insulin. *Clinical Diabetes*, 33, 175-180.

Joshi, S. R., Parikh, R. M., Das, A. K. (2007). Insulin—History, biochemistry, physiology and pharmacology. *Journal of the Association of Physicians of India*, 55, S19–S25.

Kang, C., Jin, Y. B., Lee, H., Cha, M., Sohn, E. T., Moon, J. (2010). Brown alga Ecklonia cava attenuates type 1 diabetes by activating AMPK and Akt signaling pathways. *Food & Chemical Toxicology*, 48(2), 509-516.

Kaur, J. (2014). A comprehensive review on metabolic syndrome. *Cardiology Research & Practice*, 2014, 943162.

Khalid, S., Abbas, M., Saeed, F., Bader-Ul-Ain, H., Ansar Rasul Suleria, H. (2018). Therapeutic Potential of Seaweed Bioactive Compounds. In *Seaweed Biomaterials*; IntechOpen, pp. 2-14.

Lee, S. H., Jeon, Y. J. (2013). Anti-diabetic effects of brown algae derived phlorotannins, marine polyphenols through diverse mechanisms. *Fitoterapia*, 86, 129-136.

Liu, Y., Gao, Z., Guo, Q., Wang, T., Lu, C., Chen, Y., Sheng, Q., Chen, J., Nie, Z., Zhang, Y., Wu, W., Lv, Z., Shu, J. (2014). Anti-diabetic effects of CTB-APSL fusion protein in type 2 diabetic mice. *Marine Drugs*, 13, 1512-1529.

Lordan, S., Ross, R. P., Stanton, C. (2011). Marine bioactives as functional food ingredients: potential to reduce the incidence of chronic diseases. *Marine Drugs*, 9(6), 1056-100.

Makrilakis, K. (2019). The role of DPP-4 Inhibitors in the treatment algorithm of type 2 diabetes mellitus: when to select, what to expect. *International Journal of Environmental Research Public Health*, 16, 2720.

Mayer, A. M., Glaser, K. B., Cuevas, C., Jacobs, R. S., Kem, W., Little, R. D., McIntosh, J. M., Newman, D. J., Potts, B. C., Shuster, D. E. (2010). The odyssey of marine pharmaceuticals: a current pipeline perspective. *Trends Pharmacological Science*, 31(6), 255-265.

Namvar, F., Mohamed, S., Fard, S. G., Behravan, J., Mustapha, N. M., Alitheen, N. B. M. (2012). Polyphenol-rich seaweed (Eucheuma cottonii) extract suppresses breast tumour via hormone modulation and apoptosis induction. *Food Chemistry*, 130(2), 376-382.

Newsholme, P., Cruzat, V., Arfuso, F., Keane, K. (2014). Nutrient regulation of insulin secretion and action. *Journal of Endocrinology*, 221, R105-R120.

Nuño, K., Villarruel-López, A., Puebla-Pérez, A. M., Romero-Velarde, E., Puebla-Mora, A. G., Ascencio, F. (2013). Effects of the marine microalgae *Isochrysis galbana* and *Nannochloropsis oculata* in diabetic rats. *Journal of Functional Foods*, 5(1), 106-115.

Nwosu, F., Morris, J., Lund, V. A., Stewart, D., Ross, H. A., McDougall, G. J. (2011). Anti-proliferative and potential anti-diabetic effects of phenolic-rich extracts from edible marine algae. *Food Chemistry*, 126(3), 1006-1012.

Pandey, S., Sree, A., Dash, S. S., Sethi, D. P., Chowdhury, L. (2013). Diversity of marine bacteria producing beta-glucosidase inhibitors. *Microbial Cell Factories*, 12, 1-7.

Panunti, B., Jawa, A. A., Fonseca, V. A. (2004). Mechanisms and therapeutic targets in type 2 diabetes mellitus. *Drug Discovery Today: Disease Mechanisms*, 1(2), 151-157.

Popov, A. M., Krivoshapko, O. N. (2013). Protective effects of polar lipids and redox-active compounds from marine organisms at modeling of hyperlipidemia and diabetes. *Journal of Biomedical Science & Engineering*, 6, 543–550.

Qaid, M. M., Abdelrahman, M. M. (2016). Role of insulin and other related hormones in energy metabolism—a review. *Cogent Food & Agriculture*, 2, 1267691.

Ravikumar, S., Ramanathan, G., Gnanadesigan, M., Ramu, A, Vijayakumar, V. (2011). In vitro antiplasmodial activity of methanolic extracts from seaweeds of South West Coast of India. *Asian Pacific Journal of Tropical Medicine*, 4(11), 862-865.

Reimann, M., Bonifaci, E., Solimena, M., Schwarz, P. E., Ludwig, B., Hanefeld, M., Bornstein, S. R. (2009). An update on preventive and regenerative therapies in diabetes mellitus. *Pharmacology & Therapeutics*, 121, 317-331

Rengasamy, K. R., Mahomoodally, M. F., Aumeeruddy, M. Z., Zengin, G., Xiao, J., Kim, D. H. (2020). Bioactive compounds in seaweeds: An overview of their biological properties and safety. *Food & Chemical Toxicology*, 135, 111013.

Shi, D., Guo, S., Jiang, B., Guo, C., Wang, T., Zhang, L. (2013). HPN, a synthetic analogue of bromophenol from red alga Rhodomela confervoides: synthesis and anti-diabetic effects in C57BL/KsJ-db/db mice. *Marine Drugs*, 11(2), 350-362.

Shi, D., Li, J., Jiang, B., Guo, S., Su, H., Wang, T. (2012). Bromophenols as inhibitors of protein tyrosine phosphatase 1B with antidiabetic properties. *Bioorganic & Medicinal Chemistry Letters*, 22(8), 2827-2832.

Singh, V. P., Bali, A., Singh, N., Jaggi, A. S. (2014). Advanced glycation end products and diabetic complications. *Korean journal of Physiology & Pharmacology*, 18(1), 1.

Sonksen, P., Sonksen, J. (2000). Insulin: Understanding its action in health and disease. *British Journal of Anaesthsia*, 85, 69-79.

Sudasinghe, H. P., Peiris, D. C. (2018). Hypoglycemic and hypolipidemic activity of aqueous leaf extract of Passiflora suberosa L. *PeerJ*, 6, e4389.

Tabatabaei-Malazy, O., Larijani, B., Abdollahi, M. (2013). A novel management of diabetes by means of strong antioxidants' combination. *Journal of Medical Hypotheses and Ideas*, 7(1), 25-30.

Tang, W. H., Martin, K. A., Hwa, J. (2012). Aldose reductase, oxidative stress, and diabetic mellitus. *Frontiers in Pharmacology*, 2012, 3.

Thomas, V., Spiro, T., Moomaw, W. R. (2010). Emissions and Exposure to Metals: Cadmium and Lead. In *Industrial Ecology and Global Change*; Socolow, R., Andrews, C., Berkhout, F., Thomas, V., Eds., Cambridge University Press: Cambridge; pp. 297-318.

Udayangani, R. M. A. C., Somasiri, G. D. P., Wickramasinghe, I., Kim, S. (2020). Potential Health Benefits of Sulfated Polysaccharides from Marine Algae. In *Encyclopedia of Marine Biotechnology*; Wiley, 2020; pp. 629-635.

Ustündağ, B., Canatan, H., Cinkilinç, N., Halifeoğlu, I., Bahçecioğlu, I. H. (2000). Angiotensin converting enzyme (ACE) activity levels in insulin-independent diabetes mellitus and effect of ACE levels on diabetic patients with nephropathy. *Cell Biochemistry & Function*, 18, 23-28.

Van Kaer, L. (2001). Drugs from the Sea: a marine sponge-derived compound prevents type 1 diabetes. *Scientific World Journal*, 1, 630-632.

Vieira, M. N. N., Lyra e Silva, N. M., Ferreira, S. T., De Felice, F. G. (2017). Protein tyrosine phosphatase 1B (PTP1B): a potential target for Alzheimer's therapy. *Frontiers in Aging Neuroscience*, 9, 1-9.

Vo, T., Ngo, D., Ta, Q. V., Kim, S. (2011). Marine organisms as a therapeutic source against herpes simplex virus infection. *European Journal of Pharmaceutical Science*, 44(1-2), 11-20.

Wijesekara, I., Pangestuti, R., Kim, S. K. (2011). Biological activities and potential health benefits of sulfated polysaccharides derived from marine algae. *Carbohydrate Polymers*, 84, 14-21.

Yamazaki, H., Nakazawa, T., Sumilat, D. A., Takahashi, O., Ukai, K., Takahashi, S., Namikoshi, M. (2013). Euryspongins A–C, three new unique sesquiterpenes from a marine sponge Euryspongia sp. *Bioorganic & Medicinal Chemistry Letters*, 23(7), 2151-2154.

Yasuhara-Bell, J., Lu, Y. (2010). Marine compounds and their antiviral activities. *Antiviral Research*, 86(3), 231-240.

Zaccardi, F., Webb, D. R., Yates, T., Davies, M. J. (2016). Pathophysiology of type 1 and type 2 diabetes mellitus: a 90-year perspective. *Postgraduate Medical Journal*, 92(1084), 63-69.

Zhang, Z., Zhao, M., Wang, J., Ding, Y., Dai, X., Li, Y. (2011). Oral administration of skin gelatin isolated from chum salmon (Oncorhynchus keta) enhances wound healing in diabetic rats. *Marine Drugs*, 9, 696-711.

Zhu, C. F., Peng, H. B., Liu, G. Q., Zhang, F., Li, Y. (2010). Beneficial effects of oligopeptides from marine salmon skin in a rat model of type 2 diabetes. *Nutrition*, 26, 1014-1020.

Chapter 5

Mushrooms in the Management of Diabetes Mellitus

Charu Bharti[1,*]
Shalini Jayant[1]
Neelam Gupta[2]
Surbhi Gupta[1]
and Pratibha Dwivedi[3]
[1]Department of Pharmacology, School of Pharmacy, Bharat Institute of Technology, Meerut, Uttar Pradesh, India
[2]I. T. S. College of Pharmacy, Muradnagar, Ghaziabad, Uttar Pradesh, India
[3]Krishnarpit Institute of Pharmacy, Prayagraj, Uttar Pradesh, India

Abstract

More than 1.5 million death cases worldwide each year are directly attributed to diabetes, according to a report by the World Health Organization (WHO). Diabetes mellitus is a highly complex chronic metabolic disorder caused by a decrease in insulin production or dysfunction, resulting in elevated blood glucose levels known as hyperglycemia. Despite significant advancements in medicinal chemistry, synthetic drugs have not provided a cure for diabetes due to their adverse side effects or reduced effectiveness over time. This has led to the exploration of therapeutic mushrooms as potential anti-diabetic agents, as they have long been valued as a source of natural bioactive compounds. Therapeutic mushrooms contain bioactive constituents such as terpenoids, polysaccharides, proteins, lectins,

* Corresponding Author's Email: charubhartisdmzn@gmail.com.

In: Naturally Occurring Chemicals …
Editors: A. Singh Grewal, G. Deswal, A. Kumar Dhingra et al.
ISBN: 979-8-89113-491-1

alkaloids, sterols, and phenolic compounds, which have various pharmacological benefits. The anti-diabetic action of these mushrooms has been demonstrated through in vitro and in vivo studies, as well as clinical trials. The bioactive metabolites found in mushrooms have been shown to lower blood sugar levels by blocking glucose absorption, improving pancreatic beta-cell mass, and enhancing insulin signaling pathways. In conclusion, this chapter discusses the current status and future prospects of utilizing bioactive metabolites from mushrooms for the management of diabetes.

Keywords: diabetes mellitus, mushrooms, terpenoids, natural bioactive compounds, insulin

Abbreviations

BP	Blood Pressure
DM	Diabetes Mellitus
DN	Diabetic neuropathy
IDDM	Insulin-dependent diabetes mellitus
NIDDM	Non-insulin-dependent diabetes mellitus
STZ	Streptozocin
T2DM	Type-2 diabetes mellitus.

Introduction

Historically, mushrooms or macrofungi have been added to food by civilizations such as the Romans and Greeks since ancient times, mainly because of their distinct and unique flavor. According to ancient literature, the Romans considered mushrooms as a delicacy bestowed by the gods, whereas the Chinese referred to them as the "elixir of life." Throughout the ages, different cultures have incorporated mushrooms into their cuisine, recognizing their safe and medicinal properties (Valverde et al., 2015). The word "mushroom" originated from the Greek words "fungus" and "mykes." It refers to the filamentous umbrella-shaped fruiting body of certain macrofungi. These mushrooms are rich in nutrients such as carbohydrates, proteins, vitamins (especially vitamins B and D), and minerals like potassium, copper, phosphorous, and selenium. Mushrooms are neither animals nor plants, but rather the separate sporophores of certain fungi.

Research has identified approximately 1590 mushroom species in the environment. However, only around 99 species are recognized as edible and used as food. Out of these, roughly 33 species are cultivated for food globally. Among commercially grown mushrooms, the most common types are Agaricus bisporus (white button mushrooms), Pleurotus ostreatus (oyster mushrooms), and Volvariella volvacea (paddy straw mushrooms) (Kumar et al., 2021). The taxonomic classification of mushrooms is generally divided as follows: Phylum - Basidiomycota, Division - Eumycota, and Class - Hymenomycetes. The class "mushroom" is further classified into different classes, including Agaricales, Polyporales, Sclerodermatales, Aphyllophorales, Lycoperdales, Auriculariales, and Tremellales. Mushrooms possess different medicinal values due to the presence of various secondary metabolites. However, non-edible species are not used for medicinal purposes as they can potentially cause poisonous effects on human beings. The term "mycetism" refers to mushroom poisoning, and it was first discovered among various rural populations in Africa after the ingestion of toxic mushrooms (Ukwuru et al., 2018). Some common edible mushrooms include Ganoderma lucidium (Lingzhi mushroom), Tremella fuciformis, Lentinus concentricus, Calocybe indica (Flammulina velutipes), Lentinula edodes, Hypsizygus tessellatus, Aerocybe aegerita, Coprinus comatus, Pleurotus ostreatus, Laetiporus sulphurous, Grifora frondsa, Agaricus Bisporus, Volvariella volvacea, Cordyceps sinensis, and Hericium erinaceus (Erbiai et al., 2021; Das et al., 2022). Edible mushrooms have been widely recognized for their numerous health benefits and are commonly utilized in the treatment and management of various diseases. These mushrooms possess a wide range of medicinal properties, including being used as an anti-diabetic, anti-inflammatory agent, immunity booster, anti-oxidant, anti-cancer, hypoglycemic agent, anti-bacterial, and beneficial for neurological and cardiovascular health. Additionally, they have shown promising effects as anti-androgenic, anti-depressant, and anti-microbial agents, as illustrated in Table 1.

Bio-Active Constituents Present in Mushrooms

In order to survive, macrofungi have the potential to naturally synthesize a cluster of bioactive compounds that can provide versatile therapeutic effects in various biomedical fields. Additionally, mushrooms act as a natural food product that promotes health in the market. In recent times, the population is consuming mushrooms for not only their taste but also for their extensive range of medicinal values. Research has concluded that mushrooms contain ample amounts of proteins, lipids, carbohydrates, vitamins, and minerals such as magnesium, calcium, sodium, copper, potassium, iron, selenium, etc (Lee et al., 2019; Saad et al., 2022). The bioactive chemical constituents found in edible mushrooms that are used in diabetic treatment are listed in Table 1. These constituents include various fatty acids such as linoleic, oleic, and palmitic acids. There are also carbohydrates present, such as chitosan and β-glucans, as well as proteins like lectins. Phenol-containing compounds, such as caffeine, gallic acid, p-hydroxybenzoic acid, and melatonin, are also found in mushrooms. Additionally, mushrooms contain vitamins such as vitamin B, B12, C, B6, and E. Other chemical constituents present in mushrooms include terpenoids, carotenoids (specifically β-carotene and lycopene), and molecules such as ergothioneine and glutathione, although these are present in trace amounts (Martinez Medina et al., 2021).

Carbohydrate

Mushrooms contain various types of carbohydrates that vary based on their size and can be categorized as monosaccharides, disaccharides, oligosaccharides, and polysaccharides. Chemically, they are aldehydes and ketones with multiple hydroxyl groups. Scientific literature states that mushrooms consist primarily of carbohydrates, making up around 47-81 percent of their total content (Ruthes et al., 2016; Rathore et al., 2017). Glucose, sucrose, maltose, rhamnose, arabinose, sucrose, and mannitol are commonly found carbohydrates in mushrooms (Kaliyaperumal et al., 2018) and glucans (Chemically it is linear polysaccharides integrated by glucose by different linkage like β (1–3), or β (1–6)) is the fraction of the mushrooms which is effective against treatment of diabetes. Mushrooms also contain chitin polymer as a main polysaccharide that produces stiffness and osmotic integrity to the cell wall (Kalac, 2013; Nishihara et al., 2007). Mushrooms are known to contain significant amounts of polysaccharides, which are complex carbohydrates. There are various edible and medicinal mushroom varieties that are rich in polysaccharides, some of which include Lentinus edodes (also known as shiitake mushroom), Grifola frondosa (maitake mushroom), Schizophyllum commun (split-gill mushroom), and Pleurotus ostreus (oyster mushroom).

Table 1. Various types of edible mushrooms, their bio-active compounds, and health benefits

Scientific Name/Common Name	Bioactive Chemical Compounds	Health Benefits	Reference
Ganoderma lucidum (Reishi, lingzhi)	Phenols, glycoproteins, steroids, polysaccharides (glucans)	Immuno booster, reduce stress, improve improper sleep pattern, lessen fatigue	(Veljovic et al., 2017)
Tremella Fuciformis (Snow fungus)	Ellagic acid, vanillin, luteolin, kaempferol, myricetin, and (+)-gallocatechin	Boost immune system, anti-oxidant, anti-cancer	(Wu et al., 2022)
Calocybe indica (Milky white mushrooms)	Thiamine, riboflavin, niacin and biotin, nicotinic acid, alpha-tocopherol and glucans	Anti-tumor, anti-oxidant, anti-bacterial, neurodegenerative disorders, Cardiovascular disorders	(Roy et al., 2014)
Flammulina velutipes (Enoki mushroom)	Seco-cuparane sesquiterpenes, flammu furanone L-glutamic acid, L-alanine, glycine and L-lysine	Wound healing, anti-cancer, immunity booster, anti-aging, anti-inflammatory	(Tang et al., 2016)
Lentinula edodes (Shiitake mushrooms)	Lentinan and vitamin B12, flavonoids, β-carotene, lycopene	Anti-cancer, hypocholesterolemic, hypotensive, hypoglycemic and antioxidant	(Choi et al., 2016)
Hypsizygus tessellatus (Buna shimeji)	glucans, niacin, vitamins B and D, l-ergothioneine, sterols, ergosterol	Anti-microbial, anti-oxidant, anti-bacterial	(Monira et al., 2012)
Aerocybe aegerita (Popular mushroom, chestnut mushroom)	Linoleic acid, palmitic acid, oleic acid, tocopherol	Anti-tumor, anti-fungal, anti-inflammatory	(Petrovic et al., 2015)
Coprinus comatus (Shaggy mane)	Diisobutyl phthalate, cis-9,12-octadecadienoic acid, 4-hydroxy phenethyl acetate	Anti-tumor, anti-viral, anti-inflammatory, anti-androgenic	(Chao et al., 2020; Ya-Ping et al., 2018)
Pleurotus ostreatus (Oyster mushroom)	β-Glucan proto-catechuic acid, gallic acid, homogentisic acid, rutins, myrictin, chrysin, naringin, α, γ- tocopherol, vitamin C and carotenes	Anti-diabetic, anti-viral, anti-hypercholesterolic, anti-oxidant, anti-bacterial	(Depalakshmi et al., 2014)
Laetiporous sulphurous (Sulfer shelf)	Polysaccharides, laetiporic acids, beauvericin, lectins, and triterpenes	Anti-microbial, anti-oxidant, anti-inflammatory, anti-tumor	(Katarzyna et al., 2018)
Grifora frondsa (Hen of the woods)	β-Glucan polysaccharide compounds, α-rhamnopyranose, palmitic, oleic, and linoleic acids, Grifolaone A	Anti-tumor, immunomodulation, antioxidant	(Wu et al., 2018)

Table 1. (Continued)

Scientific Name/Common Name	Bioactive Chemical Compounds	Health Benefits	Reference
Agaricus Bisporus (Button mushroom)	Polyketides, terpenoids, steroidal compounds, carotenes, and vitamins like A and C	Antimicrobial, antioxidant, anti-allergenic and dietary compounds	(Ramos et al., 2019)
Volvariella volvacea (Straw mushroom)	Volvafuranone-A, furanones	Anti-tumor, anti-oxidant, anti-bacterial, neurodegenerative disorders, Cardiovascular disorders	(Chen et al., 2018)
Cordyceps sinensis (Winter worm summer grass)	Cordycepic acid and cordycepin	hypo-glycemic activity, cellular health properties, antidepressant activity	(Liu et al., 2015)

These mushrooms have shown potential in the field of cancer treatment. (Meng et al., 2016).

Proteins

Chemically, proteins are macromolecular complexes made up of amino acids, which serve as the building blocks. They mainly consist of nitrogen components. According to literature investigations, edible mushrooms contain 19 to 40 percent of the total amount of bioactive compounds (Lin et al., 2013). Mushrooms contain various proteins with a concentration of valines and asparagine that are significantly higher. These proteins have a length of 111-114 amino acids and exhibit immunomodulatory activity (Martinez Medina et al., 2021).

Lectins

Mushrooms contain a significant amount of glycated proteins, similar to other bioactive chemical compounds found in various species such as algae, plants, and other vertebrates. Lectins make up at least 82% of the composition of mushrooms, with molecular weights ranging from 12 to 68 kDa (Varrot et al., 2013; Mishra et al., 2019).

Lipids

Mushrooms contain a variety of different lipids, including sterols, fatty acids, and phospholipids. Fatty acids such as linoleic acid, oleic acid, and palmitic acid are abundant in fungi. Macrofungi have various molecules with a cyclohexane core and a cyclopentane ring with an aliphatic addition. Research has found that ergosterol is the main sterol isolated from mushrooms and it has properties that can enhance fungal growth, hyphae formation, and sporulation (Papoutsis et al., 2020).

Others Components

The natural world is rich in diverse chemical ingredients that possess versatile properties for treating various complications. These ingredients include phenols, flavonoids, lignin, hydroxybenzoic acid, tannins, stilbene, hydroxy-cinnamic acid, and polyphenols. These components are important for their beneficial effects (Nowak et al., 2014; Martinez Medina et al., 2021).

Medicinal Importance of Mushrooms

Macrofungi, also known as mushrooms, play a crucial role in reducing total blood cholesterol levels, regulating blood lipid levels, and lowering blood glucose levels. Mushrooms are considered therapeutic ingredients due to their abundance of nutrients, a fact recognized by researchers worldwide. In fact, macrofungi contain various chemical compounds, including amino acids, polyunsaturated and saturated fatty acids, all of which have higher nutritional value than fish and other types of beef (Daba et al., 2008). The presence of various chemical components in mushrooms has shown beneficial effects in treating skin conditions such as atopic dermatitis, skin aging, and allergic reactions. Additionally, mushrooms rich in fiber, proteins, and high caloric content play a crucial role in preventing hypercholesterolemia and cardiovascular diseases (Fekadu, 2014). Due to the presence of various bioactive chemical constituents produced by mushrooms, they have been found to have significant therapeutic effects. These include being anti-inflammatory, immuno-modulators, antidiabetic, anti-oxidant, anti-viral, anti-obesity, anti-aging, and anti-microbial (Girma and Tasisa, 2018).

Importance of Mushrooms in Diabetes Mellitus

Blood Glucose Lowering Effect of Polysaccharides

Over the years, mushrooms have been extensively studied for their potential in treating various diseases and conditions, with diabetes being a particularly interesting area of research. It is widely known that different herbs contain diverse biochemical compounds, some of which are highly beneficial for treating various conditions, while others are non-beneficial for both humans and animals. Similar to other plant species, mushrooms also possess a wide range of constituents, as outlined in Table 1.

Reduction of Glucose Absorption

Recently, studies have shown that polysaccharides found in mushrooms can have positive effects on reducing high blood sugar levels, known as hyperglycemia. These polysaccharides achieve this by decreasing the efficiency of glucose absorption in the body and enhancing the insulin signaling pathway (Jelena et al., 2021). Additionally, mushrooms' polysaccharides have the potential to greatly accelerate hyperglycemia through various mechanisms and can act as supportive agents in individuals with diabetes mellitus.

Maintains Pancreatic Beta Cells Activity

It has also been reported through both in-vivo and in-vitro studies that Polysaccharides found in mushrooms can increase the number of pancreatic β-cells in the pancreas and help maintain their presence (Jelena et al., 2021). Recent research has found that natural polysaccharides extracted from mushrooms can enhance insulin sensitivity and lipid metabolism, resulting in a healthier hypoglycemic food (Siwen et al., 2019).

Blood Glucose Lowering Effect of Terpenoids

It has been reported that terpenoids found in mushrooms have the ability to inhibit α-glucosidase, an enzyme responsible for breaking down carbohydrates, and also sensitize insulin by activating PPARγ, a receptor involved in glucose and lipid metabolism. This dual action leads to the suppression of hyperglycemia in animal models of diabetes. These findings suggest that mushrooms could be a potential natural treatment for diabetes (Jelena et al., 2021).

Effect of Mushrooms on Diabetic Complications

Recent advancements in the treatment of diabetes have paved the way for innovative research on natural products, which have shown promising results in addressing diabetes and its associated complications. One such area of investigation involves mushrooms, which have demonstrated potential in addressing diabetes-related issues such as myocardial fibrosis, lipid metabolism, diabetic renal problems, bone loss, diabetic foot complications, wound healing and angiogenesis, retinopathy, obesity, and neuronal issues (Jiang et al., 2020). Obesity and complications related to abnormal lipid metabolism can be treated using polysaccharides extracted from the Pleurotus rhizome. These polysaccharides help maintain a balanced composition of fatty acids, regulate levels of hyperlipidemia, and improve conditions related to obesity by enhancing the expression of hepatic PPAR-α-mRNA-protein levels (Haung et al., 2014). According to the research conducted by Zhang et al., polysaccharides extracted from Tremella aurantialba have been found to regulate lipid metabolism and reduce oxidative stress in animals with alloxan-induced diabetes (Zhang et al., 2009). Diabetic neuropathy (DN), which is a long-term complication of diabetes, is a major cause of end-stage kidney disease. However, polysaccharides derived from Auricularia auricular (a type of edible mushroom) have shown promising potential in treating DN. These polysaccharides are able to modulate oxidative injury and the NF-κB pathway in a diabetic animal model induced by streptozotocin (STZ) (Hu et al., 2017). A study conducted by Zhang et al. showed that mycelium zinc polysaccharide obtained from Pleurotus djamor (a pink oyster mushroom) exhibits both alkaline and acidic properties. The researchers found that this polysaccharide has beneficial effects on kidney and liver protection in a mouse model of diabetes induced by STZ (streptozotocin). The polysaccharide was found to alleviate oxidative damage and improve the condition of the organs (Zhang et al., 2015). Myocardial fibrosis leads to the development of myocardial stiffness in diabetic patients which leads to dangerous cardiovascular diseases (Asbun et al., 2006). So, this chronic complication can be treated by G. lucidum polysaccharides, which can weaken collagen cross-linking in the myocardium. This is achieved by reducing the levels of advanced glycation end products (AGEs) and improving the antioxidant status in diabetic animals (Meng et al., 2011) G. lucidum polysaccharides are also utilized in the treatment of stubborn wounds in diabetic patients. It achieves this by enhancing the healing process in diabetic mice with induced diabetes through the control of mitochondrial oxidative damage, reduction of p66Shc, and MnSoD nitration, which contribute to better wound healing in diabetic patients (Tie et al., 2012). The production of Trametes versicolor polysaccharides had a significant effect on the deterioration of bones induced by diabetes in diabetic rats. It resulted in a decrease in the deficit of femoral cortical sponginess and an increase in the strength of the femoral bone, as well as an improvement in the volume of the tibia in the diabetic animal model (Chen et al., 2015).

Clinical Trials on Therapeutic Mushrooms

The clinical trial data from clinicaltrial.gov.in suggests that different edible species of mushrooms can be used for the prevention of diabetes mellitus and related issues. In a randomized placebo-controlled double-blind trial, 84 individuals with Type-2 diabetes mellitus and metabolic disorder were divided into different intervention groups. These groups received either G. lucidum, G. lucidum with Cordyceps, or placebo for sixteen weeks. The dosage of G. lucidum was 3gm/day, either alone or in combination with C. cinesis. After analyzing the primary and secondary outcome measures, it was concluded that there was no increased risk of adverse effects with any active treatment. G. lucidum, being well-tolerated, may provide benefits for various cardiovascular issues, including diabetes mellitus and its complications. This clinical trial investigation was registered with the Australian New Zealand Clinical Trials Registry on November 23, 2006, with the trial ID ACTRN12606000485538 (Klupp et al., 2016). Another study was conducted by Taiwan EC Biotech using Agaricus Blazei Murill mushroom extract for the management of type 2 diabetes mellitus (T2DM). This intervention clinical trial involved 108 participants who were given murill elixir. The primary outcomes measured were the percentage reduction of insulin resistance (HOMA-IR) and glycated hemoglobin (HbA1C). Secondary outcomes included differences in adiponectin, cholesterol, leptin, glucose, and triglyceride levels. The results of the study concluded that the mushroom elixir had a significant effect in treating diabetes in a rat model (clinicaltrial.gov.in).

Another study conducted in 2020 examined the potential of various mushroom species including Agaricus, Coprinus, Ganoderma, Grifola, and Pleurotus for treating T2DM. The results of this study also suggested that these mushroom species have potential as treatments for diabetes (Lindequist et al., 2020).

Future Perspectives

Mushrooms, also known as macrofungi, are naturally occurring species that have been found to have versatile effects in biomedical research. They have been utilized in the production of different types of pharmaceutical formulations for the treatment of various diseases and their complications. Several pharmacological investigations have been conducted on mushrooms, confirming their therapeutic efficacy and potential. One of the significant advantages of using mushrooms in medicine is their reported lack or minimal side effects, ensuring the safety of their use in diabetes treatment. Research on Ganoderma species, specifically their triterpenoids and polysaccharides, has made significant advancements in the past years due to their anti-diabetic properties. However, further investigational studies are needed in various fields related to mushrooms. For instance, the standardization of several medicinal mushroom species is necessary to ensure consistent and reliable therapeutic effects (Winska et al., 2019Additionally, more studies should be conducted to identify the specific bioactive compounds present in different species of mushrooms, as well as their potential interactions with other substances.

Furthermore, there is a need for in-vivo studies to understand the mechanism of action of these active compounds in the body, particularly in the treatment of diabetes mellitus. This would enable researchers to gather more reliable and comprehensive data, which can be used to develop more effective treatments in the future. Moreover, the toxicological profiles of mushrooms are not yet fully understood, and further research is needed to assess their safety. This includes investigating potential antagonistic or synergistic effects of active compounds with food and drug substances. Additionally, more emphasis should be placed on the structural determination of nucleic acids and proteins present in mushrooms. This would provide valuable insights into their biological functions and potential therapeutic applications. In conclusion, more clinical investigations are necessary to validate the efficacy and safety of mushrooms and their bioactive compounds. This will enhance our understanding of their potential benefits and enable the development of more targeted and efficient treatments (Winska et al., 2019, Bishop et al., 2015).

Conclusion

Therapeutic mushrooms have long been used in Asian countries as a traditional medicine due to their edible and therapeutic properties. Numerous studies have shown that mushrooms have anti-hyperglycemic, antioxidant, anti-inflammatory, anti-cancer, and immune-boosting effects, both in vitro and in vivo. However, more research is needed, particularly through prospective and retrospective studies, to better understand the potential of mushrooms in treating diabetes mellitus. These studies could include enzymatic inhibition assays, such as testing the effects of mushrooms on α-amylase, α-glucosidase, pancreatic lipase, and dipeptidyl peptidase 4. Additionally, human trials are necessary to evaluate the effectiveness of mushrooms in treating diabetes. Researchers should also focus on determining the concentration of valuable bioactive compounds in mushrooms, as well as developing formulations that can have a noticeable impact on reducing the symptoms of diabetes in patients worldwide. In conclusion, edible mushrooms have shown promise as a functional food for the treatment of diabetes, but further investigation is needed to fully understand their potential and develop effective treatments.

References

Amit, R., Prasad, P. (2014). Properties and uses of an Indigenous Mushroom: Calocybe indica. *Asian Journal of Pharmacy and Technology*, 4(1), 17-21.

Aramabasic, J., Mihailovic, J., Uskokovic, M., Melita, V. (2021). The effects of major mushroom bioactive compounds on mechanisms that control blood glucose level. *Journal of Fungi*, 7(1), 58.

Asbun, J., Villarreal, F. J. (2006). The pathogenesis of myocardial fibrosis in the setting of diabetic cardiomyopathy. *Journal of the American College of Cardiology*, 47(4), 693-700.

Bishop, K. S., Kao, C. H., Xu, Y., Glucina, M. P., Paterson, R. R. M., Ferguson, L. R. (2015). From 2000 years of Ganoderma lucidum to recent developments in nutraceuticals. *Phytochemistry*, 114, 56-65.

Brunton, S. (2016). Pathophysiology of Type 2 Diabetes: The Evolution of Our Understanding. *Journal of Family Practice*, 65(4 Suppl), supp_az_0416.

Cao, H., Qin, D., Guo, H., Cui, X., Wang, S., Wu, Y., Zheng, W., Zhong, X., Wang, H., Yu, J., Zhang, H., Han, C. (2020). The shaggy ink cap medicinal mushroom, Coprinus comatus (Agaricomycetes), a versatile functional species: a review. *International Journal of Medicinal Mushrooms*, 22(3), 245-255.

Chen, C. H., Kang, L., Lo, H. C., Hsu, T. H., Lin, F. Y., Lin, Y. S., Shen, C. L. (2015). Polysaccharides of Trametes versicolor improve bone properties in diabetic rats. *Journal of Agricultural and Food Chemistry*, 63(42), 9232-9238.

Chen, P., Qin, H., Li, Y., Ma, G., Yang, J., Wang, Q. (2018). Study on chemical constituents of an edible mushroom Volvariella volvacea and their antitumor activity in vitro. *Natural Product Research*, 34, 1417-1422.

Choi, E. J., Park, Z. Y., Kim, E. K. (2016). Chemical composition and inhibitory effect of Lentinula edodes ethanolic extract on experimentally induced atopic dermatitis in vitro and in vivo. *Molecules*, 21, 993.

Daba, A. S., Kabeil, S. S., Botros, W. A., El-Saadani, M. A. (2008). Production of mushroom (Pleurotus streatus) in Egypt as source of nutritional and Medicinal food. *World Journal of Agricultural Society*, 4(5), 630-634.

Das, A., Chen, C. M., Mu, S. C., Yang, S. H., Ju, Y. M., Li, S. C. (2022). Medicinal components in edible mushrooms on diabetes mellitus treatment. *Pharmaceutics*, 14(2), 436.

Erbiai, E. H., Da Silva, L. P., Saidi, R., Lamrani, Z., da Silva, J. C. E., Maouni, A. (2021). Chemical composition, bioactive compounds, and antioxidant activity of two wild edible mushrooms Armillaria Mellea and macrolepiota procera from two countries (Morocco and Portugal). *Biomolecules*, 11, 575-586.

Fekadu, A. (2014). Cultivation of lentinus edodes on teff straw (agricultural residue) at Dilla University, Ethiopia. *Asia Journal of Applied Microbiology*, 1(3), 49-59.

Girma, W., Tasisa, T. (2018). Application of mushroom as food and medicine. Advances in Biotechnology and Microbiology, 11(4): 555817.

Hu, X., Liu, C., Wang, X., Jia, D., Lu, W., Sun, X., Yuan, L. (2017). Hpyerglycemic and anti-diabetic nephritis activities of polysaccharides separated from Auricularia auricular in diet-streptozotocin-induced diabetic rats. *Experimental and Therapeutic Medicine*, 13(1), 352-358.

Huang, H. Y., Korivi, M., Yang, H. T., Huang, C. C., Chaing, Y. Y., Tsai, Y. C. (2014). Effect of Pleurotus tuber-regium polysaccharides supplementation on the progression of diabetes complications in obese-diabetic rats. *Chinese Journal of Physiology*, 57(4), 198-208.

Jiang, X., Meng, W., Li, L., Meng, Z., Wang, D. (2020). Adjuvant therapy with mushroom polysaccharides for diabetic complications. *Frontiers in Pharmacology*, 11, 168.

Kalac, P. (2013). A review of chemical composition and nutritional value of wild-growing and cultivated mushrooms. *Journal of the Science of Food and Agriculture*, 93(2), 209-218.

Kaliyaperumal, M., Kezo, K., Gunaseelan, S. (2018). A global overview of edible mushrooms. *Biology of Macrofungi*, 15-56.

Klupp, N. L., Kiat, H., Bensoussan, A., Steiner, G. Z., Chang, D. H. (2016). A double-blind, randomised, placebo-controlled trial of Ganoderma lucidum for the treatment of cardiovascular risk factors of metabolic syndrome. *Scientific Reports*, 6(1), 29540.

Kumar, K., Mehra, R., Guine, R. P. F., Lima, M. J., Kumar, N., Kaushik, R., Ahmed, N., Yadav, A. N., Kumar, H. (2020). Edible mushrooms: a comprehensive review on bioactive compounds with health benefits and processing aspects. *Foods*, 10, 2996.

Lee, D. H., Yang, M., Giovannucci, E. L., Sun, Q., Chavarro, J. E. (2019). Mushroom consumption, biomarkers, and risk of cardiovascular disease and type 2 diabetes: a prospective cohort study of US women and men. *American Journal of Clinical Nutrition*, 110(3), 666-674.

Li, W., Huang, E., Gao, S. (2017). Type 1 diabetes mellitus and cognitive impairments: a systematic review. *Journal of Alzheimer's Disease*, 57(1), 29-36.

Lin, J. W., Jia, J., Shen, Y. H., Zhong, M., Chen, L. J., Li, H. G., Li, T. L. (2013). Functional expression of FIP-fve, a fungal immunomodulatory protein from the edible mushroom Flammulina velutipes in Pichia pastoris GS115. *Journal of Biotechnology*, 168(4), 527-533.

Lindequist, U., Haertel, B. (2020) Medicinal mushrooms for the treatment of type-2 Diabetes: An update on clinical trials. *International Journal of Medicinal Mushrooms*, 22(9), 845-854.

Liu, Y., Wang, J., Wang, W., Zhang, H., Zhang, X., Han, C. (2015). The chemical constituents and pharmacological actions of Cordyceps sinensis. *Evidence-Based Complementary and Alternative Medicine*, 575063.

Martinez-Medina, G. A., Chavez-Gonzalez, M. L., Verma, D. K., Prado-Barragán, L. A., Martínez-Hernández, J. L., Flores-Gallegos, A. C., Aguilar, C. N. (2021). Bio-funcional components in mushrooms, a health opportunity: Ergothionine and huitlacohe as recent trends. *Journal of Functional Foods*, 77, 104326.

Meng, G., Zhu, H., Yang, S., Wu, F., Zheng, H., Chen, E., Xu, J. (2011). Attenuating effects of Ganoderma lucidum polysaccharides on myocardial collagen cross-linking relates to advanced glycation end product and antioxidant enzymes in high-fat-diet and streptozotocin-induced diabetic rats. *Carbohydrate Polymers*, 84(1), 180-185.

Meng, X., Liang, H., Luo, L. (2016). Antitumor polysaccharides from mushrooms: a review on the structural characteristics, antitumor mechanisms and immunomodulating activities. *Carbohydrate Research*, 424, 30-41.

Mishra, A., Behura, A., Mawatwal, S., Kumar, A., Naik, L., Mohanty, S. S., Dhiman, R. (2019). Structure-function and application of plant lectins in disease biology and immunity. *Food and Chemical Toxicology*, 134, 110827.

Mizukami, H., Kudoh, K. (2022). Diversity of pathophysiology in type 2 diabetes shown by islet pathology. *Journal of Diabetes Investigation*, 13(1), 6-13.

Monira, S., Haque, A., Muhit, A., Sarker N. C., Alam, A. H., Rahman A. A., Khondkar, P. (2012). Antimicrobial, antioxidant and cytotoxic properties of Hypsizygus tessulatus cultivated in Bangladesh. *Research Journal of Medicinal Plants*, 6, 300-308.

Nishihara, M., Watanabe, A., Asada, Y. (2007). Isolation and characterization of the gene encoding a chitin synthase with a myosin motor-like domain from the edible basidiomycetous mushroom, Lentinula edodes, and its expression in the course of fruit-body formation. *Mycoscience*, 48(2), 109-116.

Nowak, R., Olech, M., Nowacka, N. (2014). Plant polyphenols as chemopreventive agents. *Polyphenols in Human Health and Disease*, 1289-1307.

Papoutsis, K., Grasso, S., Menon, A., Brunton, N. P., Lyng, J. G., Jacquier, J. C., Bhuyan, D. J. (2020). Recovery of ergosterol and vitamin D2 from mushroom waste-potential valorization by food and pharmaceutical industries. *Trends in Food Science & Technology*, 99, 351-366.

Petrovic, J., Glamoclija, J., Stojkovic, D., Ciric, A., Barros, L., Ferreira, I. C., Sokovic, M. (2015). Nutritional value, chemical composition, antioxidant activity and enrichment of cream cheese with chestnut mushroom Agrocybe aegerita (Brig.) Sing. *Journal of Food Science and Technology*, 52(10), 6711-6718.

Poblete-Aro, C., Russell-Guzman, J., Parra, P., Soto-Munoz, M. (2018). Exercise and oxidative stress in type 2 diabetes mellitus. *Revista Médica de Chile*, 146(3), 362-372.

Primavera, M., Giannini, C., Chiarelli, F. (2020). Prediction and Prevention of Type 1 Diabetes. *Frontiers in Endocrinology*, 11, 248.

Ramos, M., Burgos, N., Barnard, A., Evans, G., Preece, J., Graz, M., Ruthes, A. C., Jiménez-Quero, A., Martínez-Abad, A., Vilaplana, F., Ngoc, L. P., Brouwer, A., van der Burg, B., Del Carmen Garrigós, M., Jiménez, A. (2019). Agaricus bisporus and its by-products as a source of valuable extracts and bioactive compounds. *Food chemistry*, 292, 176–187.

Rathore, H., Prasad, S., Sharma, S. (2017). Mushroom nutraceuticals for improved nutrition and better human health: A review. *PharmaNutrition*, 5(2), 35-46.

Ruthes, A. C., Smiderle, F. R., Iacomini, M. (2016). Mushroom heteropolysaccharides: A review on their sources, structure and biological effects. *Carbohydrate Polymers*, 136, 358-375.

Saad, A. Z., Sitohy, M. A., Omar, B. T., El-Saadony, M., Sitohy, B. (2022). *Mushroom; Chemistry, Bioactive Components, and Application*. IntechOpen.

Sułkowska-Ziaja, K., Muszyńska, B., Gawalska, A., Sałaciak, K. (2018). Laetiporus sulphureus – chemical composition and medicinal value. *Acta Scientiarum Polonorum, Hortorum Cultus*, 17(1), 89-98.

Tang, C., Hoo, P. C., Tan, L. T., Pusparajah, P., Khan, T. M., Lee, L. H., Goh, B. H., Chan, K. G. (2016). Golden needle mushroom: a culinary medicine with evidenced-based biological activities and health promoting properties. *Frontiers in Pharmacology*, 7, 474.

Tie, L., Yang, H. Q., An, Y., Liu, S. Q., Han, J., Xu, Y., Li, X. J. (2012). Ganoderma lucidum polysaccharide accelerates refractory wound healing by inhibition of mitochondrial oxidative stress in type 1 diabetes. *Cellular Physiology and Biochemistry*, 29(3-4), 583-594.

Ukwuru M. U., Muritala, A., Eze, L. U. (2018). Edible and non-edible wild mushrooms: nutrition, toxicity and strategies for recognition. *Journal of Clinical Nutrition and Metabolism*, 2, 2.

Valverde, M. E., Hernandez-Perez, T., Paredes-López, O. (2015). Edible mushrooms: improving human health and promoting quality life. *International Journal of Microbiology*, 2015, 376387.

Varrot, A., Basheer, S. M., Imberty, A. (2013). Fungal lectins: structure, function and potential applications. *Current Opinion in Structural Biology*, 23(5), 678-685.

Veljovic, S., Veljovic, M., Nikicevic, N., Despotovic, S., Radulovic, S., Niksic, M., Filipovic, L. (2017). Chemical composition, antiproliferative and antioxidant activity of differently processed Ganoderma lucidum ethanol extracts. *Journal of Food Science and Technology*, 54(5), 1312-1320.

Winska, K., Mączka, W., Gabryelska, K., Grabarczyk, M. (2019). Mushrooms of the Genus Ganoderma Used to Treat Diabetes and Insulin Resistance. Molecules, 24(22), 4075.

Wu, J. Y., Siu, K. C., Geng, P. (2021). Bioactive Ingredients and Medicinal Values of Grifola frondosa (Maitake). *Foods*, 10(1), 95.

Wu, Y., Ding, Y., Tanaka, Y., Zhang, W. (2014). Risk factors contributing to type 2 diabetes and recent advances in the treatment and prevention. *International Journal of Medical Sciences*, 11(11), 1185-200.

Wu, Y., Liu, Y., Wu, J., Ou, K., Huang. Q., Cao, J., Duan, T., Zhou, L., Pan, Y. (2022). Chemical profile and antioxidant activity of bidirectional metabolites from Tremella fuciformis and Acanthopanax trifoliatus as assessed using response surface methodology. *Frontiers in Nutrition*, 9, 1035788.

Yang, S., Yan, J., Yang, L., Meng, Y., Wang, Na., He, C., Fan, Y., Zhou, Y. (2019). Alkali-soluble polysaccharides from mushroom fruiting bodies improve insulin resistance. International Journal of Biological Macromolecules, 126, 466-474.

Ya-Ping, H. U., Bing-Qian, Z., Jin-Xiu, Z., Li-Qiang, Z., Li-An, W. (2018). Chemical constituents of fruiting bodies of Coprinus comatus and their activities against diabetes. *Journal of Mycosystema*, 37(3), 371-378.

Zhang, J., Meng, G., Zhang, C., Lin, L., Xu, N., Liu, M., Jia, L. (2015). The antioxidative effects of acidic-, alkalic-, and enzymatic-extractable mycelium zinc polysaccharides by Pleurotus djamor on liver and kidney of streptozocin-induced diabetic mice. *BMC Complementary and Alternative Medicine*, 15, 440.

Zhang, Z. C., Lian, B., Huang, D. M., Cui, F. J. (2009). Compare activities on regulating lipid-metabolism and reducing oxidative stress of diabetic rats of Tremella aurantialba broth's extract (TBE) with its mycelia polysaccharides (TMP). *Journal of Food Science*, 74(1), H15-H21.

Chapter 6

Carbohydrates in the Management of Diabetes Mellitus

Fatimah Jan[1,*]
Arashdeep Kaur[1]
Muneeb U. Rehman[2]
Uditi Handa[3]
Nazakat Farooq[1]
Divya Jha[4]
Vratika Jain[4]
Arpit Chowdhury[4]
Shikha Baghel Chauhan[4]
and Indu Singh[4]

[1]School of Pharmaceutical Sciences, C. T. University, Ludhiana, Punjab, India
[2]College of Pharmacy King Saud University, Riyadh, Saudi Arabia
[3]Guru Gobind Singh College of Pharmacy, Yamuna Nagar, Haryana, India
[4]Amity Institute of Pharmacy, Amity University, Noida, Uttar Pradesh, India

Abstract

Diabetes is characterized by an inadequate metabolic response to insulin, which can result in persistent hyperglycemia and microvascular problems. Due to the defining characteristic of hyperglycemia, diabetes has traditionally been considered a disease of carbohydrate metabolism.

---

[*] Corresponding Author's Email: fatimahjan0088@gmail.com.

In: Naturally Occurring Chemicals …
Editors: A. Singh Grewal, G. Deswal, A. Kumar Dhingra et al.
ISBN: 979-8-89113-491-1

Ancient Egyptian experts are credited with developing the first historical nutritional treatment, which focused on the advantages of a high-carbohydrate diet that included honey, wheat, grains, and berries from bees in managing diabetes. Previous studies have examined various approaches to managing diabetes, including sun-dried cellular membranes, very low-calorie diets, extremely low carbohydrate, high protein and fat meals, fasting, and diets with different carbohydrate, fat, and protein contents. Various biochemical studies have found that carbohydrates are significant macromolecules involved in conserving energy, acting as a structural component, and carrying out biological processes, including cell recognition. In preclinical and clinical research, oligosaccharides and polysaccharides found in plants have demonstrated hypoglycemic effects. Polyphenols, sugars, flavonoids, and other biomolecules are among the most significant active ingredients that can be isolated from herbs and used to treat illnesses.

Keywords: diabetes mellitus, carbohydrates, pregnancy, QOL, dietary changes

Introduction

Diabetes mellitus is a chronic metabolic disorder characterized by cells not functioning properly and persistent high blood sugar levels. This condition is primarily caused by defects in insulin production, insulin activity, and the insulin signaling system, which contributes to hyperglycemia. Hyperglycemia is associated with various complications including retinopathy, nephropathy, and neuropathy. It is increasingly recognized that genetic, epigenetic, and environmental factors play a role in the development of different types of diabetes. The syndrome is categorized into type-2, type-1, and gestational diabetes based on its etiology. Currently, diabetes affects 415 million individuals, and this number is projected to increase to 614 million by 2040 (Sajadimajd et al., 2019). Despite advances in our understanding of the pathophysiology and underlying causes of diabetes mellitus, patients still require personalized and targeted treatment. Therapeutic approaches, including herbal and conventional medicine, have been developed to help manage diabetes and its associated complications (Shields et al., 2010). To achieve this goal, a wide range of medicinal plants have been implicated in various aspects of diabetes pathogenesis. Specifically, Vaccinium myrtillus L., from the Ericaceae family, is a berry used as a spice in thirty-two healthy, non-diabetic subjects who are insulin-

safe. Camellia sinensis (L.) Kuntze, belonging to the Theaceae family, also known as green tea, has been tested on ninety-two subjects with type 2 diabetes mellitus and lipid abnormalities. Panax ginseng C. A. Meyer from the Araliaceae family, commonly known as ginseng, has been studied in thirty-six patients with non-insulin-dependent diabetes over an extended period. Furthermore, the plant Momordica from the Curcurbitaceae family has been investigated in twenty-four individuals with T2 diabetes. Additionally, Cinnamomum verum J. Presl from the Lauraceae family, commonly referred to as cinnamon, has been examined in fifty overweight individuals with diabetes. These medicinal plants have shown promising results in improving various aspects of diabetes pathogenesis (Kiss et al., 2018). Hepatic glucose concentrations that are higher are associated with deregulated insulin signaling and metabolism. One troubling issue related to this is the management of the enzymes that control glucose levels. Fortunately, several medicinal herbs have been shown to help with this issue. For instance, Panax ginseng, a plant in the Araliaceae family, has been found to stimulate AMPK (AMP-activated protein kinase), a protein that inhibits the activities of phosphoenolpyruvate carboxykinase (PECK) and glucose-6-phosphatase (G6Pase) enzymes. By doing so, Panax ginseng can regulate glucose metabolism. The leaves and seeds of Coccinia indica, a plant in the Curcurbitaceae family, have hypoglycemic effects when taken orally after an 18-hour fast. This is because they inhibit the enzymes glucose-6-phosphatase and fructose-1,6-bisphosphatase, leading to increased liver glycogen content and lowered glucose levels. Momordica charantia, another member of the Curcurbitaceae family, has a similar effect. Additionally, Goldenseal (Hydrastis canadensis L.), which belongs to the Ranunculaceae family, contains berberine, an Isoquinolin alkaloid. Berberine has been found to increase the expression of PPAR-gamma or insulin receptors, resulting in improved insulin sensitivity and hypoglycemia (Hui et al., 2009). An aqueous phenolic extract of green tea has been found to increase the expression levels of GLUT4, along with other insulin-signaling molecules, in adipocytes, hepatocytes, and myocytes. Given the success of herbal medicine in treating diabetes, the analysis and identification of active plant compounds are rapidly becoming an intriguing objective in research studies aimed at treating diabetics (Li et al., 2013).

Clinical Proof of Carbohydrates' Therapeutic and Protective Effects on Diabetes Mellitus

The beneficial effects of food consumption on people with diabetes were examined by comparing three different diets. These included a low-starch diet consisting of 43% carbohydrates, 22% proteins, and 34% fats; a high-starch diet consisting of 55% carbohydrates, 15% proteins, and 30% fats; and a typical American meal consisting of 40% carbohydrates, 20% proteins, and 40% fats. It was found that low-starch meals resulted in significantly lower 24-hour plasma sugar and insulin levels compared to the high-starch and American diets. Another research trial involving over 3234 participants supported these findings, suggesting that consuming meals high in fiber while limiting total and saturated fat intake can help reduce diabetic complications such as cardiovascular disease and kidney damage. Additionally, incorporating a variety of fruits, vegetables, whole grains, and lean proteins into the diet can aid in improving blood sugar control and promoting overall health for individuals with diabetes (Sylvetsky et al., 2017). The daily excretion of calcium and other minerals in urine, as well as the absorption of calcium in the intestines, have been shown to be unaffected by the use of a high-carbohydrate or high-fat diet. This suggests that conditions like nephropathy and osteoporosis, which are common consequences of diabetes, may not be present in hyperglycemic states. However, the levels of NF-B produced by a high-carbohydrate diet were found to be three times higher than those produced by a conventional meal. This indicates a connection between the glycemic index of a meal and the risk to anti-inflammatory systems. It is clear that carbohydrate consumption is essential for altering metabolism, and the levels of the hormone 3, 5, 3-triiodothyronine in the thyroid gland reflect the amount of carbohydrates in the diet. In lean, non-insulin-dependent diabetic individuals, the ingestion of carbohydrates affects the response of T3 to glucose, and this response is closely related to glucose tolerance (Koh et al., 1999).

Oligosaccharides in the Treatment of Diabetes Mellitus

The most prevalent oligosaccharides found in nature are the fructo-oligosaccharides, disaccharides, galacto-oligosaccharides, tetrasaccharides, xylo-oligosaccharides & trisaccharides (Ríos-Ríos et al., 2022).

Disaccharides are carbohydrates composed of two monosaccharide units connected together. They can be found in various sources and have different types of connections. Some examples of disaccharides include maltose, lactose, sucrose, cellubiose, mellibiose, and trehallose. Raffinose and stachyose are trisaccharides that can be directly extracted from legume seeds such as chickpeas, lentils, beans, peas, soybeans, and mustard (Xiaoli et al., 2008). Xylan, an indigestible carbohydrate, acts as a prebiotic by promoting the growth of beneficial gut bacteria. When xylan is hydrolyzed, it results in the formation of xylooligosaccharide (XOS), which is an oligomer consisting of xylopyranose residues connected by (1→4) links. XOS, along with other oligosaccharides like insulin, isomaltooligosaccharides (IOS), fructo oligosaccharides (FOS), galactooligosaccharide (GOS), and lactulose, has been found to have positive effects on the development of gut microbiota. Numerous studies have established a causal relationship between gut bacteria and the occurrence of Type-2 diabetes. Factors like obesity and insulin resistance are known to contribute to the development of Type-2 diabetes (Qin et al., 2012). Based on these data, blood sugar control seems to be influenced by non-digestible oligosaccharides such as XOS, GOS, and FOS, which contribute to the growth of beneficial gut bacteria (Figure 1). Animal studies have indicated that consuming XOS or corncob may promote longevity, while clinical evidence suggests that they may also alleviate the pathophysiology of diabetes in patients. Furthermore, T2DM patients who consumed dietary XOS experienced decreased blood glucose and lipid levels, along with increased antioxidant enzyme levels (Gobinath et al., 2010).

The presence of intestinal microbes, specifically faecal bacteria, prausnitzii, and bifidobacterium, increased in one study when FOS (fructooligosaccharide) was administered. However, the metabolism of glucose was not affected (Dewulf et al., 2013) The positive benefits of the eight-week XOS supplement on glycemic responses were examined by Shu et al., in twenty-six individuals with Type-2 DM in Taiwan. The study found that using XOS supplements for eight weeks led to a dramatic lowering of blood sugar and lipid levels. This included reductions in total cholesterol, LDL-cholesterol, and OX-LDL, while omitting SCFAs (substances produced by gut bacteria). It is worth noting that anthropometric measurements and food consumption remained constant during the experimental evaluation. Yamashita et al., conducted a similar study and also found that administering FOS for fourteen days significantly decreased fasting blood sugar levels in patients with Type-2 DM. These findings suggest that XOS and FOS supplements may have a beneficial impact on glycemic control in individuals with Type-2 DM. (Yamashita et al., 1984). To investigate the role of FOS in glucose metabolism, studies were conducted on healthy individuals.

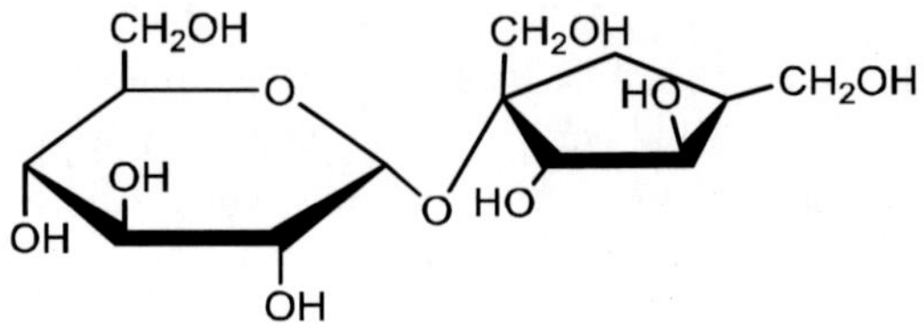

a.Sucrose

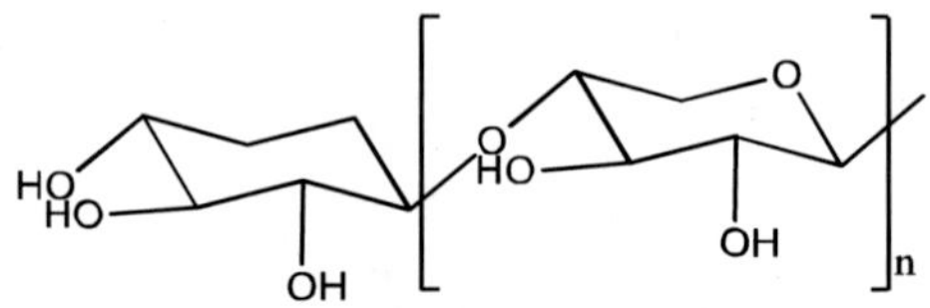

b. XOS

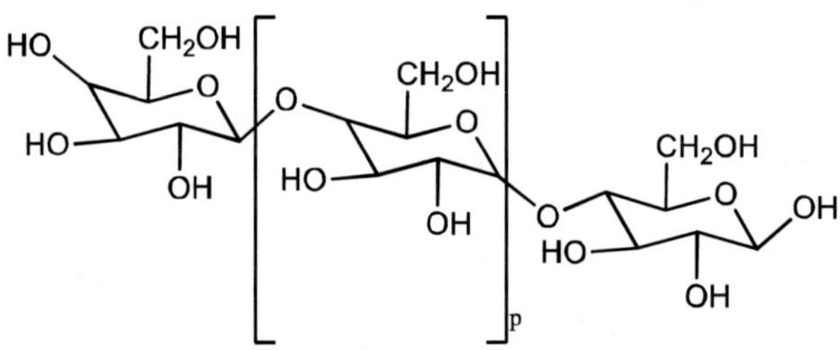

c. GOS

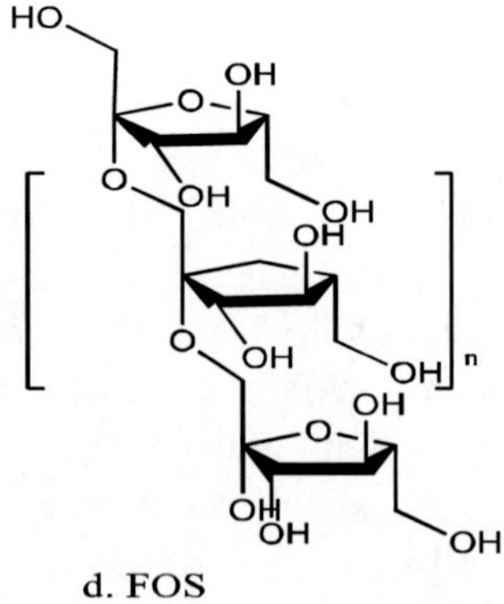

d. FOS

Figure 1. The most important oligosaccharides for controlling glycemic reactions in clinical studies. Sucrose and XOS are two examples of sugars. c. GOS: Gluco-oligosaccharide d. FOS: Fructo-oligosaccharide.

These studies also focused on a specific type of fructo-oligosaccharides known as short-chain fructo-oligosaccharides, which are present in various plants such as rye, wheat, and onions (Sajadimajd et al., 2019). Short-chain fructo-oligosaccharides significantly reduce baseline hepatic glucose synthesis when consumed over an extended period. Lipoproteins, insulin serum lipids, and fasting plasma glucose levels remained unchanged in the study participants. High fermentation potential for short-chain FOS leads to the production of short-chain fatty acids, specifically propionate and butyrate. A recent scientific investigation focused on the growth of intestinal microorganisms and the metabolism of sugar in healthy individuals, exploring the effects of popular prebiotics FOS and GOS (Luo et al., 2000). After delivery, it was found that there was a significant increase in the multiplication of intestinal bacteria. The glucose responses of the GOS volunteers, as measured by OGTT and FBS, showed a slight improvement. Moreover, the levels of short-chain fatty acids (SCFA), including butyric acid, decreased in individuals fed with FOS and GOS. Interestingly, both the GOS and FOS groups exhibited changes in the number of gut microorganisms. The growth of bacteria that produce butyrate, such as Ruminococcus for GOS and Phascolarchobacteria for FOS, was inhibited despite the increased development of Bifidobacterium in the FOS group. These findings suggest that the decreased amount of butyrate-producing bacteria could possibly be the main factor contributing to the altered glucose metabolism in individuals treated with GOS and FOS (Liu et al., 2017). n a different research study, the potential therapeutic benefits of oligofructose-enriched inulin for patients with type 2 diabetes mellitus (T2DM) were examined. It was found that oligofructose with inulin significantly reduced levels of fasting blood sugar (FBS), HbA1C, IL-6, TNF-, and plasma LPS over an 8-week period after insulin administration. This suggests that insulin may have anti-inflammatory and hypoglycemic effects in T2DM patients. Additionally, the influence of sucrose on glucose metabolism has been the subject of various studies and discussions. Sucrose, a refined carbohydrate, has been linked to the development of diabetes as it negatively affects postprandial glycaemia. In comparison, a substitute sweetener called aspartame has been studied to see how it affects metabolism in individuals with diabetes. A 6-week research study found that there were no harmful changes in insulin levels, lipid content, or glycemia in individuals who consumed either aspartame or sucrose. However, when used only as a flavoring agent, aspartame did not provide any distinct advantages over sucrose, at least in the context of T2DM (Sajadimajd et al., 2019). It has been shown that individuals with Type 2 Diabetes (T2DM) have stable levels of glycosuria, blood glucose, and glycated haemoglobin, even when there are significant changes in sucrose intake while maintaining consistent levels of carbohydrates and fats. However, T2DM individuals with pre-existing high triglyceridemia experience a reduction in postprandial triglyceride levels. In a randomised controlled trial involving healthy individuals without diabetes, comparing the effects of two different 6-week nutrition phases with a 4-week washout period, there were no significant differences in glucose response, insulin sensitivity, and vessel compliance between the eucaloric high-density diet and the low-sucrose diet (with sucrose contributing to 25% and 10% of the overall energy intake, respectively). The participants of the study were 40 normal male volunteers. It has been observed that adolescents with Type 1 Diabetes (T1DM) and normal fasting blood glucose levels had similar glycemic responses to meals with high or low levels of sucrose, indicating that other factors may influence blood glucose levels. Another study found that consuming sucrose had no impact on glucose-related metabolic reactions in children and teenagers with T1DM (Øverby et al., 2007) Furthermore, SBOS has been found to improve insulin sensitivity and regulate blood glucose levels in pregnant women with gestational diabetes. This suggests that SBOS may have potential as a natural treatment or preventive measure for gestational diabetes. Further research is needed to fully understand the mechanisms behind these beneficial effects and to determine the optimal dosage and duration of SBOS supplementation in pregnant women. Nevertheless, these findings highlight the potential of SBOS as a promising prebiotic component that can positively impact the health of pregnant women at risk of developing gestational diabetes (Fei et al., 2014).

Polysaccharide Molecules in the Diagnosed Diabetes Mellitus

There are over 30 types of carbohydrates that fall under the category of polysaccharides. This includes both homopolysaccharides, such as starch and cellulose, and heteropolysaccharides like glycosaminoglycans. These saccharides have been studied for their therapeutic hypoglycemic properties, and one example is the heteropolysaccharide called Arabino xylan (AXE) which contains xylofructose. Residues in the side chains and residues of arabinofructose in the main chain (Wang et al., 2002). Dietary fibers derived from cereal grains, such as AXE fiber, can have a significant impact on glucose responses in both healthy individuals and those with diabetes. In healthy individuals, consumption of meals rich in AXE fiber significantly reduces postprandial glucose and insulin reactions. This hypoglycemic effect can be attributed to the high viscosity of AXE fiber, which slows down the movement of the small intestine, delays glucose absorption, and results in a reduced plasma glucose response (Farina et al., 2010). The heteropolysaccharide guar gum, also known as guaran, is composed of units of galactopyranose and mannopyranose that are linked by 1, 4 and 1, 6 bonds. Gums are substances based on polysaccharides that are typically found in the seeds of woody plants. Flaxseed gum, due to its significant quantity of galacturonic acid, shows promise as a dietary hydrocolloid. It has been established that guar gum may be able to restore normalcy to the metabolic process in diabetics. This is presumed to be due to its underlying mechanism of forming a thick gel that delays the passage of stomach materials, thus increasing insulin sensitivity. Research has shown that both short-term and long-term administration of guar gum had beneficial effects on T2DM patients who required additional supplements like vitamins and minerals. The effect of guar gum on the glucose metabolism of insulin-dependent diabetic individuals has also been studied. According to the research, guar gum significantly reduced levels of blood LDL cholesterol, HbAc1, FBS, and the LDL to HDL cholesterol ratio. This demonstrates conclusively that guar gum can alleviate the symptoms of diabetes and its associated complications, including cardiovascular disease (CV) (Butt et al., 2007). The ingestion of guar gum has a positive effect on glucose and lipid breakdown. In a study by Ebeling et al., individuals with Type 1 diabetes who consumed diets containing guar gum experienced a decrease in post-prandial blood sugar, serum cholesterol, and insulin levels. Partially hydrolysed guar gum has been found to improve cardiovascular health in Type 2 diabetes patients by reducing the intensity of metabolic syndrome and cardiovascular indicators. The impact of guar gum on mineral levels in diabetic individuals was also investigated, and it was found that guar gum did not have a negative effect on mineral balance. Using guar gum as a dietary supplement for three months improved lipid and carbohydrate metabolism in Type 2 diabetes patients, although no significant changes were observed. GU-52 and glucotard, two novel derivatives of guar gum, have been shown to alter glycemic responses in diabetes patients. Diabetic individuals who took GU-052 and glucotard supplements experienced significant reductions in HbAc1, cholesterol, and triglyceride levels after 90 days of treatment. In T2DM patients, the formulation of GU-052 caused less negative side effects as compare to glucotard (Kirsten et al., 1992) in a number of studies, guar gum was recently examined in conjunction with other ingredients. Guar, wheat, and pectin have been found to significantly lower insulin and blood glucose levels in healthy individuals. Additionally, research has demonstrated that guar gum can enhance glucose metabolism synergistically when combined with a high-carbohydrate diet. Soy-soluble fibre, flaxseed gum, and guar gum have all been shown to reduce glycemic reactions compared to glucose in a study investigating the benefits of dietary fibre. However, due to its high viscosity, the gum has a considerable negative impact on the regulation of insulin and glucose responses. Furthermore, the effects of adding guar gum and microcrystalline cellulose to meals on blood sugar levels vary. The Niemi study found that both guar gum and cellulose had no significant effects on blood sugar levels in T2DM patients six weeks after administration, despite guar gum dramatically lowering fasting blood glucose levels while cellulose does not. However, the guar gum group did show a 10% decrease in serum cholesterol over a 12-week supplementation period, although serum glucose levels remained unchanged. This suggests that guar gum supplementation may help mitigate the consequences of diabetes, including cardiovascular diseases. Starch, a homopolysaccharide, is composed of α-D-glucopyranose units connected by side chains and backbones with 14 and 16 connections, respectively. Amylose and amylopectin are terms used to describe the linear and branching forms of starch, with amylopectin being the main component (Sajadimajd et al., 2019). Based on its digestibility, starch can be categorized into three types: rapidly digestible starch (RDS), slowly digestible starch (SDS), and resistant starch (RS). RDS is quickly broken down by enzymes in baked starchy foods like bread within 20 minutes. SDS takes a longer time to digest, up to 100 minutes, and contains grains with raw starch and inaccessible amorphous starch. RS, on the other hand, is not broken down by enzymes. A study compared the glycemic responses of lean and obese individuals to acute intake of banana starch. It was found that banana starch significantly decreased insulin and glucose responses in both lean and obese adults compared to digestible starch over a 5-day period. The levels of insulin and blood glucose were measured at various time points, including zero, thirty, sixty, ninety, 120, and 180 minutes. Another study examined the glycemic response and starch digestion in healthy volunteers after consuming extrusion rice noodles with a high amylose concentration. It was observed that both glycemic reaction and starch digestion were significantly reduced. The same effect was seen in T2DM groups given extruded rice noodles. RS, being an insoluble fiber and non-viscous substance, is consumed by intestinal microbial flora to produce short-chain fatty acids (SCFAs). SCFAs have been shown to play a role in regulating insulin synthesis, sensitivity, gluconeogenesis, and lipolysis. A chronic high-RS diet over a 24-hour period has been found to lower postprandial plasma glucose, improve insulin sensitivity, and inhibit the synthesis of esterified fatty acids and 5-hydroxybutyrate. The effects of RS on patients with T2DM were also investigated. In one study, blood sugar and insulin responses to RS bagels were measured in twenty-four individuals at elevated risk of T2DM. Another study verified the beneficial effects of resistant starch on glucose metabolism in T2DM patients (Kendall, Emam, Augustin, & Jenkins, 2004). Research has shown that among the five starchy items commonly consumed in the Chinese diet, Brown rice has been found to have the strongest impact on insulin and postprandial effects, including GI, GL, and insulinemic indices in healthy individuals. Compared to other starchy meals such as alday, brown rice, mung bean noodles, taro, and yam, Brown rice induces the highest levels of insulin and glycemic responses. These findings suggest that polysaccharides present in starchy meals can potentially play a significant role in the treatment of diabetes. (Lin, Wu, Lu, & Lin, 2010). Uncooked corn flour has a slow-digesting behavior in the gastrointestinal system and is composed of 73% amylopectin and 27% amylose. In a clinical study, diabetic individuals with type 1 diabetes who consumed snacks made from uncooked corn flour experienced lower levels of morning and nighttime hypoglycemia. PPB-R-203 is a product derived from retrograded starches and belongs to the resistant starch family. It is used to treat obesity in gastric bypass patients as well as diabetes. Oats and barley are two cereals that contain beta-glucan, a type of natural fiber. Beta-glucan consists of 13 and 14 linkages between its units. Patients with type 2 diabetes who consumed a functional bread high in -glucan but low in starch showed decreased HbA1C and baseline or postprandial blood glucose levels compared to a control group, indicating the potential value of -glucan in managing type 2 diabetes. In an acute randomized double-blind clinical intervention, the effects of two types of -glucan (oat-A and oat-B) with different viscosities as rheological properties were evaluated for postprandial hyperglycemia in healthy volunteers. Since oat-A has a significantly higher viscosity than oat-B, research has demonstrated that it improves postprandial glycemia compared to both the control group and oat-B (Panahi et al., 2007). It is widely accepted that carbohydrates, being a primary source of energy, have an impact on regulating metabolism. Therefore, it is recommended to carefully monitor carbohydrate intake in both normal and disordered situations.

Numerous studies have examined the effects of limiting dietary carbohydrates on metabolic illnesses. It is worth noting that reducing carb consumption in the diet seems to be beneficial in managing conditions such as diabetes (Daly et al., 2006). According to a clinical experiment, individuals with type 2 diabetes who followed a low carbohydrate diet for a short period experienced weight loss or hypoglycemia without any negative effects on their lipoprotein or glycated protein levels. Since blood sugar regulation is disrupted in both type 1 and type 2 diabetes, limiting carbohydrate intake seems necessary to reduce high blood sugar levels and improve overall glucose control (Feinman et al., 2015).

Conclusion

Diabetes is a challenging condition to treat due to its varied nature. As a result, scientists are investigating traditional medicine and herbal-based remedies as promising options to discover new and effective solutions for preventing and treating diabetes and its complications. One crucial aspect of herbal-based therapies is the identification of active hypoglycemic compounds derived from medicinal plants. The aim is to develop innovative and practical medications with fewer adverse effects compared to synthetic drugs. Oligosaccharides and polysaccharides found in plants have shown promising hypoglycemic effects in both laboratory experiments and human trials. Clinical studies have shown that certain groups of poly- and oligosaccharides can control glycemic and insulin responses in both healthy individuals and those with diabetes. However, the specific dosage and mechanisms of action for carbohydrate-based techniques are still being determined. Several anti-diabetic processes, such as enhanced expression of the GLUT4 protein, modification of insulin signaling proteins, and inhibition of PECK and G6Pase enzymes, have been considered for plant-derived oligosaccharides and polysaccharides. Regenerating beta cells, which play a crucial role in diabetes management, may be influenced by carbohydrate intake through the regulation of signaling pathways involved in their regrowth. Future research should therefore focus on understanding how plant-derived carbohydrates affect beta cell regeneration. Additionally, further investigation is needed to explore the molecular mechanisms by which dietary carbs can treat metabolic disorders such as obesity, including the inhibition of specific enzymes like alpha-glucosidase. In conclusion, the use of carbohydrates, including polysaccharides, oligosaccharides, and fibers, as medications or dietary supplements, holds great promise in the treatment of diabetes and its complications.

References

Butt, M. S., Shahzadi, N., Sharif, M. K., Nasir, M. (2007). Guar gum: a miracle therapy for hypercholesterolemia, hyperglycemia and obesity. *Critical Reviews in Food Science and Nutrition*, 47(4), 389-396.

Daly, M. E., Paisey, R., Paisey, R., Millward, B. A., Eccles, C., Williams, K., Hammersley, S., MacLeod, K. M., Gale, T. J. (2006). Short-term effects of severe dietary carbohydrate-restriction advice in Type 2 diabetes—a randomized controlled trial. *Diabetic Medicine*, 23(1), 15-20.

Dewulf, E. M., Cani, P. D., Claus, S. P., Fuentes, S., Puylaert, P. G., Neyrinck, A. M., Bindels, L. B., de Vos, W. M., Gibson, G. R., Thissen, J. P., Delzenne, N. M. (2013). Insight into the prebiotic concept: lessons from an exploratory, double blind intervention study with inulin-type fructans in obese women. *Gut*, 62(8), 1112-1121.

Farina, F., Piassi, F. G., Moyses, M. R., Bazzolli, D. M. S., Bissoli, N. S. (2010). Glycemic and urinary volume responses in diabetic mellitus rats treated with Solanum lycocarpum. *Applied Physiology, Nutrition, and Metabolism*, 35(1), 40-44.

Fei, B., Ling, L., Hua, C., Ren, S. (2014). Effects of soybean oligosaccharides on antioxidant enzyme activities and insulin resistance in pregnant women with gestational diabetes mellitus. *Food Chemistry*, 158, 429-432.

Feinman, R. D., Pogozelski, W. K., Astrup, A., Bernstein, R. K., Fine, E. J., Westman, E. C., Accurso, A., Frassetto, L., Gower, B. A., McFarlane, S. I., Nielsen, J. V., Krarup, T., Saslow, L., Roth, K. S., Vernon, M. C., Volek, J. S., Wilshire, G. B., Dahlqvist, A., Sundberg, R., Childers, A., Morrison, K., Manninen, A. H., Dashti, H. M., Wood, R. J., Wortman, J., McFarlane, S. I. (2015). Dietary carbohydrate restriction as the first approach in diabetes management: critical review and evidence base. *Nutrition*, 31(1), 1-13.

Gobinath, D., Madhu, A. N., Prashant, G., Srinivasan, K., Prapulla, S. G. (2010). Beneficial effect of xylo-oligosaccharides and fructo-oligosaccharides in streptozotocin-induced diabetic rats. *British Journal of Nutrition*, 104(1), 40-47.

Hui, H., Tang, G., Go, V. L. W. (2009). Hypoglycemic herbs and their action mechanisms. *Chinese Medicine*, 4(1), 1-11.

Kendall, C. W., Emam, A., Augustin, L. S., Jenkins, D. J. (2004). Resistant starches and health. *Journal of AOAC International*, 87(3), 769-774.

Kirsten, R., Heintz, B., Nelson, K., Oremek, G., Speck, U. (1992). Influence of two guar preparations on glycosylated hemoglobin, total cholesterol and triglycerides in patients with diabetes mellitus. *International Journal of Clinical Pharmacology, Therapy, and Toxicology*, 30(12), 582-586.

Kiss, R., Szabó, K., Gesztelyi, R., Somodi, S., Kovács, P., Szabó, Z., Németh, J., Priksz, D., Kurucz, A., Juhász, B., Szilvássy, Z. (2018). Insulin-sensitizer effects of fenugreek seeds in parallel with changes in plasma MCH levels in healthy volunteers. *International Journal of Molecular Sciences*, 19(3), 771.

Koh, H., Tsushima, M., Harano, Y. (1999). Effect of carbohydrate intake on serum 3,5,3'-triiodothyronine-response to glucose ingestion and its relation to glucose tolerance in lean non-insulin-dependent diabetic patients. *Arzneimittel-Forschung*, 49(1), 30-34.

Li, G. Q., Kam, A., Wong, K. H., Zhou, X., Omar, E. A., Alqahtani, A., Li, K. M., Razmovski-Naumovski, V., Chan, K. (2012). Herbal medicines for the management of diabetes. *Advances in Experimental Medicine and Biology*, 771, 396-413.

Lin, M.- H. A., Wu, M.- C., Lu, S., Lin, J. (2010). Glycemic index, glycemic load and insulinemic index of Chinese starchy foods. *World Journal of Gastroenterology*, 16(39), 4973.

Sylvetsky, A., Edelstein, S., Walford, G., Boyko, E., Horton, E. S., Ibebuogu, U., Knowler, W., Montez, M., Temprosa, M., Hoskin, M., Rother, K., Delahanty, L., Diabetes Prevention Program Research Group. (2017). A high-carbohydrate, high-fiber, low-fat diet results in weight loss among adults at high risk of type 2 diabetes. *Journal of Nutrition*, 147(11), 2060-2066.

Liu, F., Li, P., Chen, M., Luo, Y., Prabhakar, M., Zheng, H., He, Y., Qi, Q., Long, H., Zhang, Y., Sheng, H., Zhang, Y. (2017). Fructooligosaccharide (FOS) and galactooligosaccharide (GOS) increase Bifidobacterium but reduce butyrate producing bacteria with adverse glycemic metabolism in healthy young population. *Scientific Reports*, 7(1), 11789.

Luo, J., Van Yperselle, M., Rizkalla, S. W., Rossi, F., Bornet, F. R., Slama, G. (2000). Chronic consumption of short-chain fructooligosaccharides does not affect basal hepatic glucose production or insulin resistance in type 2 diabetics. *Journal of Nutrition*, 130(6), 1572-1577.

Øverby, N., Margeirsdottir, H., Brunborg, C., Andersen, L., Dahl-Jørgensen, K. (2007). The influence of dietary intake and meal pattern on blood glucose control in children and adolescents using intensive insulin treatment. *Diabetologia*, 50, 2044-2051.

Panahi, S., Ezatagha, A., Temelli, F., Vasanthan, T., Vuksan, V. (2007). β-Glucan from two sources of oat concentrates affect postprandial glycemia in relation to the level of viscosity. *Journal of the American College of Nutrition*, 26(6), 639-644.

Qin, Q., Yan, S., Yang, Y., Chen, J., Li, T., Gao, X., Yan, H., Wang, Y., Wang, J., Wang, S., Ding, S. (2021). A metagenome-wide association study of the gut microbiome and metabolic syndrome. *Frontiers in Microbiology*, 12, 682721.

Ríos-Ríos, K. L., Rémond, C., Dejonghe, W., Van Roy, S., Vangeel, S., Van Hecke, W. (2022). Production of tailored xylo-oligosaccharides from beechwood xylan by different enzyme membrane reactors and evaluation of their prebiotic activity. *Biochemical Engineering Journal*, 185, 108494.

Sajadimajd, S., Bahrami, G., Daglia, M., Nabavi, S. M., Naseri, R., Farzaei, M. H. (2019). Plant-derived supplementary carbohydrates, polysaccharides and oligosaccharides in management of diabetes mellitus: a comprehensive review. *Food Reviews International*, 35(6), 563-586.

Shields, B., Hicks, S., Shepherd, M., Colclough, K., Hattersley, A. T., Ellard, S. (2010). Maturity-onset diabetes of the young (MODY): how many cases are we missing? *Diabetologia*, 53, 2504-2508.

Wang, M., Hamer, R. J., van Vliet, T., Oudgenoeg, G. (2002). Interaction of water extractable pentosans with gluten protein: effect on dough properties and gluten quality. *Journal of Cereal Science*, 36(1), 25-37.

Xiaoli, X., Liyi, Y., Shuang, H., Wei, L., Yi, S., Hao, M., Jusong, Z., Xiaoxiong, Z. (2008). Determination of oligosaccharide contents in 19 cultivars of chickpea (Cicer arietinum L) seeds by high performance liquid chromatography. *Food Chemistry*, 111(1), 215-219.

Yamashita, K., Kawai, K., Itakura, M. (1984). Effects of fructo-oligosaccharides on blood glucose and serum lipids in diabetic subjects. *Nutrition Research*, 4(6), 961-966.

Chapter 7

Glycosides for the Management of Diabetes Mellitus

Fatimah Jan[1]
Arashdeep Kaur[1,*]
Saika Bashir[1]
Swati Pahwa[2]
Binu Raina[3]
Abhimanyu[3]
Prabhjot Singh Bajwa[3]
and Kumar Guarve[2]

[1]School of Pharmaceutical Sciences, C. T. University, Ludhiana, Punjab, India
[2]Guru Gobind Singh College of Pharmacy, Yamuna Nagar, Haryana, India
[3]Ch. Devi Lal College of Pharmacy, Jagadhri, Haryana, India

Abstract

Diabetes is a chronic metabolic disorder characterized by elevated blood glucose levels stemming from issues with insulin action, synthesis, or both. Effective management of diabetes is crucial, as prolonged uncontrolled diabetes can result in complications such as neuropathy, retinopathy, cardiomyopathy, and nephropathy. Studies have highlighted its classification among the top five global causes of mortality. Pharmaceutical substances within medical practice are grappling with challenges including numerous undesirable effects, ineffectiveness in a broad population, and patient compliance. Hence,

* Corresponding Author's Email: ad357754@gmail.com.

In: Naturally Occurring Chemicals …
Editors: A. Singh Grewal, G. Deswal, A. Kumar Dhingra et al.
ISBN: 979-8-89113-491-1

the quest for novel effective treatments is imperative. A noteworthy solution in this context could be natural products, which have long been recognized as a legitimate therapeutic approach. In this review, a multitude of plant-derived glycosides exhibiting antidiabetic properties are explored. These effects are orchestrated through various mechanisms. The utilization of glycosides as antidiabetic interventions holds potential for unveiling novel and beneficial therapeutic agents.

Keywords: diabetes mellitus, glycosides, natural products, management

Introduction

A metabolic disorder with diverse etiologies, diabetes mellitus is defined by the World Health Organization (WHO) as "a metabolic disorder of multiple etiologies characterized by sustained high blood sugar levels with disruptions in lipid, protein, and carbohydrate metabolism, arising from irregularities in insulin secretion, insulin action, or both." Projections for the year 2040 indicate a global diabetic population of 642 million individuals (Skyler et al., 2017). The International Diabetes Federation, also known as IDF, reported that diabetes affected approximately 366 million people globally in 2011, with an estimated annual death toll of around 4.6 million due to the condition. The focal point of this diabetes epidemic has been pinpointed to the Indian subcontinent. According to data, individuals aged 20 to 79 in this region have the following diabetes prevalence rates: India, Bangladesh, Nepal, Sri Lanka, and Pakistan are all among the top five countries by population percentage affected: 8.31%, 9.85%, 7.77%, and 6.72%, respectively (Rizvi & Mishra, 2013). Diabetes exerts significant impacts while also heightening risk factors for atherosclerosis, hypertension, dyslipidemia, elevated blood sugar, and platelet aggregation. It has evolved into a critical public health concern, substantially diminishing both the longevity and quality of life for affected individuals. Diabetes mellitus, a chronic disorder, stems from inadequate insulin production by the pancreas, and it can result from inherited factors, acquired influences, or a combination of both. The resulting elevated blood glucose levels, triggered by this insufficiency, exert adverse effects on our physical well-being, particularly affecting the neurological system and blood vessels. Termed hyperglycemia, the abnormally high level of glucose in the blood associated with diabetes mellitus is a metabolic condition. According to data, over 90% of individuals with diabetes are diagnosed with type 2 diabetes (Yadav et al., 2015). The unrestricted expense and negative consequences of synthetic hypoglycemic agents may be to blame for this practice (Chen et al., 2015). Given their effectiveness, non-toxic nature, minimal to no side effects, and suitability for oral administration, the World Health Organization (WHO) has recommended the evaluation of traditional plant remedies for diabetes. Herbal treatments have proven beneficial for patients with both insulin-dependent and non-insulin-dependent forms of diabetes mellitus, as well as conditions like diabetic retinal degeneration and diabetic neuropathy. However, it's important to note that several of the currently used herbal treatments lack comprehensive scientific validation, and some may carry serious toxic risks or trigger significant drug interactions. The growing prevalence of diabetes mellitus has spurred the development of numerous innovative therapies for hyperglycemia, with the aim of maintaining blood sugar levels as close to normal as possible while averting complications. To date, a wide range of diabetes medications & the mechanisms of actions exist as through oral tradition drugs, including alpha-glucosidase inhibitors, sulfa glitazones, meglitinides, biguanides, a class of drugs a dopamine D2-receptor agonists, or inhibitors of DPP-4 (Tong and Adler, 2018), & glucagon-like peptide receptor agonists, or injected therapies involve GLP-1 agonists, amylin analogues, insulin, insulin analogues, and so forth. The rehabilitation of diabetes patients is considerably affected by the unfavorable side effects and limited efficacy of numerous medications. Metformin, for instance, is associated with gastrointestinal disturbances, such as nausea, loss of appetite, diarrhea, and mild abdominal discomfort, constituting the majority of its potential side effects. Dipeptidyl peptidase-IV inhibitor (DPP-4 inhibitors) can lead to other adverse reactions like nasopharyngitis, headaches, hypersensitivity, and skin responses (Gooßen and Gräber, 2012). Although linked with numerous benefits, incretin-based medications are still associated with severe gastrointestinal side effects, including vomiting, nausea, acid reflux, indigestion, and diarrhea. Diabetes is a chronic condition necessitating lifelong management. Consequently, the cost of diabetes medication has emerged as a significant obstacle to patient adherence. Researchers have calculated and examined the expenses of pharmaceutical treatments based on the patient's medication regimen. The findings revealed a high cost per prescription, believed to be a primary factor contributing to patients' non-adherence to therapy (Acharya et al., 2013). Hence, there is an urgent imperative to develop medicinal products that are both more effective and safer. Plants such as Acacia arabica (babul), Aegle marmelos (bael), Agrimonia eupatoria (church steeples), Allium cepa (onions), Allium sativum (garlic), Mangifera indica (mango), Morus alba (mulberry), Mucuna pruriens (fever nut or kiwach), Ocimum sanctum (tulsi), Pterocarpus marsupium (Indian kino or bisasar), Punica granatum (pomegranate or anar), Syzygium cumini (jamun), Tinospora cordifolia (giloy), and Trigonella foenum-graecum (fenugreek or methi) hold botanical significance. These plants are abundant sources of various plant-based chemicals (Mukherjee et al., 2006).

Phytochemicals in Diabetic Mellitus Management

Active constituents for the management of various ailments encompass compounds with diverse structures but similar therapeutic effects, derived from a multitude of plant species. The utilization of these plants or phytoconstituents, through various mechanisms, serves to thwart the onset of diabetic complications and regulate metabolic anomalies (Mukherjee et al., 2006). Furthermore, over the past few years, numerous phytochemicals with anti-diabetic properties have been identified from various plants. Examples include dietary fibers, alkaloid compounds, saponins, flavonoids, polymers, glycolipids, amino acids, peptides, and other plant-derived compounds.

Glycosides in Diabetes

The leaves of Myrcia multiflora DC. (Myrtaceae) yielded additional compounds, namely flavanone glucosides known as Myrciacitrins I & II, along with novel substances named glucosides (myrciaphenones A & B). These compounds exhibited inhibitory effects on aldose reductase and alpha-glucosidase activities. Moreover, in experiments with sucrose-loaded rats and alloxan-induced diabetic mice, the herb effectively curbed the rise in blood glucose levels (Gaikwad et al., 2014). Upon the purification of myrciacitrins 1 and 2, as well as myrciaphenones A and B, three additional new flavanone glucosides—myrciacitrins III, IV, and V—were identified from the leaves of M. multiflora. Research by Matsuda et al., (2002) showcased the substantial inhibitory effect of myrciacitrins on aldose reductase. Extracted from the primary barks of Kalopanax pictus Nakai (Araliaceae), seven chemical constituents were identified, including hederagenin glycosides and phenolic glycosides. In streptozotocin-induced diabetes rats, the antidiabetic effects of these isolated compounds revealed that kalopanax (saponin A) exhibited significant antidiabetic activity, while hederagenin displayed a more modest effect (Narender et al., 2009). Before the discovery of insulin, the stems and leaves of Vaccinium myrtillus L. (Ericaceae) were commonly employed as a treatment for diabetes. Allen identified neomyrtillin, an active glycoside compound, from V. myrtillus leaf tissue. This compound proved beneficial in reducing glycosuria and postprandial hyperglycemia in most adult-onset diabetic patients, albeit less effective in juvenile-onset diabetics. The substance was found to enhance the hypoglycemic effect of external insulin while reducing insulin requirements, possibly aiding insulin activity. Allen proposed that "myrtillin performs some auxiliary role in carbohydrate breakdown and, if used effectively, can be a valuable adjunct to diabetic treatment." Similarly, Kato et al., isolated two steroidal glycosides, PO-1 and PO-2, from the rhizome of Polygonatum sp. (Liliaceae), testing them as novel hypoglycemic agents in mice. The roots of Anemarrhena asphodeloides Bunge (Asparagaceae) yielded pseudoprototinosaponin AIII and prototinosaponin AIII. Both glycosides were found to modify glucose absorption and insulin release in KK-Ay mice, suggesting their hypoglycemic effects are linked to the liver's glucose production or glycogenolysis. Furthermore, the glycoside jamboline (antimellin), discovered in the seed pods of Syzygium cumini (Eugenia jambolana), possesses anti-diabetic properties. Jamboline exerts a hypoglycemic impact by inhibiting starch conversion into sugar, reducing glucose levels in urine, and curbing appetite. (Yarnell et al., 2009; Sagrawat et al., 2006). The effects of three flavonoids glycosides found in the stems and leaves of the species Microcos paniculata L. (Tiliaceae) on -glucosidase were investigated (Table 1). The inhibitory effects of three different flavonoids tested positive: vitexin, isovitexin, and isorhamnetin 3-O--Drutinoside.

Citrus flavonoids have demonstrated various biological advantages through both in vitro and in vivo studies, particularly in the context of chronic-degenerative conditions such as cancer, diabetes, and cardiovascular disease. Additionally, the flavonoids present in citrus fruits act as antioxidants, providing protection against oxidative stress—a process linked to inflammation—and thereby reducing the risk of damage to macromolecules caused by the activity of reactive species. This antioxidant action contributes to defense against several diseases, particularly diabetes. Furthermore, mechanistic investigations suggest that flavonoids found in fruits can potentially reduce glycemia while enhancing insulin secretion and sensitivity. Hesperidin, chemically known as (3,5,7-trihydroxyflavanone-7-rhamnoglucoside), is an abundant and cost-effective primary dietary flavone glycoside extracted from citrus species like sweet orange and lemon. It is often referred to as "Vitamin P." Interestingly, the group treated with hesperidin exhibited significantly elevated levels of glucokinase mRNA.

Table 1. Glycosides used to treat diabetes

Plants Name	Glycosides	Parts used	References
Kalopanax pictus	Kalopanax	Stem bark	(Gaikwad et al., 2014)
Syzygium cumini	Jamboline & antimellin	Seeds	(Yarnell et al., 2009)
Myrcia multiflora	Myrciacitrins I & II; myrciaphenones A and B	Leave	Matsuda et al., 2002)
Vaccinium myrtillus	Neomyrtillin	Leaves	(Gaikwad et al., 2014)
Ficus bengalensis	Perlargonidin 3-o- l rhamnoside	Bark	(Gaikwad et al., 2014)
Anemarrhena asphodeloides	Pseudoprototinosaponin AIII & prototinosaponin AIII	Rhizome	(Gaikwad et al., 2014)
Microcos paniculata	Vitexin, isovitexin and isorhamnetin 3-O-D-rutinoside	Leaves	(Matsuda et al., 2002)

Conclusion

Undoubtedly, diabetes stands out as the metabolic condition experiencing the most rapid global expansion. As our understanding of the complexities of the disorder deepens, so does the demand for novel treatments. Traditional plant remedies have been employed worldwide to manage diabetes, owing to their wide availability and affordability. Through systematic examination of numerous plant species, the beneficial effects of botanicals in diabetes control have been substantiated through various approaches. However, many of the herbal remedies currently in use lack thorough scientific evaluation, and only a small fraction of them possesses the potential for significant drug interactions and potentially adverse outcomes. Comprehensive research and advancements in drug delivery techniques are essential to elucidate the pharmacological activities of the herbal therapies employed for diabetes management today. The exploration of these therapeutic avenues may eventually unveil a natural solution within the realm of diabetology.

References

Acharya, K. G., Shah, K. N., Solanki, N. D., Rana, D. A. (2013). Evaluation of antidiabetic prescriptions, cost and adherence to treatment guidelines: A prospective, cross-sectional study at a tertiary care teaching hospital. *Journal of Basic and Clinical Pharmacy*, 4(4), 82.

Chen, X. W., He, Z. X., Zhou, Z. W., Yang, T., Zhang, X., Yang, Y. X., Duan, W., Zhou, S. F. (2015). (2015). An update on the clinical pharmacology of the dipeptidyl peptidase 4 inhibitor alogliptin used for the treatment of type 2 diabetes mellitus. *Clinical and Experimental Pharmacology and Physiology*, 42(12), 1225-1238.

Fort, D. M., Ubillas, R. P., Mendez, C. D., Jolad, S. D., Inman, W. D., Carney, J. R., Chen, J. L., Ianiro, T. T., Hasbun, C., Bruening, R. C., Luo, J., Reed, M. J., Iwu, M., Carlson, T. J., King, S. R., Bierer, D. E., Cooper, R. (2000). Novel antihyperglycemic terpenoid-quinones from Pycnanthus angolensis. *The Journal of Organic Chemistry*, 65(20), 6534-6539.

Gaikwad, S. B., Mohan, G. K., Rani, M. S. (2014). Phytochemicals for diabetes management. *Pharmaceutical Crops*, 2014, 5(Suppl 1: M2), 11-28.

Gooßen, K., Gräber, S. (2012). Longer term safety of dipeptidyl peptidase-4 inhibitors in patients with type 2 diabetes mellitus: systematic review and meta-analysis. *Diabetes, Obesity and Metabolism*, 14(12), 1061-1072.

Matsuda, H., Nishida, N., Yoshikawa, M. (2002). Antidiabetic principles of natural medicines. V. Aldose reductase inhibitors from Myrcia multiflora DC.(2): Structures of myrciacitrins III, IV, and V. *Chemical and Pharmaceutical Bulletin*, 50(3), 429-431.

Mukherjee, P. K., Maiti, K., Mukherjee, K., Houghton, P. J. (2006). Leads from Indian medicinal plants with hypoglycemic potentials. *Journal of Ethnopharmacology*, 106(1), 1-28.

Narender, T., Khaliq, T., Singh, A. B., Joshi, M. D., Mishra, P., Chaturvedi, J. P., Srivastava, A. K., Maurya, R., Agarwal, S. C. (2009). Synthesis of α-amyrin derivatives and their in vivo antihyperglycemic activity. *European Journal of Medicinal Chemistry*, 44(3), 1215-1222.

Ragasa, C. Y., Tsai, P.- W., Shen, C.- C. (2009). Terpenoids and sterols from the endemic and endangered Philippine trees, Ficus pseudopalma and Ficus ulmifolia. *Philippine Journal of Science*, 138(2), 205-209.

Rizvi, S. I., Mishra, N. (2013). Traditional Indian medicines used for the management of diabetes mellitus. *Journal of Diabetes Research*, 2013, 712092.

Sagrawat, H., Mann, A., Kharya, M. (2006). Pharmacological potential of Eugenia jambolana: A review. *Pharmacognosy Magazine*, 2(6), 96-105.

Skyler, J. S., Bakris, G. L., Bonifacio, E., Darsow, T., Eckel, R. H., Groop, L., Groop, P. H., Handelsman, Y., Insel, R. A., Mathieu, C., McElvaine, A. T., Palmer, J. P., Pugliese, A., Schatz, D. A., Sosenko, J. M., Wilding, J. P., Ratner, R. E. (2017). Differentiation of diabetes by pathophysiology, natural history, and prognosis. *Diabetes*, 66(2), 241-255.

Tong, L., Adler, S. (2018). Glycemic control of type 2 diabetes mellitus across stages of renal impairment: information for primary care providers. *Postgraduate Medicine*, 130(4), 381-393.

Yadav, M. K., Tripathi, J., Tripathi, P. (2015). Ethno medicinal plants with antidiabetic activity: a review. *International Journal of Pharmaceutical Sciences and Research*, 6(12), 4570-4578.

Yarnell, E., Abascal, K., Rountree, R. (2009). *Clinical Botanical Medicine*. Mary Ann Liebert, Inc., Publishers.

Chapter 8

Alkaloids in the Management of Diabetes Mellitus

Shikha Kamboj[1,*]
Sweta Kamboj[1]
Rohit Kamboj[1]
Priyanka Kriplani[1]
Kumar Guarve[1]
Sweta Pundir[2]
Raj Kumari[2]
Meenakshi Sharma[2]
and Rohit Malik[3]
[1]Guru Gobind Singh College of Pharmacy, Yamuna Nagar, Haryana, India
[2]I. T. S. College of Pharmacy, Muradnagar, Ghaziabad, Uttar Pradesh, India
[3]Veer Kunwar College of Pharmacy, Bijnor, Uttar Pradesh, India

Abstract

Diabetes mellitus (DM) is an alternate term for an enduring metabolic disorder that is currently witnessing a significant surge in prevalence and causing thousands of deaths annually. Type 1 DM is characterized by insufficient insulin due to the decline of β-cells. Conversely, type 2 DM, a more prevalent form, is linked with insulin resistance and β-cell dysfunction. To manage glucose homeostasis and forestall the development of late-stage diabetic complications, various synthetic

* Corresponding Author's Email: shikhakamboj21@gmail.com.

In: Naturally Occurring Chemicals …
Editors: A. Singh Grewal, G. Deswal, A. Kumar Dhingra et al.
ISBN: 979-8-89113-491-1

medications have been developed. However, many of these chemical agents either yield suboptimal effects or carry the potential for adverse side effects. In recent times, herbal remedies have emerged as a potential therapeutic avenue alongside conventional medicine for diabetes mellitus. These herbal treatments encompass biological macromolecules with diverse anti-diabetic properties. These naturally occurring substances might play a role in averting or regulating diabetes and are generally considered benign phytochemicals. Core mechanisms of their anti-diabetic effects encompass enhanced insulin secretion, diminished insulin resistance, and heightened hepatic glycogen synthesis activities. What's intriguing is the potential therapeutic impact of alkaloids on blood glucose anomalies, orchestrated through diverse signaling cascades and pathways. These encompass hindering or propelling an array of systems, such as inhibiting the -glucosidase enzyme, obstructing PTP-1B, deactivating DPP-IV, amplifying insulin sensitivity, and mitigating oxidative stress. Alkaloids from a wide spectrum of species have undergone clinical trials and animal model studies to showcase their effectiveness in reducing blood glucose levels.

Keywords: diabetes mellitus, alkaloids, anti-diabetic action

Abbreviations

AMPK	Activation of AMP-activated protein kinase
AR	Aldose reductase
DM	Diabetes mellitus
DPP-4	Dipeptidyl peptidase-4
DPP-IV	Dipeptidyl peptidase IV
FDA	Food and drug administration
GLP-1	Glucagon-like peptide-1 receptor agonists
PAs	Pyrrolizidine alkaloids
PTP-1B	Protein tyrosine phosphatase 1B
ROS	Reactive oxygen species
SGLT2	Sodium-glucose cotransporter-2.

Introduction

Diabetes, also referred to as diabetes mellitus, is an enduring metabolic condition that interferes with the body's processing of blood sugar (glucose)

(Verma et al., 2006). Glucose serves as the primary energy source for cells, and insulin is the hormone responsible for regulating blood glucose levels (Pang et al., 2021). Type 1 diabetes develops when the immune system targets and eliminates the cells in the pancreas that produce insulin (Bouillon et al., 2012). Individuals with type 1 diabetes need to administer insulin injections or use insulin pumps daily to regulate their blood sugar levels. Type 2 diabetes develops when the body becomes resistant to insulin or doesn't produce enough insulin to maintain normal blood sugar levels. Managing type 2 diabetes usually entails adopting a healthy lifestyle, including balanced nutrition, regular physical activity, and, at times, medication or insulin therapy (Adhikari, 2021). Between 2023 and 2045, it is predicted that there would be 578 million adults living with diabetes worldwide (Lee, 2018). A variety of drug targets exist for diabetes treatment, each with its distinct mechanism of action. Among the frequently utilized medications for diabetes management are insulin, biguanides, GLP-1 receptor agonists, SGLT2 inhibitors, DPP-4 inhibitors, and alpha-glucosidase inhibitors (Amar et al., 2022).

Chemistry of Alkaloids

"Alkaloids" refers to naturally occurring organic nitrogen-containing substances with a basic pH. These compounds, categorized as alkaloids, are distinguished by their alkaline properties and the inclusion of at least one nitrogen atom in a heterocyclic ring structure. They can be found in various plants, fungi, and animals, often exerting potent pharmacological effects. Alkaloids represent a prominent category of secondary metabolites, demonstrated to yield crucial biological effects such as analgesic, muscle relaxation, and antioxidative properties. They serve to bring about advantages for humankind and exhibit efficacy against certain life-threatening diseases. In particular severe instances, a few alkaloids have led to patient fatality through suffocation, paralysis, or other adverse outcomes. The development of numerous methods for extracting and quantifying alkaloids has simplified the progress of scientific research beyond previous methodologies (Roy, 2017). The chemistry of alkaloids is intricate and varies based on the specific compound. A distinctive characteristic of alkaloids is their inherent alkaline nature. This results from the inclusion of one or more nitrogen atoms within the molecule, enabling them to function as proton acceptors or bases. These nitrogen atoms might form components of a heterocyclic ring, a ring containing atoms other than carbon alongside carbon atoms. While the structure of alkaloids can display substantial diversity, a significant number originate from amino acids, which serve as the fundamental constituents of proteins (Beniddir et al., 2021). Alkaloids frequently exhibit intricate structures encompassing multiple rings, functional groups, and stereochemistry. Several familiar classes of alkaloids encompass indole alkaloids (present in plants like the opium poppy and the hallucinogenic Ayahuasca plant), quinoline alkaloids (occurring in plants like cinchona), and pyridine alkaloids (found in plants like tobacco). The pharmacological effects of alkaloids can diverge considerably, contingent on the individual compound (Funayama et al., 2014). Certain alkaloids, like caffeine and theobromine (discovered in chocolate), produce stimulating effects, whereas others, including morphine and codeine (found in opium), induce pain relief and sedation. Some alkaloids, like quinine (found in cinchona), possess antimalarial properties, whereas others, such as atropine (found in deadly nightshade), manifest anticholinergic effects. They can be classified as primary amines (R-NH2; e.g., norephedrine), secondary amines (R2-NH; e.g., ephedrine), tertiary amines (R3-N; e.g., atropine), or quaternary ammonium salts (R4-N; e.g., d-tubocurarine) (Kukula et al., 2017). The class of secondary metabolites known as pyrrolizidine alkaloids (PAs) encompasses a wide array of uniquely structured compounds. It is estimated that over the past several decades, more than 12,000 PAs have been identified. They possess a pungent taste. PAs are found in various types of plants, with prevalence ranging from 14-20%. Consequently, amino acids play a pivotal role as intermediates in the biosynthesis pathways of PAs, and these substances are prevalent in the natural world. Alkaloids are categorized into three primary groups: true, pseudo-, and proto-alkaloids, based on their distinct chemical structures. Each subgroup of PAs within this classification displays specific biological traits, and thus, the complexity of their molecular makeup can impact their in vivo functions. The following sections delve into recently isolated PAs from diverse plant and tree sources, showcasing noteworthy anti-diabetic properties. (Beato et al., 2021).

Anti-Diabetic Alkaloids from Different Families

Anti-Diabetic Alkaloids from Moraceae

Research indicates that plants belonging to the Moraceae family possess potent anti-diabetic attributes. Several secondary metabolites originating from the mulberry plant Morus atropurpurea, such as phenolic acids, flavonoids, and alkaloids, exhibit anti-diabetic effects. Among these, alkaloids and their associated structures show potential for diabetes treatment. Notably, six inhibitory alkaloids, which are derivatives of piperidine, pyrimidine, and pyrazine, have been identified. The literature details the isolation of -5-(1," 2," 3," 4"-tetrahydroxybutyl)-pyrazine from M. atropurpurea leaves, elucidating its activity against -glucosidase (Abdel et al., 2023). As per the study, inhibitory effects were observed in the leaves of both M. bombycis and M. alba, attributed to tropane and polyhydroxylated alkaloids. Remarkably, potent glucosidase inhibitors were identified, including calystegines B1 and B2, 6-O-D-glucopyranosyl-1-deoxynojirimycin, compound, and 2-hydroxynortropane. These compounds were isolated from distinct aerial parts of M. alba.

Anti-Diabetic Alkaloids from Acanthaceae, Piperaceae, Fabaceae, and Portulacaceae

In a distinct study, researchers examined the efficacy of trigonelline in inhibiting the activity of DPP-4, -glucosidase, and ACE enzymes. The results highlighted that trigonelline significantly impeded the function of DPP-4 and -glucosidase enzymes in both the plasma and small intestine of diabetic rats. Furthermore, this compound ameliorated metabolic indices and ACE activity. The investigation conducted by Beato et al., in 2021 revealed that the behavior of these compounds in diabetic rats exhibited variation based on the glucose concentration. These substances primarily showcased their anti-diabetic attributes by augmenting insulin secretion. Notably, the compound Lupanine displayed its capacity to stimulate insulin secretion at lower glucose concentrations, whereas the other two compounds manifested effects solely at higher glucose concentrations.

Castanospermine and 6-epi castanospermine, indoline alkaloids originating from the seeds of the Australian tree Castanospermum australe

(Fabaceae), were identified as inhibitors of glycosidase activity. These findings were reported by Beato et al., in 2021.

Anti-Diabetic Alkaloids from Euphorbiaceae and Apocynaceae Species

The Euphorbiaceae family of flowering plants, which thrives in regions beyond the tropics such as the southern United States, the Middle East, and the Mediterranean Basin, offers potential for enhancing health. From the Chrozophora plicata plant, Mathe isolated Pyrrole alkaloids named plicatanins A–C (18-20) and speranberculatine A in 2020. These compounds exhibited promising effects in diabetes management by impeding the activity of enzymes responsible for carbohydrate digestion. Notably, among these compounds, plicatain C emerged as the most effective inhibitor of the yeast - glucosidase enzyme.

Anti-Diabetic Alkaloids from Rutaceae Species

Within this group of medicinal plants, there exist around 2,070 species and 160 genera. The fruit pulp of Murraya koenigii has been discovered to encompass several alkaloids, including bisgerayafoline D, bismahanimbinol, O-methyl mahanine, O-methyl mukonal, bispyrayafoline, and mahanine. Notably, these compounds displayed notable inhibitory effects on α-glucosidase. Of these, mahanine stood out due to its remarkable cytotoxicity against the α-glucosidase enzyme, evident from its IC50 value of 21.40 μM. The reported IC50 values for compounds 28-30 were measured as 46.10, 77.50, and 29.10 μM, respectively. Moreover, the leaves of Murraya koenigii were found to harbor a carbazole alkaloid known as mahanimbine. This compound has demonstrated anti-diabetic and hypolipidemic properties in rats induced with STZ. In contrast to previously studied alkaloids, mahanimbine exhibited a modest inhibitory profile against α-glucosidase. However, it displayed potent activity against α-amylase when compared to the drug acarbose. (Rasouli et al., 2020).

Mechanism of Action of Alkaloids as Antidiabetic Agents

In the past year, several categories of anti-hyperglycemic drugs have been introduced. According to Drug Bank, more than 95% of FDA-approved anti-diabetic drugs are linked to Type 2 Diabetes (T2D) by promoting insulin production, thereby reducing blood glucose levels. Typically, these medications are administered alone or in combination with other diabetes drugs. Synthetic anti-diabetic medications work by increasing peripheral glucose disposal, reducing liver glucose production, enhancing insulin sensitivity, decreasing liver glucose output, and limiting carbohydrate intake. These include various drugs that often target intestinal glucosidase inhibition, such as acarbose, voglibose, and miglitol. It's important to note that they have minimal to no impact on insulin production. In contrast, drugs based on sulfonylureas, like glimepiride and glyburide, directly stimulate insulin synthesis, alongside a moderate impact on enzymatic hydrolysis. The most prevalent side effects of glucosidase inhibitors are diarrhea and abdominal discomfort. Furthermore, thiazolidinediones (such as pioglitazone and rosiglitazone) have been associated with adverse effects like anemia, heart failure, and weight gain. Additional diabetes medications have also been connected to negative side effects, including vaginal and bladder infections, fatigue, dyspepsia, nausea, vomiting, headache, hypoglycemia, dizziness, nausea, and vomiting (Liu et al., 2023). Long-term use of conventional medications may not be acceptable due to the likelihood of negative effects.

Restriction of Digestive Enzymes

Increased blood glucose levels result from the degradation of dietary polysaccharides by digestive enzymes. An enzyme known as -amylase, which is abundant in pancreatic juice and saliva, facilitates the hydrolysis of 1,4-glycosidic bonds present in starch, glycogen, and other oligosaccharides. Similarly, -glucosidase, released by cells in the brush borders of the epithelial cells in the small intestine, participates in the breakdown of oligosaccharides into readily absorbable monosaccharides. This process contributes to postprandial hyperglycemia, as explained by (Yang et al., 2023). A frequently utilized strategy to lower post-meal blood glucose levels involves the inhibition of these digestive enzymes using secondary metabolites present in plants. Alkaloids, for instance, can bind to competitive or noncompetitive sites on these enzymes, hindering the creation of enzyme-substrate complexes and thereby reducing enzyme activity.

Aldose Reductase and Protein Tyrosine Phosphatase-1b Inhibition

When the principal enzyme of the polyol pathway, aldose reductase (AR), initiates the conversion of glucose into sorbitol, an excessive quantity of reactive oxygen species (ROS) is produced. AR transforms cytosolic glucose into sorbitol, a compound that is sometimes metabolized at a sluggish pace and possesses limited ability to traverse cell membranes. Due to hyperglycemia, sorbitol and its derivative, fructose, might amass within cells, potentially leading to osmotic swelling and cellular dysfunction (Sawant et al., 2015). Under typical glycemic conditions, aldose reductase serves to diminish levels of steroids and catecholamines, generate fructose for sperm, uphold equilibrium in the kidney's osmoregulatory system, and neutralize toxic aldehydes in extrahepatic tissues. However, heightened polyol metabolism in hyperglycemic conditions leads to an escalation in sorbitol levels, promoting osmotic stress that is particularly conducive to cataract formation. Furthermore, this process contributes to glycative stress and elevates reactive oxygen species through receptor interactions. (Kousaxidis et al., 2020).

Elevation in Insulin Secretion

The islets of Langerhans within the pancreas play a role in controlling blood sugar levels by producing insulin and glucagon, which exert opposing effects on the body's peripheral organs. Insulin works to lower blood sugar levels by enhancing glucose absorption in skeletal muscles, while simultaneously inhibiting hepatic glucose synthesis and slowing down lipolysis (Tsuchiya et al., 2023). Conversely, glucagon elevates blood glucose levels by stimulating gluconeogenesis and lipolysis. Within the small intestinal L-cells, the proglucagon gene generates GLP-1, which enhances insulin production and release, lowers glucagon levels, curbs hunger, retards gastric emptying, and hampers the regenerative and differentiating capacity of pancreatic islet -cells in response to food (Zhao et al., 2023). Numerous alkaloidal drugs, including berberine, metformin, and galegine, have demonstrated antidiabetic effects. The mechanism of action of alkaloidal drugs as antidiabetic agents may involve several pathways, including:

Activation of AMP-Activated Protein Kinase (AMPK)

AMPK is an enzyme that holds a pivotal role in regulating cellular energy metabolism. Alkaloidal drugs like berberine and metformin have been demonstrated to activate AMPK, resulting in heightened glucose uptake and reduced glucose production by the liver (Li et al., 2023).

Increased Insulin Sensitivity

Alkaloidal drugs like berberine and metformin have demonstrated the ability to augment insulin sensitivity. This facilitates more efficient utilization of insulin to facilitate the transport of glucose into cells for energy generation (Purwaningsih et al., 2023).

Modulation of Gut Microbiota

Alkaloids such as berberine have been shown to modulate the gut microbiota, which may contribute to their antidiabetic effects (Tong et al., 2023).

Clinical Studies

A progressively growing body of research suggests that pyrrolizidine alkaloids (PAs) hold promise as potential enhancers for routine DM treatment. The biological impact of these compounds is delineated by their chemical composition. Some PAs are already undergoing clinical trials to evaluate their potential benefits for individuals with type 2 diabetes (T2D) in terms of blood sugar levels, serum HbA1c, and management of dyslipidemia (Table 1) (https://clinicaltrials.gov) (Pathak et al., 2019). Both trigonelline (ID: NCT03166540) and berberine (ID: NCT00462046) belong to this category. Additionally, a root extract from Sida cordifolia, abundant in alkaloids (registered under ID NCT02107469), displayed considerable promise in alleviating diabetic polyneuropathy (Zhou et al., 2012, Mukhtar et al., 2020).

Table 1. Several ongoing clinical trials on alkaloids

Alkaloids	On going Clinical trials	References
Kratom	several clinical trials of kratom alkaloids were ongoing, including studies on their safety and efficacy for pain relief	Saengow et al., 2022
Ibogaine (root bark)	several clinical trials of ibogaine were ongoing, including studies on its safety and efficacy for treating opioid addiction	Noller et al., 2017
Vinflunine (periwinkle plant)	several clinical trials of vinflunine were ongoing, including studies on its safety and efficacy for the treatment of other types of cancer	Hoimes et al., 2022
Psilocybin (species of mushrooms)	several clinical trials of psilocybin were ongoing, including studies on its safety and efficacy for the treatment of depression and alcohol use disorder.	Ziff et al., 2022
Nicotine (tobacco)	several clinical trials of nicotine-based therapies were ongoing, including studies on their safety and efficacy for smoking cessation and the treatment of other conditions, such as attention deficit hyperactivity disorder	Almahasneh et al., 2023.

Conclusion

Naturally occurring compounds derived from plants are now widely utilized to address various ailments and extend lifespans. These natural products encompass an array of metabolites, notably alkaloids, which combat infectious diseases through diverse avenues while mitigating adverse effects. Alkaloids have emerged as promising contenders, as evidenced by numerous in vitro and in vivo studies; however, only a few, if any, of these bioactive agents have progressed to clinical trials. It is imperative to meticulously evaluate the bioactivity of pure compounds that can function independently or synergistically for enhanced effects. Alkaloids, with their multifaceted roles in diabetes treatment, warrant further exploration to potentially become optimal medication candidates or dietary supplements. While alkaloids exhibit potential as antidiabetic agents, thorough investigation is required to comprehensively comprehend their mechanisms of action and potential side effects. Consequently, additional research is necessary to develop alkaloid-based drugs that are both efficacious and safe, while also exhibiting favorable bioavailability. In conclusion, alkaloids have demonstrated encouraging outcomes as antidiabetic agents through diverse mechanisms of action.

References

Abdel Razek, M. M., Elissawy, A. M., Mostafa, N. M., Moussa, A. Y., Elanany, M. A., Elshanawany, M. A., Singab, A. N. B. (2023). Chemical and biological review of endophytic fungi associated with Morus sp. *Molecules*, 28(4), 1718.

Adhikari, B. (2021). Roles of alkaloids from medicinal plants in the management of diabetes mellitus. *Journal of Chemistry*, 2691525, 1-10.

Almahasneh, F., Gerges, R. H., Abu-El-Rub, E., Khasawneh, R. R. (2023). Nicotine abuse and neurodegeneration: novel pharmacogenetic targets to aid quitting and reduce the risk of dementia. *CNS & Neurological Disorders-Drug Targets*, 23(1), 2-8.

Beato, A., Gori, A., Boucherle, B., Peuchmaur, M., Haudecoeur, R. (2021). β-Carboline as a privileged scaffold for multitarget strategies in Alzheimer's disease therapy. Journal of Medicinal Chemistry, 64(3), 1392-1422.

Beniddir, M. A., Kang, K. B., Genta-Jouve, G., Huber, F., Rogers, S., Van Der Hooft, J. J. (2021). Advances in decomposing complex metabolite mixtures using substructure-and network-based computational metabolomics approaches. *Natural Product Reports*, 38(11), 1967-1993.

Funayama, S., Cordell, G. A. (2014). *Alkaloids: A Treasury of Poisons and Medicines*. Elsevier Science.

Hoimes, C. J., Flaig, T. W., Milowsky, M. I., Friedlander, T. W., Bilen, M. A., Gupta, S., Srinivas, S., Merchan, J. R., McKay, R. R., Petrylak, D. P., Sasse, C., Moreno, B. H., Yu, Yao., Carret, A. S., Rosenberg, J. E. (2023). Enfortumab vedotin plus pembrolizumab in previously untreated advanced urothelial cancer. *Journal of Clinical Oncology*, 41, 22-31.

Kousaxidis, A., Petrou, A., Lavrentaki, V., Fesatidou, M., Nicolaou, I., Geronikaki, A. (2020). Aldose reductase and protein tyrosine phosphatase 1B inhibitors as a promising therapeutic approach for diabetes mellitus. *European Journal of Medicinal Chemistry*, 207, 112742.

Kukula-Koch, W. A., Widelski, J. (2017). Alkaloids. In *Pharmacognosy* (pp. 163-198). Academic Press.

Linn, A. K. H. (2014). Diabetic nephropathy - complications and treatment. *International Journal of Nephrology and Renovascular Disease*, 15(7), 361-381.

Liu, Y., Niu, Z., Yang, J., Yang, X., Chen, Y., Li, Y., Liang, X., Zhang, J., Fan, F., Wu, P., Peng, C., Shen, B. (2023). Rapid metabolic reprogramming mediated by the AMP-activated protein kinase during the lytic cycle of Toxoplasma gondii. *Nature Communications*, 14(1), 422.

Mukhtar, Y., Galalain, A., Yunusa, U. (2020). A modern overview on diabetes mellitus: a chronic endocrine disorder. *European Journal of Biology*, 5(2), 1-14.

Neag, M. A., Mocan, A., Echeverría, J., Pop, R. M., Bocsan, C. I., Crişan, G., Buzoianu, A. D. (2018). Berberine: botanical occurrence, traditional uses, extraction methods, and relevance in cardiovascular, metabolic, hepatic, and renal disorders. *Frontiers in Pharmacology*, 9, 557.

Noller, G. E., Frampton, C. M., Yazar, K. B. (2017). Ibogaine treatment outcomes for opioid dependence from a twelve-month follow-up observational study. *American Journal of Drug and Alcohol Abuse*, 44(1), 37-46.

Pagni, B. A., Hill, E., Walsh, M. J., Delaney, S., Ogbeama, D., Monahan, L., Braden, B. B. (2023). Distinct and shared therapeutic neural mechanisms of mindfulness-based and social support stress reduction groups in adults with autism spectrum disorder. *Journal of Psychiatry and Neuroscience*, 48(2), 102-114.

Purwaningsih, I., Maksum, I. P., Sumiarsa, D., Sriwidodo, S. (2023). A review of Fibraurea tinctoria and its component, berberine, as an antidiabetic and antioxidant. *Molecules*, 28(3), 1294.

Rasouli, H., Yarani, R., Pociot, F., Popovic-Djordjevic, J. (2020). Anti-diabetic potential of plant alkaloids: Revisiting current findings and future perspectives. *Pharmacological Research*, 155, 104723.

Roy, A. (2017). A review on the alkaloids an important therapeutic compound from plants. *International Journal of Plant Biotechnology*, 3(2), 1-9.

Saengow, U. Aramrattana, A., Chaichan, W., Wongrith, P., La-up, A., (2022). Association between kratom (Mitragyna speciosa) use and metabolic syndrome. *Heliyon*, 8(5), e09468.

Sawant, L., Singh, V. K., Dethe, S., Bhaskar, A., Balachandran, J., Mundkinajeddu, D., Agarwal, A. (2015). Aldose reductase and protein tyrosine phosphatase 1B inhibitory active compounds from Syzygium cumini seeds. *Pharmaceutical Biology*, 53(8), 1176-1182.

Tong, A., Wu, W., Chen, Z., Wen, J., Jia, R., Liu, B., Zhao, C. (2023). Modulation of gut microbiota and lipid metabolism in rats fed high-fat diets by Ganoderma lucidum triterpenoids. *Current Research in Food Science*, 6, 100427.

Tsuchiya, Y., Yoshimoto, J., Kobayashi, H., Ishii, S., Kishi, M. (2023). Yellow Pea Pasta Enhances the Saltiness and Suppression of Postprandial Blood Glucose Elevation. *Nutrients*, 15(2), 283.

Verma, M., Paneri, S., Badi, P., Raman, P. G. (2006). Effect of increasing duration of diabetes mellitus type 2 on glycated hemoglobin and insulin sensitivity. *Indian Journal of Clinical Biochemistry*, 21(1), 142-146.

Wu, H., Norton, V., Cui, K., Zhu, B., Bhattacharjee, S., Lu, Y. W., Wang, B., Shan, D., Wong, S., Dong, Y., Chan, S. L., Cowan, D., Xu, J., Bielenberg, D. R., Zhou, C., Chen, H. (2022). Diabetes and its cardiovascular complications: comprehensive network and systematic analyses. *Frontiers in Cardiovascular Medicine*, 9, 841928.

Yang, J. J., Zhang, X., Dai, J. F., Ma, Y. G., Jiang, J. G. (2023). Effect of fermentation modification on the physicochemical characteristics and anti-aging related activities of Polygonatum kingianum polysaccharides. *International Journal of Biological Macromolecules*, 235, 123661.

Zhao, X., Deng, L., Ren, L., Yang, H., Wang, B., Zhu, X., Zhang, X., Guo, C., Zhang, Y., Liu, Y. (2023). VPAC2 receptor mediates VIP-potentiated insulin secretion via ion channels in rat pancreatic β cells. *Experimental Cell Research*, 423, 113471.

Zhou, J., Chan, L., Zhou, S. (2012). Trigonelline: A Plant Alkaloid with Therapeutic Potential for Diabetes and Central Nervous System Disease. *Current Medicinal Chemistry*, 19(21), 3523-3531.

Ziff, S., Stern, B., Lewis, G., (2022). Analysis of psilocybin-assisted therapy in medicine: a narrative review. *Cureus*, 14(2), e21944.

Chapter 9

Phenolic Compounds in the Management of Diabetes Mellitus

Nisham Rani[1]
Jyoti[1]
Meena Devi[1]
Ritu Kataria[1,*]
Sangya Dubey[2]
Chaitanay Vinayak Narayan[2]
Janhavi Singh[2]
Sarika Chaudhary[3]
and Snigdha Bhardwaj[2]

[1]G. V. M. College of Pharmacy, Sonepat, Haryana, India
[2]I. T. S. College of Pharmacy, Muradnagar, Ghaziabad, Uttar Pradesh, India
[3]One Beat College of Medical Sciences, Sant Garh Nagar, Bhira, Uttar Pradesh, India

Abstract

Type 2 diabetes mellitus (T2DM) is a complex metabolic condition influenced by several contributing factors, including genetics, epigenetics, the environment, and lifestyle choices, including nutrition. T2DM, along with other chronic metabolic conditions, is expected to benefit significantly from the utilization of polyphenolic compounds. Polyphenols have the potential to offer anti-diabetic benefits due to their ability to regulate oxidative stress, inflammation, and other

* Corresponding Author's Email: drritukataria17@gmail.com.

In: Naturally Occurring Chemicals …
Editors: A. Singh Grewal, G. Deswal, A. Kumar Dhingra et al.
ISBN: 979-8-89113-491-1

pathways that protect β-cells and enhance insulin sensitivity. One major contributor to decreased β-cell function and disrupted insulin signaling is intracellular reactive oxygen species (ROS)-induced stress. This stress is primarily activated by hyperlipidemia and chronic hyperglycemia. ROS can disrupt intracellular signaling networks and alter the expression of genes involved in insulin production and signaling. Recent investigations have shown that diets rich in polyphenols can modify the expression of genes related to insulin release pathways, insulin signaling, and liver gluconeogenesis. This chapter explores the modifying effects of various polyphenols and phenolic compounds on genes associated with cellular signaling pathways in the context of T2DM pathogenesis. These effects are examined through studies conducted in humans, animals, and cell models, both *in vitro* and *in vivo*.

Keywords: type 2 diabetes, pancreatic β-cell function, insulin resistance, insulin signaling

Abbreviations

AMPK	AMP-activated protein kinase
DM	Diabetes mellitus
PTPI	Protein tyrosine phosphatase inhibitors
ROS	Reactive oxygen species
T1DM	Type 1 diabetes mellitus
T2DM	Type 2 diabetes mellitus.

Introduction

Diabetes mellitus (DM) is one of the most chronic and severe diseases due to its disruption of glucose homeostasis. It can lead to either insulin resistance or insufficient glucose utilization, resulting in conditions such as hypertension, chronic hyperglycemia, and hyperlipidemia. These factors are hallmark characteristics of type 2 diabetes mellitus (T2DM) (Holman et al., 2015). T2DM is a leading cause of adult mortality globally and significantly impacts the quality of life (Saeedi et al., 2020). Furthermore, diabetes mellitus is associated with an increased risk of various malignancies, including gastrointestinal and women-specific cancers (Tomic et al., 2022).

Individuals with diabetes often experience decreased bone density and strength, which can increase their lifetime risk of fractures, even if they have normal bone mass. In T2DM, this heightened fracture risk is particularly noteworthy. While T2DM typically develops in adulthood, type 1 diabetes mellitus (T1DM) more commonly presents in childhood and early life, often before individuals reach their peak bone mass. T1DM is also associated with an increased risk of fractures that can persist throughout a person's life (Hofbauer et al., 2022). Chronic tissue inflammation is a significant aspect of obesity and T2DM and is observed in insulin-target tissues like adipose tissue, liver, skeletal muscle, and pancreatic islets. This concept has led to the term "immune metabolism," which recognizes the intricate interaction between immune processes and metabolic abnormalities (Rohm et al., 2022). Polyphenols are the most common type of phytochemicals found in plant-based foods. Diets rich in polyphenols have been associated with numerous health benefits (Tsao et al., 2010; Alara et al., 2021). These compounds have been studied for their potential to mitigate oxidative stress, inflammation, and other processes that are relevant to the management and prevention of diabetes and its complications. Incorporating a diet rich in polyphenol-containing foods may be a valuable component of a diabetes management plan.

Phenolic Compounds

Phenolic or phenol carboxylic acids constitute a significant subgroup of plant phenolic compounds, which themselves belong to the broader category of phytochemicals known as polyphenols. These compounds are widely distributed across various plant-based foods, with their highest concentrations typically found in seeds, fruit and vegetable skins, as well as leaves (Perrenira et al., 2009). Phenolic compounds serve crucial roles in plants as secondary metabolites and are produced as part of the plant's defense mechanisms (Albuquerque et al., 2021). These compounds are involved in diverse biological functions, including protection against pathogens, UV radiation, and oxidative stress. In the context of the human diet, phenolic compounds have garnered attention due to their potential health benefits, primarily stemming from their antioxidant and anti-inflammatory properties, among other potentially beneficial bioactive effects.

Classification and Chemistry of Polyphenols

Phenolic acids are divided into two main groups: hydroxybenzoic and hydroxycinnamic acids. Hydroxybenzoic acids are relatively rare in the human diet, and it's believed that they have little impact on health. These acids are derivatives of benzoic acid and cinnamic acid, with carbon backbones of C1-C6 and C3-C6, respectively. While some phenolic acids are naturally present in fruits and vegetables, they can also be found in bound forms within the hull, bran, and seeds of various plants (Hussain et al., 2004). Flavonoids are compounds formed by linking two benzene rings with a chain of three carbon atoms from a neighboring pyran ring. Flavonoids typically have a basic structure of C6-C3-C6, containing two phenolic units (C6). Flavonoids are further classified into subclasses such as flavonols, flavones, flavanones, and anthocyanidins based on their hydroxylation patterns. In isoflavones, the B ring is connected to the C ring at its C3 position (Sachez et al., 2001). Flavonoids are the most common type of polyphenols in the human diet. They consist of two phenolic rings joined by a heterocyclic ring with oxygen. In a plant-based human diet, you can find various types of flavonoids, including flavonols, flavanones, flavones, flavan-3-ols, anthocyanidins, and isoflavones. Many of these flavonoids contain a 3-hydroxypyran-4-one group on the C ring, especially in foods like tea, fruits, and vegetables (Xiao et al., 2017). Dietary flavonoids are primarily found in nature as glycosides, including galactosides, glucosides, rhamnosides, rutinosides, and arabinosides. Among these, flavonol O-glycosides and flavone O/C-glycosides are the more commonly occurring plant flavonoid glycosides (Xiao et al., 2020). Polyphenols, a broad and diverse class of phytochemicals with phenol rings, can be further categorized into flavonoids, phenolic acids, stilbenes, and lignans (Walther et al., 2019).

Polyphenols as Anti-Diabetic Agents

T2DM is a complex condition characterized by several factors, including insulin resistance, dysfunction of β-cells, impaired insulin signaling, abnormal glucose and fatty acid metabolism, and increased oxidative stress (Santguida et al., 2008). There are various techniques that can be employed to improve glycemic control in individuals with T2DM. One approach is to protect pancreatic β-cells from glucose-induced toxicity and oxidative stress

(Heinviwa et al., 2010). Flavonoids, which are commonly found in vegetables and fruits, have been suggested as key phenolic compounds that may help reduce the risk of diabetes (Andrade et al., 2011; Shah et al., 2012). Some specific phenolic substances, such as procyanidin from grape seeds and naringin from orange peel, have been studied for their potential to inhibit the action of DPP-IV, an enzyme involved in glucose regulation (Blay et al., 2012; Chauhan et al., 2012). Dietary polyphenols play a role in managing diabetes by enhancing insulin secretion in the pancreas, reducing oxidative stress, improving glucose uptake in muscle cells, and regulating carbohydrate metabolism (Dias et al., 2022). Curcumin, a type of polyphenol derived from turmeric (Curcuma longa), which belongs to the curcuminoid class of compounds, has a long history of medicinal use (Abdollahi et al., 2018). Phenolic acids can be classified into hydroxybenzoic acids with seven carbon atoms and hydroxycinnamic acids with nine carbon atoms. Some examples of phenolic acids include caffeic acid, ellagic acid, gallic acid, and chlorogenic acids. These compounds have various roles in managing diabetes mellitus, as discussed in Table 1 (Kumar et al., 2019).

Table 1. Mechanism of action of phenolic compounds

Phenolic compounds	Sources	MOA	References
Chlorogenic acid	Tea, coffee	↑se glucose uptake, inhibit α-glucosidase, activate AMPK	Ong et, al., 2013
Ellagic acid	Pomegranate, grapes (*Vitis vinifera*)	↑se signalling by insulin, ↑es glucose converter	Amim et al., 2017
Caffeic acid	Tea, coffee	↓se glucose-6-phosphatase, ↑se glucokinase activity	Jung et al., 2006
Gallic acid	Pomegranate, oak bark	↑se glucose absorption ↑ Phosphatidylinositol-3 kinase, Akt/protein kinase B	Haung et al., 2016
Quercetin	Tea, fennel	↑se glycogen synthase	Eid et al., 2015
Genistein	Soy food	↑se cAMP signalling ↑ PKA activation	Babu et al., 2012
Kaempferol	Spinach, dill	↓se apoptosis, ↓escaspase-3	Zhang et al., 2011
Tangeretin	Peel	Activate AMPK pathway	Kim et al., 2012
Rutin	Lemons, grapes	α-Glucosidase and α-amylase inhibition, ↑se hexokinase, ↓se G6Pase, PEPCK, glycogen phosphorylase	Ghorbani et al., 2017
Resveratrol	Grapes, barriers	AMPK activation, SIRT1, inhibition of PTP1B	Ohenihi et al., 2016

Health Benefits and Pharmacological Effects of Spices Derived Phenolic Compounds

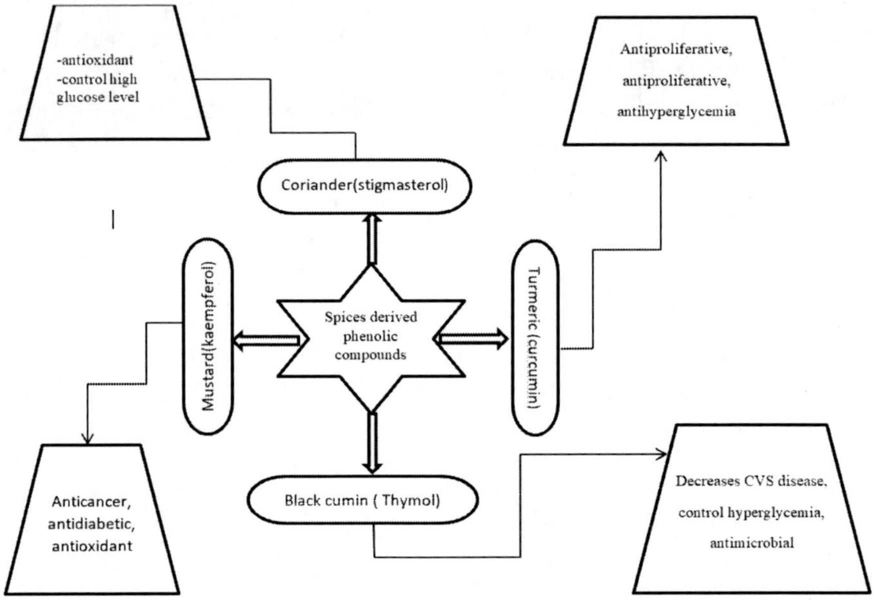

Figure 1. Pharmacological properties of polyphenols.

Table 2. Recent advancement of polyphenols in diabetes management

Compounds	Site of action (mechanism)	Reference
Plant derived phenolic compounds	Activation of the AMPK pathway, inhibition of glucosidase and amylase, and absorption of glucose and Enhanced insulin sensitivity	Ananta et al., 2022
Polyphenols	protecting pancreatic β-cells, altering the digestion of glucose, absorption, and uptake, and stimulating the pathways of fat and glucose metabolism	Chen et al., 2022
Polyphenols	deregulate pancreatic -cells' ability to produce insulin, increasing the risk of hyperglycemia	Clement et al., 2022

Amylase absorption can indeed be inhibited by certain chemical components of plants known as phenolic compounds. This inhibition can be particularly relevant in managing conditions related to carbohydrate absorption, such as diabetes (Mejia et al., 2013). Many spices contain polyphenols with potential health benefits and various pharmacological activities. There are many spices derived from polyphenols like curcumin (turmeric), coriander, mustard and thymol (black cumin) which have many pharmacological activities and health benefits as shown in Figure 1.

Polyphenols exhibit their actions on various sites, with recent advancements focusing on their ability to protect pancreatic β-cells, activate the AMPK pathway, and modulate insulin production, as indicated in Table 2.

Conclusion

Over the past few decades, there has been a growing consumer interest in natural products due to increased awareness. Polyphenols are regarded as a valuable resource within the realm of food, as they contain a wide array of compounds with highly diverse compositions. These compounds are known for their numerous bioactive properties, and their biological effects and potential applications have been extensively researched. Polyphenols are secondary metabolites of plant origin, and they have gained significant attention due to their widespread presence in plant-based diets. Compelling research data has also established a connection between the consumption of polyphenols and their potential benefits in relation to conditions like diabetes.

References

Abdel-Moneim, A., Yousef, A. I., Abd El-Twab, S. M., Abdel Reheim, E. S., Ashour, M. B. (2017). Gallic acid and p-coumaric acid attenuate type 2 diabetes-induced neurodegeneration in rats. *Metabolic Brain Disease*, 32, 1279-1286.

Alara, O. R., Abdurahman, N. H., Ukaegbu, C. I. (2021). Extraction of phenolic compounds: a review. *Current Research in Food Science*, 4, 200-214.

Albuquerque, B. R., Heleno, S. A., Oliveira, M. B. P., Barros, L., Ferreira, I. C. (2021). Phenolic compounds: Current industrial applications, limitations and future challenges. *Food & Function*, 12(1), 14-29.

Amin, M. M., Arbid, M. S. (2017). Estimation of ellagic acid and/or repaglinide effects on insulin signaling, oxidative stress, and inflammatory mediators of liver, pancreas, adipose tissue, and brain in insulin resistant/type 2 diabetic rats. *Applied Physiology, Nutrition, and Metabolism*, 42(2), 181-192.

Babu, P. V. A., Si, H., Fu, Z., Zhen, W., Liu, D. (2012). Genistein prevents hyperglycemia-induced monocyte adhesion to human aortic endothelial cells through preservation of the cAMP signaling pathway and ameliorates vascular inflammation in obese diabetic mice. *Journal of Nutrition*, 142(4), 724-730.

Chen, L., Pu, Y., Xu, Y., He, X., Cao, J., Ma, Y., Jiang, W. (2022). Anti-diabetic and anti-obesity: Efficacy evaluation and exploitation of polyphenols in fruits and vegetables. *Food Research International*, 111202.

Dias, M., Romaní-Pérez, M., Romaní, A., De La Cruz, A., Pastrana, L., Fuciños, P., Amado, I. R. (2022). Recent technological advances in phenolic compounds recovery and applications: source of nutraceuticals for the management of diabetes. *Applied Sciences*, 12(18), 9271.

Ditano-Vázquez, P., Torres-Peña, J. D., Galeano-Valle, F., Pérez-Caballero, A. I., Demelo-Rodríguez, P., Lopez-Miranda, J., Katsiki, N., Delgado-Lista, J., Alvarez-Sala-Walther, L. A. (2019). The fluid aspect of the Mediterranean diet in the prevention and management of cardiovascular disease and diabetes: the role of polyphenol content in moderate consumption of wine and olive oil. *Nutrients*, 11(11), 2833.

Eid, H., Nachar, A., Thong, F., Sweeney, G., Haddad, P. (2015). The molecular basis of the antidiabetic action of quercetin in cultured skeletal muscle cells and hepatocytes. *Pharmacognosy Magazine*, 11(41), 74.

Fan, J., Johnson, M. H., Lila, M. A., Yousef, G., De Mejia, E. G. (2013). Berry and citrus phenolic compounds inhibit dipeptidyl peptidase IV: Implications in diabetes management. *Evidence-Based Complementary and Alternative Medicine*, 2013, 479505.

Ghorbani, A. (2017). Mechanisms of antidiabetic effects of flavonoid rutin. *Biomedicine & Pharmacotherapy*, 96, 305-312.

Gonzalez-Abuin, N., Martinez-Micaelo, N., Blay, M., Pujadas, G., Garcia-Vallve, S., Pinent, M., Ardevol, A. (2012). Grape seed-derived procyanidins decrease dipeptidyl-peptidase 4 activity and expression. *Journal of Agricultural and Food Chemistry*, 60(36), 9055-9061.

Grace, M. H., Ribnicky, D. M., Kuhn, P., Poulev, A., Logendra, S., Yousef, G. G., Raskin, I., Lila, M. A. (2009). Hypoglycemic activity of a novel anthocyanin-rich formulation from lowbush blueberry, Vaccinium angustifolium Aiton. *Phytomedicine*, 16(5), 406-415.

Hanhineva, K., Törrönen, R., Bondia-Pons, I., Pekkinen, J., Kolehmainen, M., Mykkänen, H., Poutanen, K. (2010). Impact of dietary polyphenols on carbohydrate metabolism. *International Journal of Molecular Sciences*, 11(4), 1365-1402.

Hofbauer, L. C., Busse, B., Eastell, R., Ferrari, S., Frost, M., Müller, R., Burden, A. M., Rivadeneira, F., Napoli, N., Rauner, M. (2022). Bone fragility in diabetes: novel concepts and clinical implications. *Lancet Diabetes & Endocrinology*, 10(3), 207-220.

Holman, N., Young, B., Gadsby, R. (2015). Current prevalence of type 1 and type 2 diabetes in adults and children in the UK. *Diabetic Medicine*, 9(32), 1119-1120.

Hussain, T., Gupta, S., Adhami, V., Mukhtar, H. (2005). Green tea constituent epigallocatechin-3-gallate selectively inhibits COX-2 without affecting COX-1 expression in human prostate carcinoma cells. *International Journal of Cancer*, 113(4), 660-669.

Jadav, P., Bahekar, R., Shah, S. R., Patel, D., Joharapurkar, A., Kshirsagar, S., Jain, M., Shaikh, M., Sairam, K. V. (2012). Long-acting peptidomimetics based DPP-IV inhibitors. *Bioorganic & Medicinal Chemistry Letters*, 22(10), 3516-3521.

Jung, U. J., Lee, M. K., Park, Y. B., Jeon, S. M., Choi, M. S. (2006). Antihyperglycemic and antioxidant properties of caffeic acid in db/db mice. *Journal of Pharmacology and Experimental Therapeutics*, 318(2), 476-483.

Kim, M. S., Hur, H. J., Kwon, D. Y., Hwang, J. T. (2012). Tangeretin stimulates glucose uptake via regulation of AMPK signaling pathways in C2C12 myotubes and improves glucose tolerance in high-fat diet-induced obese mice. *Molecular and Cellular Endocrinology*, 358(1), 127-134.

Kumar, N., Goel, N. (2019). Phenolic acids: Natural versatile molecules with promising therapeutic applications. *Biotechnology Reports*, 24, e00370.

Ong, K. W., Hsu, A., Tan, B. K. H. (2013). Anti-diabetic and anti-lipidemic effects of chlorogenic acid are mediated by ampk activation. *Biochemical pharmacology*, 85(9), 1341-1351.

Oyenihi, O. R., Oyenihi, A. B., Adeyanju, A. A., Oguntibeju, O. O. (2016). Antidiabetic effects of resveratrol: the way forward in its clinical utility. *Journal of Diabetes Research*, 2016, 9737483.

Parmar, H. S., Jain, P., Chauhan, D. S., Bhinchar, M. K., Munjal, V., Yusuf, M., Choube, K., Tawani, A., Tiwari, V., Manivannan, E., Kumar, A. (2012). DPP-IV inhibitory potential of naringin: an in silico, in vitro and in vivo study. *Diabetes Research and Clinical Practice*, 97(1), 105-111.

Pereira, D. M., Valentão, P., Pereira, J. A., Andrade, P. B. (2009). Phenolics: From chemistry to biology. *Molecules*, 14(6), 2202-2211.

Rohm, T. V., Meier, D. T., Olefsky, J. M., Donath, M. Y. (2022). Inflammation in obesity, diabetes, and related disorders. *Immunity*, 55(1), 31-55.

Saeedi, P., Salpea, P., Karuranga, S., Petersohn, I., Malanda, B., Gregg, E. W., Unwin, N., Wild, S. H., Williams, R. (2020). Mortality attributable to diabetes in 20–79 years old adults, 2019 estimates: results from the International Diabetes Federation Diabetes Atlas. *Diabetes Research and Clinical Practice*, 162, 108086.

Salehi, B., Ata, A., V Anil Kumar, N., Sharopov, F., Ramírez-Alarcón, K., Ruiz-Ortega, A., Abdulmajid Ayatollahi, S., Tsouh Fokou, P. V., Kobarfard, F., Amiruddin Zakaria, Z., Iriti, M., Taheri, Y., Martorell, M., Sureda, A., Setzer, W. N., Durazzo, A., Lucarini, M., Santini, A., Capasso, R., Ostrander, E. A., Atta-ur-Rahman, Choudhary, M. I., Cho, W. C, Sharifi-Rad, J. (2019). Antidiabetic potential of medicinal plants and their active components. *Biomolecules*, 9(10), 551.

Schewe, T., Sadik, C., Klotz, L. O., Yoshimoto, T., Kühn, H., Sies, H. (2001). Polyphenols of cocoa: inhibition of mammalian 15-lipoxygenase. *Biological Chemistry*, 382(12), 1687-1696.

Semighini, E. P., Resende, J. A., de Andrade, P., Morais, P. A., Carvalho, I., Taft, C. A., Silva, C. H. (2011). Using computer-aided drug design and medicinal chemistry strategies in the fight against diabetes. *Journal of Biomolecular Structure and Dynamics*, 28(5), 787-796.

Seyyedebrahimi, S., Khodabandehloo, H., Nasli Esfahani, E., Meshkani, R. (2018). The effects of resveratrol on markers of oxidative stress in patients with type 2 diabetes:

a randomized, double-blind, placebo-controlled clinical trial. *Acta Diabetologica*, 55, 341-353.

Sun, C., Zhao, C., Guven, E. C., Paoli, P., Simal-Gandara, J., Ramkumar, K. M., Wang, S., Buleu, F., Pah, A., Turi, V., Damian, G., Xiao, J. (2020). Dietary polyphenols as antidiabetic agents: Advances and opportunities. *Food Frontiers*, 1(1), 18-44.

Tomic, D., Shaw, J. E., Magliano, D. J. (2022). The burden and risks of emerging complications of diabetes mellitus. *Nature Reviews Endocrinology*, 18(9), 525-539.

Türkan, F., Taslimi, P., Saltan, F. Z. (2019). Tannic acid as a natural antioxidant compound: Discovery of a potent metabolic enzyme inhibitor for a new therapeutic approach in diabetes and Alzheimer's disease. *Journal of Biochemical and Molecular Toxicology*, 33(8), e22340.

Zhang, H., Tsao, R. (2016). Dietary polyphenols, oxidative stress and antioxidant and anti-inflammatory effects. *Current Opinion in Food Science*, 8, 33-42.

Zhang, Y., Liu, D. (2011). Flavonol kaempferol improves chronic hyperglycemia-impaired pancreatic beta-cell viability and insulin secretory function. *European Journal of Pharmacology*, 670(1), 325-332.

Chapter 10

Terpenoids in the Management of Diabetes Mellitus

Anjali Sharma[1,*]
Shabnam Faridi[2]
Devkant Sharma[3]
and Deepshi Arora[1]

[1]Guru Gobind Singh College of Pharmacy, Yamuna Nagar, Haryana, India
[2]Guru Nanak Institute of Technology, Ambala, Mullana, Haryana, India
[3]Ch. Devi Lal College of Pharmacy, Jagadhri, Haryana, India

Abstract

Diabetes mellitus is a chronic metabolic condition that ranks among the leading global causes of death. Currently affecting approximately 285 million individuals, this number is expected to double over the next two decades. By 2030, the World Health Organization predicts that diabetes will affect 300 million people worldwide, making up 7.8% of the global population. In India, diabetes is a prevalent and growing issue, impacting 10% of rural populations and a striking 20% of urban populations. This condition arises from inadequate insulin secretion or action, often due to abnormalities within the metabolic, genetic, and hemodynamic systems. Terpenoids, a class of natural compounds, have gained attention for their potential anti-diabetic properties. Some of these terpenoids are currently under evaluation in various pre-clinical and clinical phases as potential antidiabetic drugs. They work by influencing enzymes that play critical roles in normalizing plasma glucose and insulin levels, as well as regulating glucose metabolism.

* Corresponding Author's Email: sharma.sharmaa.anjali@gmail.com.

In: Naturally Occurring Chemicals …
Editors: A. Singh Grewal, G. Deswal, A. Kumar Dhingra et al.
ISBN: 979-8-89113-491-1

Additionally, triterpenes, a subset of terpenoids, show promise as therapeutic agents for managing complications associated with diabetes, such as diabetic retinopathy, neuropathy, nephropathy, and impaired wound healing. They achieve this by targeting various pathways linked to diabetes and its consequences. This chapter delves into the subject of terpenoids and their applications in the treatment of diabetes mellitus, shedding light on their potential as valuable tools in managing this widespread and growing health challenge.

Keywords: diabetes mellitus, terpenoids, insulin, retinopathy, clinical phases, anti-diabetic agents

Abbreviations

AMP	Adenosine monophosphate
AMPK	AMP-activated Protein Kinase
FXR	Farnesoid X receptor
GLUT 4	Glucose transporter 4
NLRP3	Nucleotide-binding domain, leucine-rich-containing family, pyrin domain–containing-3
Nrf2	Nuclear factor erythroid 2-related factor 2
P 38 MAPK	p38 mitogen-activated protein kinases
PPAR-α	peroxisomes proliferator-activated receptor alpha
SREBP	Sterol regulatory element binding protein
STZ	streptozotocin.

Introduction

Diabetes mellitus is one of the most prevalent metabolic disorders, currently affecting approximately 2.8% of the global population, with a projected increase to 5.4% by 2025 (Rao et al., 2010). By 2030, it is estimated that up to 4.4% of the world's population will have diabetes (Preethi et al., 2013). While several antidiabetic medications are available to help manage and control diabetes, they come with limitations such as pharmacokinetic characteristics, secondary failure rates, and potential side effects like abdominal pain, weight gain, and low blood sugar (Donath and Ehses, 2006). Due to these drawbacks associated with oral hypoglycemic drugs, there is growing interest in herbal therapies for diabetes management. Traditional herbal remedies for diabetes have proven to be effective because they are derived from plants (Khan et al., 2012; Prabhakar and Doble, 2011). Throughout history, herbs have been a reliable source of medicine, and they continue to play a vital role in modern medicine. Medicinal plants have been extensively studied for their potential in treating diabetes mellitus, given their rich content of compounds such as flavonoids, terpenoids, coumarins, phenolic compounds, and others, many of which exhibit promising anti-diabetic properties. These substances work by lowering blood sugar levels and improving insulin sensitivity. Ethnobotanical information suggests that approximately 800 plants have potential antidiabetic properties, but only a limited number of them have received scientific validation. Therefore, it is essential to assess the therapeutic potential of medicinal plants through experimental research to support their effectiveness (Ghorbani, 2013). Medicinal plants are favored because they are effective, non-toxic, have minimal to no side effects, and are considered excellent candidates for oral therapy. The World Health Organization (WHO) has recommended the evaluation of traditional plant treatments for diabetes due to these favorable qualities (Halberstein, 2005). Plants with antidiabetic properties typically contain a variety of bioactive compounds, including glycosides, alkaloids, terpenes, flavonoids, and carotenoids (Malviya et al., 2010). The management of diabetes mellitus increasingly relies on traditional remedies derived from plant sources (Khan et al., 2012).

Overview of Terpenoids

Triterpenoids are a significant class of secondary metabolites found in a wide range of plant tissues, including leaves, stem bark, fruits, and roots. Nature boasts around 20,000 different triterpenoids (Dzubak et al., 2006). Some well-known plant sources of terpenoids include citrus fruits (like lemon, orange, and mandarin), tea, thyme, cannabis, Spanish sage, and thyme (Cox et al., 2019). Triterpenoids come in various forms, such as free compounds, triterpene glycosides, saponins, or their esters. Structurally, they can be categorized into tetracyclic and pentacyclic triterpenoids. These can be further divided into subgroups like friedelanes, lupanes, leananes, ursanes, cycloartanes, lanostanes, cucurbitanes (tetracyclic triterpenoids), and others (Bis et al., 2011). Triterpenes hold immense healing potential, although this potential is still not fully recognized. Numerous in vitro and in vivo studies have unveiled their multifaceted properties, including anti-inflammatory effects (Yasukawa et al., 1996). Terpenoids have also emerged as potential natural agents for diabetes management. Several studies indicate that various terpenoids possess anti-diabetic properties. They can stimulate insulin secretion, reduce insulin resistance, and enhance glucose uptake (Ramachandran and Prasad, 2008). One such terpenoid is β-caryophyllene, which is present in various plants like black pepper, cloves, and hops (Sudhahar et al., 2007). Studies have demonstrated that β-caryophyllene can enhance glucose tolerance and decrease insulin resistance by activating the peroxisome proliferator-activated receptor alpha (PPAR-α). Another terpenoid with anti-diabetic effects is oleanolic acid, found in olive leaves and other plants. Oleanolic acid has been shown to lower blood glucose levels and improve insulin sensitivity by activating the AMPK pathway (Alqahtani et al., 2013). Additionally, several triterpenoids found in medicinal plants exhibit anti-diabetic effects. For example, asiatic acid, a triterpenoid from *Centella asiatica*, enhances glucose uptake in muscle cells and increases insulin sensitivity by activating the AMPK pathway. Similarly, maslinic acid, a pentacyclic triterpenoid found in olives and other plants, improves insulin sensitivity and reduces inflammation in diabetic mice (Laszczyk, 2009). Although the potential benefits of terpenoids in diabetes management are promising, more research is needed to determine the optimal dosages and safety profiles of these compounds, as well as their potential interactions with other medications. Consulting a healthcare professional before using terpenoids or any other natural remedies for diabetes management is essential. Most bioactive terpenes are extracted from medicinal plants, with larger molecular weight terpenes like triterpenes primarily found in balsam and resin, while monoterpenes and sesquiterpenes are prevalent in the essential oils of medicinal plants.

Molecular Target of Terpenoids

Terpenoids indeed form a diverse group of natural compounds with a wide range of therapeutic properties, including their potential anti-diabetic effects. Multiple molecular targets have been identified for terpenoids concerning diabetes mellitus (Gowri et al., 2007).

Peroxisome Proliferator-Activated Receptors (PPARs)

PPARs are nuclear receptors that play a pivotal role in glucose and lipid metabolism. Terpenoids such as carnosic acid, rosiglitazone, and thymoquinone have demonstrated the ability to activate PPARs, thereby enhancing insulin sensitivity.

AMP-Activated Protein Kinase (AMPK)

AMPK functions as a cellular energy sensor, regulating glucose uptake and metabolism. Terpenoids like ginsenoside Rg3, oleanolic acid, and ursolic acid have been observed to activate AMPK, leading to improved glucose uptake in skeletal muscle cells (Uddin et al., 2012).

Glucose Transporter 4 (GLUT4)

GLUT4 serves as a crucial mediator of glucose uptake in muscle and fat cells. Terpenoids such as betulin, lupeol, and maslinic acid have been found to enhance GLUT4 translocation, resulting in improved glucose uptake in these cells (De Sales et al., 2012).

α-Glucosidase

α-Glucosidase is an enzyme involved in carbohydrate digestion. Inhibiting α-glucosidase can reduce the absorption of glucose from the gut, leading to improved blood glucose control. Terpenoids such as asiatic acid, oleanolic acid, and ursolic acid have demonstrated the ability to inhibit α-glucosidase activity (Lai et al., 2012).

Inflammation

Chronic low-grade inflammation plays a role in the development of insulin resistance and type 2 diabetes. Terpenoids such as curcumin, resveratrol, and quercetin have been shown to possess anti-inflammatory effects by inhibiting pro-inflammatory cytokines and signaling pathways (Hou et al., 2009).

Anti-Diabetic Activity of Terpenoids

Insulin Mimetic Action

Insulin, a crucial hormone responsible for regulating glucose homeostasis, plays a pivotal role in maintaining balanced blood sugar levels. Its deficiency or resistance is associated with various metabolic disorders, notably type 2 diabetes. Several terpenoids have been identified for their insulin-mimetic activity, meaning they can replicate the effects of insulin within the body (Jeppesen et al., 2002, 2003). Ursolic acid has demonstrated the capacity to enhance insulin sensitivity and promote glucose uptake by activating the PI3K/Akt pathway, a crucial mediator in insulin signaling within muscle cells. Oleanolic acid improves insulin sensitivity through the activation of the PI3K/Akt pathway. Additionally, it engages the AMPK pathway, which plays a vital role in energy metabolism. Betulin stimulates glucose uptake and utilization by activating the PI3K/Akt pathway and facilitating the translocation of GLUT4 to the cell membrane. Ginsenosides have been found to enhance glucose uptake and utilization by activating the AMPK pathway and promoting increased translocation of GLUT4. Maslinic acid contributes to improved insulin sensitivity and glucose uptake by activating the PI3K/Akt pathway while concurrently reducing inflammation within adipose tissue (Jeppesen et al., 2000).

Stimulation of Insulin Secretion

Terpenoids, a diverse group of natural compounds, have demonstrated various therapeutic properties, including the ability to stimulate insulin secretion. Insulin, a hormone produced by the pancreas, plays a pivotal role in regulating blood glucose levels (Bansal et al., 2008). Several terpenoids have been identified for their capacity to enhance insulin secretion from pancreatic beta cells. Here are some examples: Pinene has been shown to stimulate insulin secretion and improve glucose tolerance in animal models of diabetes (Gilon et al., 2001). Pulegone stimulates insulin secretion by activating the cAMP/PKA pathway in pancreatic beta cells (Lee et al., 2006; Hsu et al., 2006). Citronellal stimulates insulin secretion by activating the intracellular calcium signaling pathway in beta cells. Caryophyllene oxide stimulates insulin secretion by activating the PI3K/Akt pathway in beta cells. Squalene stimulates insulin secretion by modulating the activity of ATP-sensitive potassium channels in beta cells (Lee et al., 2006; Hsu et al., 2006).

Blocking of Gluconeogenesis

Gluconeogenesis is a metabolic process in which the body synthesizes glucose from non-carbohydrate sources. In individuals with type 2 diabetes, there is often an increase in gluconeogenesis. Potential therapeutic approaches for diabetes treatment include the development of gluconeogenesis inhibitors (Kashiwagi, 1995). Corosolic acid has shown promise in reducing gluconeogenesis. In isolated hepatocytes and perfused rat liver, corosolic acid has been found to reduce gluconeogenesis at doses ranging from 20 to 100 M. This suggests that corosolic acid may have the potential as a therapeutic agent for managing diabetes (Yamada et al., 2008).

Increasing the Activity of AMP-Activated Protein Kinase

AMPK is a critical energy-sensing enzyme in the body that regulates glucose and lipid metabolism. Activation of AMPK has the potential to enhance glucose uptake and utilization, stimulate fatty acid oxidation, and reduce hepatic glucose production. This makes it an attractive target for the development of anti-diabetic agents. Several terpenoids have been identified as activators of AMPK, including ginsenosides, oleanolic acid, ursolic acid from *Ganoderma lucidum*, and maslinic acid (Ha et al., 2009). These terpenoids can activate AMPK in various cell types, such as skeletal muscle cells and adipocytes, resulting in improved glucose uptake and increased insulin sensitivity. Ginsenosides have been demonstrated to enhance glucose uptake and utilization by activating AMPK in skeletal muscle cells and adipocytes. Similarly, oleanolic acid has been found to activate AMPK, leading to improved insulin sensitivity in both skeletal muscle cells and adipocytes (Winder et al., 1999).

Promoting Glycogen Synthesis and Inhibiting Glycogen Degradation

Glycogen synthesis and degradation are crucial processes in maintaining glucose homeostasis in the body. Several terpenoids have been identified for their potential to influence these processes, offering promise as candidates for the development of anti-diabetic agents. Astragaloside IV, a triterpenoid saponin, found in *Astragalus membranaceus*, has been shown to promote glycogen synthesis by activating the PI3K/Akt in liver cells (Luo et al., 2008). Ganoderic acid A inhibits glycogen degradation by reducing the activity of glycogen phosphorylase, an enzyme involved in glycogen breakdown (Gong et al., 1991). Berberine promotes glycogen synthesis by activating the AMPK pathway and inhibits glycogen degradation by reducing the activity of glycogen phosphorylase (Praly et al., 2010). β-Caryophyllene oxide promotes glycogen synthesis by activating the PI3K/Akt pathway and inhibits glycogen degradation by reducing the activity of glycogen phosphorylase (Guan et al., 2009). Curcumin promotes glycogen synthesis by activating the AMPK pathway and inhibits glycogen degradation by reducing the activity of glycogen phosphorylase (Yokozawa et al., 1985; Lee et al., 2014).

Reduction of Blood Glucose Level

In comparison to glibenclamide, the triterpene betulin, isolated from the root bark of the *Euclea undulata* plant, has shown significant effects in reducing blood sugar levels (Deutschlander et al., 2011). Betulin appears to be a promising natural compound for glycemic control. Additionally, blocking the transcription factor responsible for activating genes involved in the production of fatty acids, cholesterol, and triglycerides can lead to reduced cellular lipid levels, potentially improving insulin resistance (Tang et al., 2011). Moreover, in STZ-nicotinamide-induced diabetic mice, lower blood glucose levels, decreased α-amylase activity, and improved insulin sensitivity was observed, along with improvements in renal parameters, lipid profiles, and blood glucose levels (Arvindeker et al., 2014). These findings indicate that certain interventions or compounds may have multifaceted effects on various aspects of diabetes management.

Reduction of Oxidative Stress

Antioxidant drugs that can reduce oxidative damage have the potential to be used as treatments for diabetes. Safranal, a monoterpene found in saffron essential oil, has demonstrated a protective effect against oxidative damage in diabetic rats (Samarghandian et al., 2013). This suggests that safranal may have antioxidant properties that could help mitigate oxidative stress associated with diabetes. D-limonene, a monocyclic monoterpene primarily found in citrus fruit essential oils, has been shown to have a protective impact on the antioxidant defense system of streptozotocin (STZ)-induced diabetic rats (Murali et al., 2013). This indicates that d-limonene may support the body's natural antioxidant defenses, which can be compromised in diabetes.

Hypolipidemic Activity

Dyslipidemia, characterized by abnormal lipid levels in the bloodstream, is a condition associated with elevated levels of cholesterol and triglycerides. Several terpenoids have demonstrated potential in reducing serum cholesterol and triglyceride levels, making them candidates for natural anti-dyslipidemia agents. Limonene has been shown to reduce serum cholesterol and triglyceride levels by inhibiting hepatic lipogenesis (the production of lipids in the liver) and increasing fatty acid oxidation. This suggests that limonene may help regulate lipid metabolism (Gudr 2016). Citral has been found to decrease serum cholesterol and triglyceride levels by reducing hepatic lipogenesis and increasing bile acid synthesis. These actions contribute to improved lipid profile regulation (Gudr 2016). Guggulsterone reduces serum cholesterol and triglyceride levels by activating the farnesoid X receptor (FXR) and inhibiting the sterol regulatory element-binding protein (SREBP) pathway. FXR activation plays a role in cholesterol and bile acid homeostasis (Tan et al., 2008). Ursolic acid reduces serum cholesterol and triglyceride levels by inhibiting hepatic lipogenesis and promoting cholesterol efflux from macrophages. This compound may help prevent the accumulation of lipids in the liver and support the removal of cholesterol from cells (Bustanji et al., 2011). Betulinic acid reduces serum cholesterol and triglyceride levels by inhibiting hepatic lipogenesis and promoting cholesterol efflux from macrophages. This dual action can contribute to improved lipid regulation (Bustanji et al., 2011).

Inhibition of Aldose Reductase

Aldose reductase (AR) is the primary and most crucial enzyme in the polyol pathway, catalyzing the reduction of carbonyl compounds in a manner that contributes to the emergence of diabetic complications. Inhibitors of AR slow the progression of long-lasting diabetes-related problems (Panigrahy et al., 2016). Various types of sesquiterpenes, such as acylated eudesmane sesquiterpene (salasol A), friedelane type (salasones A, B, and C), norfriedelane triterpene sala quinone A and the abietane diterpenoids panthenol A and B isolated from the roots and rhizome of *Salvia miltiorrhiza* exhibit AR inhibitory effects (Kishi et al., 2003). D-limonene prevented the progress of diabetic cataracts in rats with STZ-induced diabetes by inhibiting AR activity (Kumar et al., 2020).

Reduction of Diabetes Mellitus Complications

Various important terpenoids, including palbinone, oleanolic acid, ursolic acid, betulinic acid, eugenol, and zerumbone, exhibit a wide range of biological activities. According to Nazaruk and Borzym-Kluczyk (2015), triterpenes play a preventive role in the formation of advanced glycation end products (AGEs) implicated in diabetic nephropathy, embryopathy, neuropathy, and impaired wound healing. Furthermore, research by Shi et al. (2019) suggests that palbinone can hinder the production of NLRP3 inflammasomes in diabetic retinopathy and activate the antioxidative Nrf2 pathway. In the case of STZ-induced diabetic mice, both oleanolic acid and ursolic acid have been shown to reduce renal aldose reductase (AR) activity (Wang et al., 2010). They also enhance glyoxalase activity, which reduces the formation of renal AGEs and improves renal function. Ursolic acid has been found to ameliorate kidney damage in type 2 diabetes, particularly in db/db mice. It accomplishes this by reducing oxidative stress, extracellular matrix production, and renal inflammation through the downregulation of enzymes in the ARAp1/AT1R signaling pathway (Ma et al., 2019). Additionally, ursolic acid promotes SIRT1 overexpression in STZ-induced diabetic mice, resulting in cell regeneration. In the case of STZ-NA-induced diabetic mice, betulinic acid has been shown to significantly reduce liver damage by increasing levels of leptin, adiponectin, liver enzymes, and lipids. Eugenol, a major component of clove oil, has demonstrated the ability to mitigate vascular and neurological problems in Sprague-Dawley rats (Ahangarpour et al., 2018). Its antioxidant and anti-inflammatory properties are thought to contribute to these observed effects (Nangle et al., 2005). Zerumbone, a sesquiterpene, has been found to mitigate retinal damage in STZ-induced diabetic mice by suppressing AGEs and their receptor system. It also reduces retinal inflammation and angiogenesis by inhibiting the p38 MAPK and NF-kB signaling pathways (Liu et al., 2016).

Future of Terpenoids as Antidiabetic Agents

The future of terpenoids as antidiabetic agents is promising due to their diverse therapeutic properties and potential mechanisms of action. As natural compounds, terpenoids offer a distinct advantage over synthetic drugs in terms of safety and tolerability. Several terpenoids have been identified for their ability to stimulate insulin secretion, activate AMPK, promote glycogen synthesis, inhibit glycogen degradation, and reduce serum cholesterol and triglyceride levels. These actions make terpenoids attractive candidates for the development of natural anti-diabetic agents. However, there are challenges that must be addressed before terpenoids can be widely used as anti-diabetic agents. One major challenge is the lack of standardized methods for extracting and analyzing terpenoids from various plant sources. This variability in extraction methods can result in differences in the quality and quantity of terpenoids obtained, which may impact their therapeutic efficacy. Another challenge is the need for more research to better understand the pharmacokinetics and pharmacodynamics of terpenoids and their potential interactions with other medications. Additionally, more clinical studies are needed to evaluate the safety and efficacy of terpenoids as anti-diabetic agents in humans. Despite these challenges, the use of terpenoids as anti-diabetic agents offers several benefits. Terpenoids are generally well-tolerated and have fewer side effects compared to conventional anti-diabetic drugs. With the increasing demand for natural and safe therapies, the future of terpenoids as anti-diabetic agents looks promising. Advancements in technology and analytical methods are likely to enhance our understanding of the pharmacology of these compounds and their potential therapeutic applications. Furthermore, improvements in drug delivery systems may help overcome some of the challenges associated with the use of terpenoids as anti-diabetic agents, including issues related to bioavailability and variable quality.

Conclusion

Natural products have proven to be a rich source of bioactive compounds for drug development due to their diverse structures and involvement in various physiological processes. Terpenes, derived from numerous natural sources, have shown potential as hypolipidemic agents, glucosidase inhibitors, and hypoglycemic compounds, among others. Additionally, they have demonstrated the ability to reduce oxidative stress and lower plasma glucose levels, which can help in mitigating complications associated with diabetes. One standout terpene, ursolic acid, possesses the unique potential to both increase insulin secretion and reduce insulin resistance. Its mechanisms of action include stimulating the insulin signaling pathway, inhibiting enzymes like PTP1B, GP, 11-HSD1, α-glucosidase, and α-amylase, and activating AMPK and PPARs. These multifaceted actions contribute to its effectiveness in managing diabetes. Triterpenoids, a subset of terpenes, hold promise for the development of novel diabetes treatments, as supported by existing experimental data. They have exhibited not only the ability to reduce body fat but also strong antidiabetic efficacy in both laboratory and animal studies. Importantly, terpenoids are readily available in nature and cost-effective, further emphasizing their potential as therapeutic agents. While these terpenes have shown encouraging antidiabetic properties, clinical investigations are lacking. To establish their clinical status, unexplored terpenes require more rigorous clinical research to assess their effectiveness, potency, and safety in real-world scenarios. Some terpenoids, including β-caryophyllene, limonene, myrcene, linalool, and α-pinene, have undergone research in relation to diabetes. Nevertheless, additional studies are needed to determine optimal dosages, safety profiles, and potential interactions with other medications. As with any natural remedy, it is essential to seek guidance from healthcare professionals before considering terpenoids for diabetes management. This precaution ensures the safe and effective integration of terpenoids into diabetes treatment plans, ultimately benefiting individuals living with this condition.

References

Ahangarpour, A., Shabani, R., Farbood, Y. (2018). The effect of betulinic acid on leptin, adiponectin, hepatic enzyme levels, and lipid profiles in streptozotocin–

nicotinamide-induced diabetic mice. *Research in Pharmaceutical Sciences*, 13(2), 142–148.

Alarcon-Aguilara, F. J., Roman-Ramos, R., Perez-Gutierrez, S., Aguilar-Contreras, A., Contreras-Weber, C. C., Flores-Saenz, J. L. (1998). Study of the antihyperglycemic effect of plants used as antidiabetics. *Journal of Ethnopharmacology*, 61(2), 101–110.

Alqahtani, A., Hamid, K., Kam, A., Wong, K. H., Abdelhak, Z., Razmovski-Naumovski, V., Chan, K., Li, K. M., Groundwater, P. W., Li, G. Q. (2013). The pentacyclic triterpenoids in herbal medicines and their pharmacological activities in diabetes and diabetic complications. *Current Medicinal Chemistry*, 20(7), 908–931

Bansal, P., Wang, Q. (2008). Insulin as a physiological modulator of glucagon secretion. American Journal of Physiology. *Endocrinology and Metabolism*, 295(4), E751–E761.

Bustanji, Y., Al-Masri, I. M., Mohammad, M., Hudaib, M., Tawaha, K., Tarazi, H., AlKhatib, H. S. (2011). Pancreatic lipase inhibition activity of tri lactone terpenes of Ginkgo biloba. *Journal of Enzyme Inhibition and Medicinal Chemistry*, 26(4), 453–459.

Deutschländer, M. S., Lall, N., Van de Venter, M., Hussein, A. A. (2011). Hypoglycaemic evaluation of a new triterpene and other compounds isolated from Euclea undulata Thunb. var. myrtina (Ebenaceae) root bark. *Journal of Ethnopharmacology*, 133(3), 1091–1095.

do Ha, T., Tuan, D. T., Thu, N. B., Nhiem, N. X., Ngoc, T. M., Yim, N., Bae, K. (2009). Palbinone and triterpenes from the moutan Cortex (Paeonia suffruticosa, Paeoniaceae) stimulate glucose uptake and glycogen synthesis via activation of AMPK in insulin-resistant human HepG2 Cells. *Bioorganic and Medicinal Chemistry Letters*, 19(19), 5556–5559.

Donath, M. Y., Ehses, J. A. (2006). Type 1, type 1.5, and type 2 diabetes: NOD diabetes we thought it was. *Proceedings of the National Academy of Sciences of the United States of America*, 103(33), 12217–12218.

Dzubak, P., Hajduch, M., Vydra, D., Hustova, A., Kvasnica, M., Biedermann, D., Markova, L., Urban, M., Sarek, J. (2006). Pharmacological activities of natural triterpenoids and their therapeutic implications. *Natural Product Reports*, 23(3), 394–411.

Ghorbani, A. (2013). Best herbs for managing diabetes: A review of clinical studies. *Brazilian Journal of Pharmaceutical Sciences*, 49(3), 413–422.

Gilon, P., Henquin, J. C. (2001). Mechanisms and physiological significance of the cholinergic control of pancreatic beta-cell function. *Endocrine Reviews*, 22(5), 565–604.

Gong, Y. H., Jiang, J. X., Li, Z., Zhu, L. H., Zhang, Z. Z. (1991). Hypoglycemic effect of sanchinoside C1 in alloxan-diabetic mice. *Yao Xue Xue Bao*, 26(2), 81–85.

Gowri, P. M., Tiwari, A. K., Ali, A. Z., Rao, J. M. (2007). Inhibition of αglucosidase and amylase by bartogenic acid isolated from Barringtonia racemosa Roxb. seeds. *Phytotherapy Research*, 21(8), 796–799.

Guan, T., Li, Y., Sun, H., Tang, X., Qian, Y. (2009). Effects of maslinic acid, a natural triterpene, on glycogen metabolism in cultured cortical astrocytes. *Planta Medica*, 75(10), 1141–1143.

Güdr, A. (2016). Influence of total anthocyanins from bitter melon (Momordica charantia linn.) as antidiabetic and radical scavenging agents. *Iranian Journal of Pharmaceutical Research*, 15(1), 301–309.

Halberstein, R. A. (2005). Medicinal plants: Historical and cross-cultural usage patterns. *Annals of Epidemiology*, 15(9), 686–699.

Hou, W., Li, Y., Zhang, Q., Wei, X., Peng, A., Chen, L., Wei, Y. (2009). Triterpene acids isolated from Lagerstroemia speciosa leaves as a-glucosidase inhibitors. *Phytotherapy Research*, 23(5), 614–618.

Hsu, J. H., Wu, Y. C., Liu, I. M., Cheng, J. T. (2006). Release of acetylcholine to raise insulin secretion in Wistar rats by oleanolic acid, one of the active principles contained in Cornus officinalis. *Neuroscience Letters*, 404(1–2), 112–116.

Jeppesen, P. B., Gregersen, S., Poulsen, C. R., Hermansen, K. (2000). Stevioside acts directly on pancreatic β cells to secrete insulin: Actions independent of cyclic adenosine monophosphate and adenosine triphosphate-sensitive K+ channel activity. *Metabolism: Clinical and Experimental*, 49(2), 208–214.

Jeppesen, P. B., Gregersen, S., Rolfsen, S. E., Jepsen, M., Colombo, M., Agger, A., Xiao, J., Kruhøffer, M., Orntoft, T., Hermansen, K. (2003). Antihyperglycemic and blood pressure reducing effects of stevioside in the diabetic Goto Kakizaki rat. *Metabolism: Clinical and Experimental*, 52(3), 372–378.

Kashiwagi, A. (1995). Rationale and hurdles of inhibitors of hepatic gluconeogenesis in treatment of diabetes mellitus. *Diabetes Research and Clinical Practice*, 28, Suppl., S195–S200.

Khan, V., Najmi, A. K., Akhtar, M., Aqil, M., Mujeeb, M., Pillai, K. K. (2012). A pharmacological appraisal of medicinal plants with antidiabetic potential. *Journal of Pharmacy and Bioallied Sciences*, 4(1), 27–42.

Kishi, M. T., Matsuda, H., Yoshikawa, M. (2003). Structures of new f riedelane and no r friedelane type triterpenes and polyacylatedeudesmanetype sesquiterpene from Salacia chinensis Linn. (S. prinoides DC., Hippocrateaceae) and radical scavenging activities of principal constituents. *Chemical and Pharmaceutical Bulletin*, 51, 10515.

Kumar, M. P., Mamidala, E., Al-Ghanim, K., Al-Misned, F., Ahmed, Z., Mahboob, S. (2020). Effects of D-limonene on aldose reductase and protein glycation in diabetic rats. *Journal of King Saud University*, 32(3), 1953-1958.

Lai, Y. C., Chen, C. K., Tsai, S. F., Lee, S. S. (2012). Triterpenes as α-glucosidase inhibitors from Fagus hayatae. *Phytochemistry*, 74, 206–211.

Laszczyk, M. N. (2009). Pentacyclic triterpenes of the lupane, oleanane and ursane group as tools in cancer therapy. *Planta Medica*, 75(15), 1549–1560.

Lee, J., Lee, H. I., Seo, K. I., Cho, H. W., Kim, M. J., Park, E. M., Lee, M. K. (2014). Effects of ursolic acid on glucose metabolism, the polyol pathway and dyslipidemia in non-obese type 2 diabetic mice. *Indian Journal of Experimental Biology*, 52(7), 683–691.

Lee, W. K., Kao, S. T., Liu, I. M., Cheng, J. T. (2006). Increase of insulin secretion by ginsenoside Rh2 to lower plasma glucose in Wistar rats. *Clinical and Experimental Pharmacology and Physiology*, 33(1–2), 27–32.

Liu, W. Y., Tzeng, T. F., Liu, I. M. (2016). Zerumbone, a bioactive sesquiterpene, Ameliorates diabetes-induced retinal microvascular damage through inhibition of phospho-p38 mitogen-activated protein kinase and nuclear factor-κB pathways. *Molecules*, 21(12), 708.

Luo, J. G., Liu, J., Kong, L. Y. (2008). New pentacyclic triterpenes from Gypsophila oldhamiana and their biological evaluation as glycogen phosphorylase inhibitors. *Chemistry and Biodiversity*, 5(5), 751–757.

Ma, T. K., Xu, L., Lu, L. X., Cao, X., Li, X., Li, L. L., Wang, X., Fan, Q. L. (2019). Ursolic acid treatment alleviates diabetic kidney injury by regulating the ARAP1/AT1R signaling pathway. *Diabetes, Metabolic Syndrome and Obesity: Targets and Therapy*, 12, 2597–2608.

Malviya, N., Jain, S., Malviya, S. (2010). Antidiabetic potential of medicinal plants. *Acta Poloniae Pharmaceutica*, 67(2), 113–118.

Murali, R., Karthikeyan, A., Saravanan, R. (2013). Protective effects of DLimonene on lipid peroxidation and antioxidant enzymes in streptozotocin-induced diabetic rats. *Basic and Clinical Pharmacology and Toxicology*, 112(3), 175–181.

Nangle, M. R., Gibson, T. M., Cotter, M. A., Cameron, N. E. (2006). Effects of eugenol on nerve and vascular dysfunction in streptozotocin diabetic rats. *Planta Medica*, 72(6), 494–500.

Nazaruk, J., Borzym-Kluczyk, M. (2015). The role of triterpenes in the management of diabetes mellitus and its complications. *Phytochemistry Reviews: Proceedings of the Phytochemical Society of Europe*, 14(4), 675–690.

Panigrahy, S. K., Bhatt, R., Kumar, A. (2017). Reactive oxygen species: Sources, consequences and targeted therapy in type 2 diabetes. *Journal of Drug Targeting*, 25(2), 93–101.

Prabhakar, P. K., Doble, M. (2011). Mechanism of action of natural products used in the treatment of diabetes mellitus. *Chinese Journal of Integrative Medicine*, 17(8), 563–574.

Praly, J. P., Vidal, S. (2010). Inhibition of glycogen phosphorylase in the context of type 2 diabetes, with focus on recent inhibitors bound at the active site. *Mini Reviews in Medicinal Chemistry*, 10(12), 1102–1126.

Preethi, P. J. (2013). Herbal medicine for diabetes mellitus: A review. *Asian Journal of Pharmaceutical Research*, 3(2), 57–70.

Ramachandran, S., Prasad, N. R. (2008). Effect of ursolic acid, a triterpenoid antioxidant, on ultraviolet-B radiation-inducedcytotoxicity, lipid peroxidation and DNA damage in human lymphocytes. *Chemico-Biological Interactions*, 176(2–3), 99–107.

Rao, M. U., Sreenivasulu, M., Chengaiah, B., Reddy, K. J., Chetty, C. M. (2010). Herbal medicines for diabetes mellitus: A review. *International Journal of PharmTech Research*, 2(3), 1883–1892.

Sales, P. M., Souza, P. M., Simeoni, L. A., Magalhães, P. O., Silveira, D. (2012). a-amylase inhibitors: A review of raw material and isolated compounds from plant source. *Journal of Pharmacy and Pharmaceutical Sciences*, 15(1), 141–183.

Samarghandian, S., Borji, A., Delkhosh, M. B., Samini, F. (2013). Safranal treatment improves hyperglycemia, hyperlipidemia and oxidative stress in streptozotocin-induced diabetic rats. *Journal of Pharmacy and Pharmaceutical Sciences*, 16(2), 352–362.

Shi, Q., Wang, J., Cheng, Y., Dong, X., Zhang, M., Pei, C. (2019). Palbinone alleviates diabetic retinopathy in STZ-induced rats by inhibiting NLRP3 inflammatory activity. *Journal of Biochemical and Molecular Toxicology*, 2019, e22489.

Sudhahar, V., Kumar, S. A., Sudharsan, P. T., Varalakshmi, P. (2007). Protective effect of lupeol and its ester on cardiac abnormalities in experimental hypercholesterolemia. *Vascular Pharmacology*, 46(6), 412–418.

Tan, M. J., Ye, J. M., Turner, N., Hohnen-Behrens, C., Ke, C. Q., Tang, C. P., Chen, T., Weiss, H. C., Gesing, E. R., Rowland, A., James, D. E., Ye, Y. (2008). Antidiabetic activities of triterpenoids isolated from bitter melon associated with activation of the AMPK pathway. *Chemistry and Biology*, 15(3), 263–273.

Tang, J. J., Li, J. G., Qi, W., Qiu, W. W., Li, P. S., Li, B. L., Song, B. L. (2011). Inhibition of SREBP by a small molecule, Betulin, improves hyperlipidemia and insulin resistance and reduces atherosclerotic plaques. *Cell Metabolism*, 13(1), 44–56.

Uddin, G., Rauf, A., Al-Othman, A. M., Collina, S., Arfan, M., Ali, G., Khan, I. (2012). Pistagremic acid, a glucosidase inhibitor from Pistacia integerrima. *Fitoterapia*, 83(8), 1648–1652.

Wang, Z. H., Hsu, C. C., Huang, C. N., Yin, M. C. (2010). Anti-glycative effects of oleanolic acid and ursolic acid in kidney of diabetic mice. *European Journal of Pharmacology*, 628(1–3), 255–260.

Winder, W. W., Hardie, D. G. (1999). AMP-activated protein kinase, a metabolic master switch: Possible roles in type 2 diabetes. *American Journal of Physiology*, 277(1), E1–E10.

Yamada, K., Hosokawa, M., Fujimoto, S., Fujiwara, H., Fujita, Y., Harada, N., Yamada, C., Fukushima, M., Ueda, N., Kaneko, T., Matsuyama, F., Yamada, Y., Seino, Y., Inagaki, N. (2008). Effect of corosolic acid on gluconeogenesis in rat liver. *Diabetes Research and Clinical Practice*, 80(1), 48–55.

Yasukawa, K., Akihisa, T., Oinuma, H., Kasahara, Y., Kimura, Y., Yamanouchi, S., Kumaki, K., Tamura, T., Takido, M. (1996). Inhibitory effect of di- and trihydroxy triterpenes from the flowers of Compositae on 12-O-tetradecanoylphorbol-13-acetate-induced inflammation in mice. *Biological and Pharmaceutical Bulletin*, 19(10), 1329–1331.

Yokozawa, T., Kobayashi, T., Oura, H., Kawashima, Y. (1985). Studies on the mechanism of the hypoglycemic activity of ginsenoside-Rb2 in streptozotocin-diabetic rats. *Chemical and Pharmaceutical Bulletin*, 33(2), 869–872.

Chapter 11

The Role of Gingerols in the Management of Diabetes Mellitus

Hemlata Nimesh*

Amity Institute of Pharmacy, Amity University, Noida, Uttar Pradesh, India

Abstract

Diabetes mellitus is a chronic metabolic disorder of the endocrine system characterized by disruptions in insulin secretion or insufficiency, along with impaired metabolism of glucose, lipids, and proteins. The global prevalence of diabetes, currently affecting approximately 382 million individuals, is projected to rise to 471 million by 2035. Natural compounds have exhibited a range of promising medicinal properties. Among these compounds, ginger (*Zingiber officinale*) stands out due to its potent and abundant bioactive constituent, gingerol, belonging to the Zingiberaceae family. The gingerol derivatives, namely 10-gingerol, 8-gingerol, and 6-gingerol, which confer ginger's characteristic pungency, are believed to be the driving force behind ginger's medicinal effects in diabetes management. Through a series of distinct mechanisms, gingerols have demonstrated noteworthy anti-diabetic attributes, encompassing: Activation of 5′ adenosine monophosphate-activated protein kinase phosphorylation; Enhancement of glucose absorption; Suppression of reactive oxygen species (ROS) levels induced by glycation end products in pancreatic β-cells; Facilitation of translocation of glucose transporter 4 to the cytoplasm; Optimization of hepatic enzyme expression linked to glucose metabolism, culminating in reduced blood glucose levels. Reduction in fasting blood glucose levels and

* Corresponding Author's Email: hemlatanimesh@gmail.com; hnimesh@amity.edu.

In: Naturally Occurring Chemicals …
Editors: A. Singh Grewal, G. Deswal, A. Kumar Dhingra et al.
ISBN: 979-8-89113-491-1

improvement of glucose intolerance. This chapter centers on the bioactive constituents of ginger, specifically gingerols, both in their isolated form and as part of ginger extracts enriched with gingerol. It offers a comprehensive understanding of their therapeutic potential, particularly their role in mitigating diabetes, while shedding light on the intricate mechanisms that underlie their anti-diabetic effects.

Keywords: ginger, gingerol, hyperglycemia, insulin, diabetes mellitus

Introduction

Diabetes mellitus (DM) is a condition that affects a staggering 100 million individuals worldwide. It falls within a diverse category of diseases that ultimately result in elevated blood glucose levels (hyperglycemia), leading to the excretion of glucose in urine. Distinctive signs of DM include polydipsia (excessive thirst), polyphagia (excessive eating), and polyuria (increased urine production). It is a chronic metabolic disorder of the endocrine system characterized by deficiencies in insulin secretion, as well as abnormalities in protein, lipid, and glucose metabolism. Projections indicate a concerning rise in diabetes cases to 471 million by 2035, a significant increase from the current 382 million cases, underscoring its profound impact on global health (Bi et al., 2017; Ogurtsova et al., 2017). Various forms of diabetes exist, encompassing gestational diabetes mellitus, the autoimmune disorder type 1 diabetes marked by damage to pancreatic β-cells, and the more prevalent type 2 diabetes characterized by impaired glucose regulation due to a combination of insulin resistance and pancreatic β-cell dysfunction. In the realm of diabetes management, the current arsenal includes pharmacotherapy, dietary interventions, and insulin administration, each showcasing antidiabetic effects through diverse mechanisms. Mechanistically, drugs like sulfonylureas and meglitinides stimulate insulin secretion, while biguanides and thiazolidinediones enhance peripheral glucose absorption. Alpha-glucosidase inhibitors, on the other hand, delay intestinal carbohydrate absorption, and biguanides contribute to the reduction of gluconeogenesis in the liver (Bathaie et al., 2012; Kooti et al., 2016). Despite the ongoing advancements in disease management through conventional drug utilization and other strategies, diabetes and its associated consequences continue to present a substantial medical challenge, with an escalating disease burden. Synthetic oral hypoglycemic agents, while contributing to disease control, carry significant drawbacks including serious side effects, drug resistance, and limited usage during pregnancy, exacerbated by their toxicity and high costs (Haque et al., 2011). Herbs and spices have left an indelible mark on human civilization and history across the globe. Spices, in particular, serve not only as flavor enhancers but also hold diverse medicinal and pharmacological properties, contributing to the creation of numerous medicines. A variety of species within the Zingiberaceae plant family find application as culinary herbs and spices. One such notable member, *Zingiber officinale* (Ginger), boasts a rich and diverse historical lineage in both traditional and alternative medicine. Ginger has played a crucial role in alternative and complementary medicinal formulations, addressing an array of ailments. Prominent among ginger's medicinal attributes are its proven benefits in alleviating nausea, asthma, arthritis, gastrointestinal distress, headaches, and other maladies. It has also demonstrated effectiveness against nausea, vomiting, and motion sickness induced by chemotherapy (Semwal et al., 2015; Packer et al., 2004; Butt & Sultan, 2011; Sharma et al., 2022). The intricate chemical composition of ginger encompasses phenolic and terpene compounds, with the principal and abundant bioactive constituent being gingerol. This compound bestows ginger with its distinctive mild pungency and therapeutic properties, stemming from a trio of active derivatives collectively referred to as gingerols - (10)-gingerol, (8)-gingerol, and (6)-gingerol (Ma et al., 2021).

Central to ginger's pharmacological activity is the aromatic polyphenol known as (6)-gingerol, scientifically designated as (S)-5-hydroxy-1-(4-hydroxy-3-methoxyphenol)-3-decanone (Kubra et al., 2012; Wand et al., 2018). Among these derivatives, the most potent, 6-gingerol, was first identified and acknowledged in 1917. The synthesis of gingerol follows the phenylpropanoid pathway (Alharbi et al., 2022). In the realm of chemistry, gingerol has relatives in capsaicin and piperine, forming a group depicted in Figure 1 (Beltran et al., 2013). With a robust aroma, gingerol takes the form of a low-melting crystalline solid. Upon heating, gingerol undergoes a reverse aldol process, resulting in the formation of zingerone—a molecule possessing a milder spiciness and a sweet fragrance. Furthermore, exposure of gingerol to heat, drying, or prolonged storage prompts a dehydration reaction, giving rise to corresponding shogaols. These shogaols, characterized by a more intense pungency than gingerol (Jung et al., 2018). Research findings highlight the mutagenic properties of both shogaols and gingerols (Mao et al., 2019). Additionally, ginger harbors a variety of other phenolic compounds, including gingerenone-A, zingerone, quercetin, and 6-

dehydrogingerdione (Shadich et al., 2016; Ji et al., 2017). Within ginger, one also finds an array of terpene compounds, such as curcumene, bisabolene, zingiberene, sesquiphellandrene, and farnesene, recognized as the principal constituents of ginger essential oils (Yeh et al. in 2014). Complementing this diverse chemical profile, ginger also contains organic acids, polysaccharides, lipids, and dietary fibers. The quantification of various gingerols per gram of ginger powder has been established (Schwertner et al., 2007).

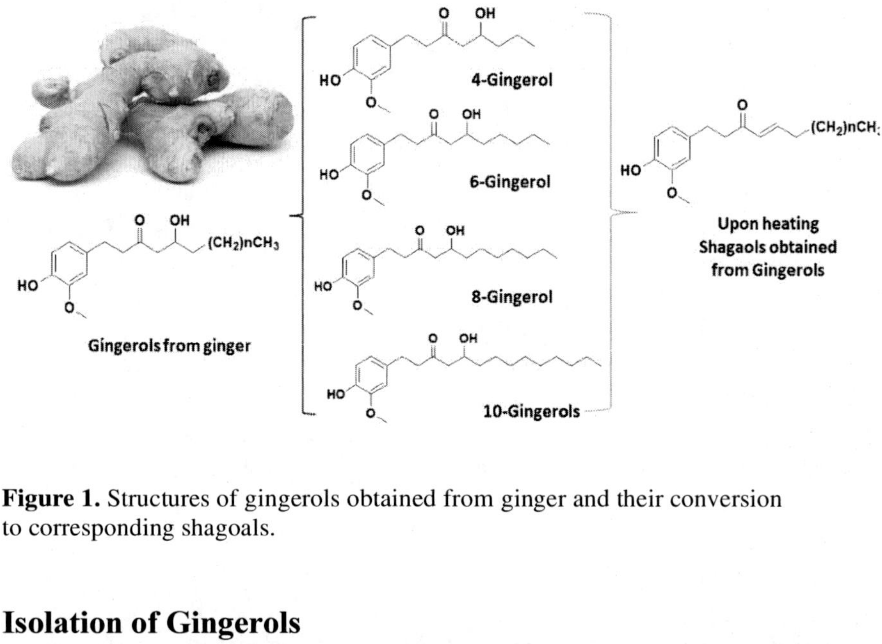

Figure 1. Structures of gingerols obtained from ginger and their conversion to corresponding shagoals.

Isolation of Gingerols

The separation of gingerols from powdered ginger root was accomplished through counter current chromatography. With minor adjustments to the procedure, (4)-gingerol was also successfully extracted using this method. These techniques leveraged diol-bonded columns to isolate interfering constituents, effectively obtaining individual gingerols from crude methanolic extracts. A fractionation strategy, combined with normal phase High-Performance Liquid Chromatography (HPLC), facilitated the extraction of distinct gingerols using crude extracts from fresh ginger rhizomes dissolved in methylene chloride. Furthermore, the molecules were characterized through mass spectrum analyses (Farthing and O'Neill, 1990). An alternative approach (Hiserodt et al., 1998), employed 95% ethanol for the extraction of *Zingiber officinale* rhizomes, employing a straightforward maceration procedure. For the extraction of gingerol and related compounds from ginger rhizomes, dichloromethane was utilized, followed by a subsequent substitution with alkyl groups (Gaikwad et al., 2017). In a distinct study, chemical modifications were applied to 6-gingerol post-isolation from ginger rhizomes. Upon assessing the therapeutic effects of these modified compounds on diabetic mice, it was observed that insulin signaling was significantly enhanced (Masuda et al., 2004).

Synthesis of Gingerols

Synthesis of (10)-, (8)-, and (6)-gingerols in one-step can be done (Figure 2). In order to produce gingerol, vanillylacetone was first reacted with butyl lithium, followed by lithium diisopropylamide and the appropriate aldehyde (Fleming et al., 1999). Dennif et al. (1980) used phenylalanine to create (6)-gingerol in 1980. This precursor generated *p*-coumaric acid, which then produce dihydroferulic acid, (6)-gingerdione, and the final product. In another study phenylalanine was used along with other enzymes (del Carmen Ramirez-Ahumada et al., 2006). Eugenol converted into nitro molecule and upon reaction with terminal alkenes to obtain isoxazolines, that resulted in (6)-, (7)-, and (9)]-gingerols. Respective gingerols were produced via catalytic hydrogenation with Raney nickel (Kumar et al., 2012). In order to achieve desired products, a research team chose a different strategy in 2009 to synthesise (+)-(S)-(6), (8), and (10)-gingerols using an enantioselective technique (Ma et al., 2009).

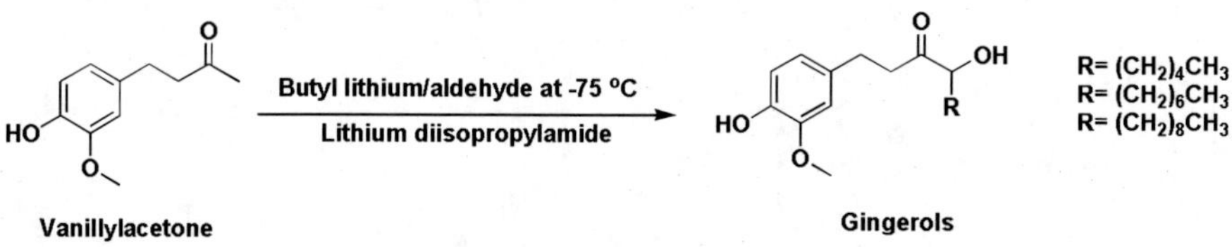

Figure 2. Synthesis of (6)-, (8)-, (10)-gingerols from vanillylacetone.

Mechanism of Antidiabetic Action of Gingerols

The anti-diabetic and hypoglycemic properties of medicinally important compounds of plant origin have been explained by a number of different mechanisms. Peripheral glucose uptake, increased synthesis of liver glycogen due to enhanced liver expression of glycogen regulation enzymes, carbohydrate metabolising enzymes inhibition, pancreatic insulin release stimulation, insulin mimetic effects, and inhibition of hepatic glucose production are some of those processes (Sharma et al., 2022; Bnouham et al., 2006; Yatoo et al., 2017). In some studies, ginger's bioactive components can increase uptake of glucose in murine skeletal muscle cells and promote the GLUT-4 glucose transporter's enhanced expression and translocation to the cells' plasma membranes, are credited with having anti-diabetic properties (Anfenan, 2014). Another approach involved ginger's phenolic components (gingerols and shogaols), which block the primary enzymes, α-glucosidase and α-amylase related to carbohydrate metabolism (Nammi et al., 2009; Sattar et al., 2012) Other researchers, however, have shown that ginger boosts liver and muscle glycogen stores by improving peripheral glucose utilisation, which inhibits gluconeogenesis in kidney and liver like insulin (Iranloye et al., 2011). Overall gingerols exhibited antidiabetic action via six distinct types of mechanisms (Figure 3) (Bin et al., 2009; Son et al., 2015).

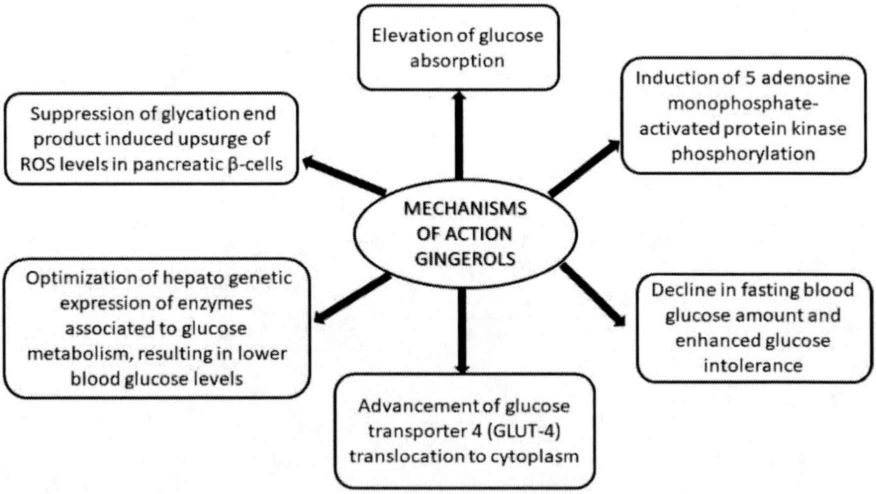

Figure 3. Different mechanism of potential antidiabetic action of gingerols.

Antidiabetic Action of Gingerols: *In Vitro* and *In Vivo*

Numerous researchers have undertaken extensive investigations into the antidiabetic properties of ginger, exploring its key active constituents. The underlying factor in the disease is believed to be insulin resistance or insufficiency. Sustained hyperglycemia can accelerate the formation of advanced glycation end products (AGEs) and protein glycation. Notably, (6)-gingerol and (6)-shogaol were found to hinder the emergence of diabetic complications in vitro by curbing the generation of AGEs through the sequestration of methylglyoxal, an AGE precursor (Zhu et al., 2015). Through the activation of Nrf2, (6)-gingerol was also able to reduce N-carboxymethyl-lysine (Sampath et al., 2017). The potential antidiabetic effects of (6)-gingerol were evaluated based on various parameters, including glucose uptake in L6 myocytes, protection of pancreatic β-cells from oxidative stress caused by reactive oxygen species, and more. Intriguingly, (6)-gingerol employed distinct mechanisms, such as initiating 5' AMP-activated protein kinase phosphorylation, enhancing glucose uptake, and promoting translocation of glucose transporter 4 to the plasma membrane in L6 myotubes, even in the absence of insulin. This array of in vitro findings strongly supports the notion that (6)-gingerol exerts its antidiabetic efficacy through multiple pathways (Bin et al., 2009; Son et al., 2015). Notably, (6)-gingerol appears to play a significant role in glucose metabolism by modulating the trafficking of glucose transporters within skeletal muscle cells. Research demonstrated that 6-gingerol induced AMPK phosphorylation in mouse skeletal muscle C2C12 cells. This effect relied on AMPKα2, as inhibition or knockdown of AMPKα2 halted the glucose uptake stimulated by (6)-gingerol (Lee et al., 2015). Effective intracellular vesicular transport is crucial for the secondary phase of biphasic insulin release in response to glucose, a process vital for maintaining glucose homeostasis (Wang & Thurmond, 2009). A different study indicated that (6)-gingerol activated the GLP-1-mediated insulin secretion pathway. This activation led to the upregulation of glycogen synthase 1 and an increase in GLUT4 membrane presentation, ultimately facilitating glucose disposal in skeletal muscle (Bin et al., 2017).

The core attributes of a potent antidiabetic drug encompass insulin secretion, antihyperglycemic effects, lipid-lowering capabilities, and antioxidant properties. In a type-2 diabetic animal model, (6)-gingerol displayed a notable reduction in fasting glucose levels and an enhancement in glucose tolerance. A multitude of biomarkers, including insulin, free fatty acids, low-density lipoprotein cholesterol, total cholesterol, and triglycerides, exhibited substantial decreases. Moreover, the generation of reactive oxygen species (ROS) was curtailed, and antioxidant enzymes saw recovery in db/db mice (Singh et al., 2009; Bin et al., 2017). Notably, (6)-gingerol demonstrated its potential by elevating hepatic expression of vital metabolic genes and ameliorating the serum lipid profile in a high-fat fed rat model, leading to diminished diabetes-related complications (de Las Heras et al., 2017). Type 2 diabetes primarily arises from two factors: lack of insulin production due to pancreatic β-cell dysfunction and insulin resistance (Pajvani & Accili, 2015). Mediated by endocrine hormones, the incretin effect, also known as nutrient-stimulated insulin production, plays a pivotal role (D'Alessio, 2016). In a study exploring the protective benefits of a 6-gingerol-rich fraction from Zingiber officinale against carbendazim-induced reproductive toxicity in rats, it was discerned that (6)-gingerol reinstated disrupted endocrine signaling in the testes and epididymis. This restoration was attributed to a significant reduction in oxidative damage and an elevation in glutathione levels and antioxidant enzyme activity (Salihu et al., 2017). Moreover, (6)-gingerol facilitated glucose-stimulated insulin secretion, improving glucose tolerance by increasing glucagon-like peptide 1 levels in a diabetic animal model. Furthermore, (6)-gingerol treatment led to the activation of glycogen synthase 1 and an increase in glucose transporter type 4 (GLUT4) presentation on cell membranes, contributing to enhanced glycogen storage in skeletal muscles (Samad et al., 2017). Notably, (6)-gingerol exhibited anti-hyperglycemic properties and improved impaired insulin signaling in arsenic-intoxicated mice due to its stress-mediated mechanism induction of type 2 diabetes. This effect was attributed to reduced oxidative stress, lower blood glucose levels, and elevated plasma insulin levels post-(6)-gingerol treatment. Additionally, (6)-gingerol countered the cyto-degenerative effects and reactive oxygen species (ROS) accumulation in pancreatic beta-cells and hepatocyte primary cell cultures induced by arsenic exposure. The expression levels of several pivotal signaling molecules related to insulin signaling were restored through (6)-gingerol intervention (Chakraborty et al., 2012). In an assessment of glucose absorption using radioactively tagged 2-[1,2-^{3}H]-deoxy-D-glucose in L6 myotubes, (S)-(6)-gingerol emerged as the most abundant gingerol component, with (S)-(8)-gingerol demonstrating the highest potency in glucose uptake (Li et al., 2012). Clinical trials involving individuals with hypercholesterolemia and diabetes revealed that a 3 g/day dose of ginger over 30 days resulted in reduced blood glucose and lipid levels (Andallu et al., 2003; Mahluji et al., 2013). Gingerols were found to delay diabetes complications in another clinical study (Saraswat et al., 2010). Additionally, ginger's main pungent constituents, gingerols, were shown to aid in diabetes management. These compounds also exhibited the potential to inhibit α-amylase and α-glucosidase, key enzymes associated with type 2 diabetes (Rani et al., 2011). (10)-Gingerol's robust anti-diabetic effects, resulting in decreased blood glucose levels, were identified in another investigation (Yadav & Garg, 2019). Furthermore, ginger consumption was linked to lower levels of insulin, total cholesterol, triglycerides, and fasting plasma glucose in individuals with type 2 diabetes mellitus (Arablou et al., 2014).

Antidiabetic Activity of Ginger Extracts: *In Vivo* and *In Vitro* Experiments

Numerous comprehensive studies have delved into the antidiabetic potential of ginger extracts. For instance, in an investigation by Rani et al. (2012), it was revealed that ginger extract in ethyl acetate at a concentration of 5 g/mL enhanced glucose uptake by stimulating glucose transporters. Clinical studies with individuals afflicted by type 2 diabetes unveiled significant reductions in glucose levels and improvements in insulin sensitivity check scores upon ginger supplementation (Li et al., 2014). Moreover, ginger extract demonstrated its efficacy in mitigating streptozotocin-induced diabetes in rats. This extract led to decreased levels of TNF-α, vascular endothelial growth factor, and NF-kB in retinal tissue (Dongare et al., 2014). The impact of ginger's hydro-alcoholic extract on arginase I activity in the rat retina was explored, revealing notable reductions in body weight increase, blood glucose concentration, arginase I expression and activity, and elevated serum insulin in diabetic rats upon extract administration (Lamuchi-Deli et al., 2017). In a separate study by de Las Heras et al. (2017), the hydro-ethanolic extract of ginger exhibited insulin-sensitizing and lipid-lowering effects in the livers of high-fat diet (HFD) fed rats, ameliorating the lipid profile, glucose, leptin, and insulin levels in plasma. Cooked and raw ginger extracts were evaluated in healthy and streptozotocin-induced diabetic rats for their impact on plasma glucose levels. Both extracts effectively lowered fasting glucose in diabetic rats to normal levels, akin to glibenclamide (Oludoyin et al., 2014). Similarly, a comprehensive assessment of ginger powder, methanolic and aqueous extracts, and essential oil on streptozotocin-induced diabetic rats demonstrated reduced levels of various markers and improved liver glycogen and triglyceride levels. Ginger oil showcased more potent anti-diabetic effects than extracts (Nammi et al., 2009). Furthermore, research by Anfenan (2014) exhibited the protective effects of ginger extract against insulin resistance in male Sprague-Dawley diabetic rats. Additionally, the aqueous ginger extract demonstrated efficacy in reducing serum glucose, restoring haematological indices to normal, and repairing damaged pancreas in rats with alloxan-induced diabetes (Al-Qudah et al., 2016). Fresh ginger extracts were found to significantly lower serum total cholesterol and low-density lipoprotein in alloxan-induced diabetic rats, with similar outcomes to atorvastatin (Abdulrazaq et al., 2012). Furthermore, ginger juice administration to streptozotocin-induced Type I diabetic rats led to increased insulin levels, decreased fasting glucose levels, and improved glucose tolerance (Akhani et al., 2004). Raw ginger at a dosage of 500 mg/kg proved effective in reducing serum cholesterol, triacylglycerol, glucose, and proteinuria in rats with diabetes induced by streptozotocin (Bhandari et al., 2005; Al-Amin et al., 2006). In a distinct study, ethanol-based ginger extracts at a dosage of 200 mg/kg displayed significant anti-hyperglycemic effects, elevating HDL cholesterol levels and lowering serum total cholesterol and triglycerides (Otunola & Afolayan, 2015). Furthermore, the hypoglycemic effect of intraperitoneally administered ginger (4 and 8 g/kg) became more pronounced 2 hours after diabetes induction in rats (Otunola & Afolayan, 2015).

Role of Gingerol in Diabetes Associated Problems

In myocardia isolated from mice with diabetic produced by streptozotocin, the effects of gingerol, on the contraction and Ca^{2+} transient was assessed and compared to control mice. It was shown that streptozotocin-treated animals required significantly more time for the ventricular wall to relax. The SERCA inhibitor cyclopiazonic acid reduced Ca^{2+} transient decay and relaxation rates. Gingerol accelerated the rate of Ca^{2+} transient decay and relaxation, although their effects were more pronounced in mice given streptozotocin. Cyclopezionic acid completely prevented the gingerol-induced acceleration. These findings imply that reduced SERCA function contributes to the myocardial diastolic dysfunction induced by diabetes mellitus and can be treated with SERCA activators (Namekata et al., 2013). Diabetes has been linked to lower bone mass and higher fracture rates. The indicators of osteoblast function and oxidised protein were tested to assess the (6)-gingerol effects on osteoblast dysfunction caused by 2-deoxy-D-ribose. With 30 mM 2-deoxy-D-ribose presence, 6-gingerol (10^{-7} M) stimulated the proliferation of MC3T3-E1 cells. By using 6-gingerol, the cells' alkaline phosphatase activity, collagen content, and osteocalcin production were all markedly increased. Additionally, in osteoblastic cells 6-gingerol increased osteoprotegerin secretion which is significant for diabetes-related bone diseases (Kim et al., 2007). Pre-treatment with (6)-gingerol and (6)-shogaol significantly reduced the downregulation of adiponectin expression mediated by TNF-α in 3T3-L1 adipocytes. While c-Jun-$NH_{(2)}$-terminal kinase signalling activation caused by TNF-α is effectively inhibited by 6-gingerol, despite the fact that it is not a PPAR-γ agonist, this inhibitory effect is the basis of 6-gingerol's inhibitory mechanism. PPAR-γ transactivation explains how 6-shaagaol's inhibitory mechanism acts as a PPAR-γ agonist (Isa et al., 2008).

Conclusion

This chapter underscores the therapeutic significance of the active phytoconstituents in ginger for diabetes mellitus. Ginger and its active constituents are widely regarded as a safe alternative for treating various ailments, owing to their minimal side effects. While numerous in vitro and in vivo reports are available, there is a relatively limited number of clinical trial studies. These studies exhibit variations in doses, outcomes, and mechanisms of antidiabetic action. Ginger's antidiabetic effects operate through multifaceted mechanisms, including the restoration of pancreatic beta-cell function, enhancement of insulin sensitivity, promotion of peripheral glucose uptake, and insulin-like actions. Additionally, the mechanisms encompass improved hepatic glycogen synthesis through heightened liver expression of glycogen-regulating enzymes, inhibition of carbohydrate-metabolizing enzymes, stimulation of pancreatic insulin release, and reduction of hepatic glucose production. Further research is warranted, especially involving human subjects, considering that ginger is a common spice widely perceived as safe. Additionally, it is crucial to ascertain the safety of prolonged oral consumption of various ginger extracts over extended periods.

References

Abdulrazaq, N. B., Cho, M. M., Win, N. N., Zaman, R., Rahman, M. T. (2012). Beneficial effects of ginger (Zingiber officinale) on carbohydrate metabolism in streptozotocin-induced diabetic rats. *British Journal of Nutrition*, 108(7), 1194-1201.

Akhani, S. P., Vishwakarma, S. L., Goyal, R. K. (2004). Anti-diabetic activity of Zingiber officinale in streptozotocin-induced type I diabetic rats. *Journal of Pharmacy and Pharmacology*, 56(1), 101-105.

Al-Amin, Z. M., Thomson, M., Al-Qattan, K. K., Peltonen-Shalaby, R., Ali, M. (2006). Anti-diabetic and hypolipidaemic properties of ginger (Zingiber officinale) in streptozotocin-induced diabetic rats. *British Journal of Nutrition*, 96(4), 660-666.

Alharbi, K. S., Nadeem, M. S., Afzal, O., Alzarea, S. I., Altamimi, A. S. A., Almalki, W. H., Mubeen, B., Iftikhar, S., Shah, L., Kazmi, I. (2022). Gingerol, a natural antioxidant, attenuates hyperglycemia and downstream complications. *Metabolites*, 12(12), 1274.

Al-Noory, A. S., Amreen, A. N., Hymoor, S. (2013). Antihyperlipidemic effects of ginger extracts in alloxan-induced diabetes and propylthiouracil-induced hypothyroidism in (rats). *Pharmacognosy Research*, 5(3), 157.

Al-Qudah, M. M., Haddad, M. A., EL-Qudah, J. M. (2016). The effects of aqueous ginger extract on pancreas histology and on blood glucose in normal and alloxan monohydrate-induced diabetic rats. *BioMed Research*, 27(2), 350-356.

Andallu, B., Radhika, B., Suryakantham, V. (2003). Effect of aswagandha, ginger and mulberry on hyperglycemia and hyperlipidemia. *Plant Foods for Human Nutrition*, 58, 1-7.

Anfenan, M. L. K. (2014). Evaluation of nutritional and antidiabetic activity of different forms of ginger in rats. *Middle-East Journal of Scientific Research*, 21(1), 56-62.

Arablou, T., Aryaeian, N., Valizadeh, M., Sharifi, F., Hosseini, A., Djalali, M. (2014). The effect of ginger consumption on glycemic status, lipid profile and some inflammatory markers in patients with type 2 diabetes mellitus. *International Journal of Food Sciences and Nutrition*, 65(4), 515-520.

Bathaie, S. Z., Mokarizade, N., Shirali, S. (2012). An overview of the mechanisms of plant ingredients in the treatment of diabetes mellitus. *Journal of Medicinal Plants*, 11(44), 1-24.

Beltrán, L. R., Dawid, C., Beltrán, M., Gisselmann, G., Degenhardt, K., Mathie, K., Hofmann, T., Hatt, H. (2013). The pungent substances piperine, capsaicin, 6-gingerol and polygodial inhibit the human two-pore domain potassium channels TASK-1, TASK-3 and TRESK. *Frontiers in Pharmacology*, 4, 141.

Bhandari, U., Pillai, K. K. (2005). Effect of ethanolic extract of Zingiber officinale on dyslipidaemia in diabetic rats. *Journal of Ethnopharmacology*, 97(2), 227-230.

Bi, X., Lim, J., Henry, C. J. (2017). Spices in the management of diabetes mellitus. *Food Chemistry*, 217, 281-293.

Bnouham, M., Ziyyat, A., Mekhfi, H., Tahri, A., Legssyer, A. (2006). Medicinal plants with potential antidiabetic activity-A review of ten years of herbal medicine research (1990-2000). *Dubai Diabetes and Endocrinology Journal*, 14, 1-25.

Butt, M. S., Sultan, M. T. (2011). Ginger and its health claims: molecular aspects. *Critical Reviews in Food Science and Nutrition*, 51(5), 383-393.

Chakraborty, D., Mukherjee, A., Sikdar, S., Paul, A., Ghosh, S., Khuda-Bukhsh, A. R. (2012). [6]-Gingerol isolated from ginger attenuates sodium arsenite induced oxidative stress and plays a corrective role in improving insulin signaling in mice. *Toxicology Letters*, 210(1), 34-43.

D'Alessio, D. (2016). Is GLP-1 a hormone: Whether and When? *Journal of Diabetes Investigation*, 7, 50-55.

de Las Heras, N., Valero-Muñoz, M., Martín-Fernández, B., Ballesteros, S., López-Farré, A., Ruiz-Roso, B., Lahera, V. (2017). Molecular factors involved in the hypolipidemic-and insulin-sensitizing effects of a ginger (Zingiber officinale Roscoe) extract in rats fed a high-fat diet. *Applied Physiology, Nutrition, and Metabolism*, 42(2), 209-215.

del Carmen Ramirez-Ahumada, M., Timmermann, B. N., Gang, D. R. (2006). Biosynthesis of curcuminoids and gingerols in turmeric (Curcuma longa) and ginger (Zingiber officinale): identification of curcuminoid synthase and hydroxycinnamoyl-CoA thioesterases. *Phytochemistry*, 67(18), 2017-2029.

Denniff, P., Macleod, I., Whiting, D. A. (1980). Studies in the biosynthesis of [6]-gingerol, pungent principle of ginger (Zingiber officinale). *Journal of the Chemical Society*, Perkin Transactions 1, 2637-2644.

Dongare, S., Gupta, S. K., Mathur, R., Saxena, R., Mathur, S., Agarwal, R., Nag, T. C., Srivastava, S., Kumar, P. (2016). Zingiber officinale attenuates retinal microvascular changes in diabetic rats via anti-inflammatory and antiangiogenic mechanisms. *Molecular Vision*, 22, 599.

Farthing, J. E., O'neill, M. J. (1990). Isolation of gingerols from powdered root ginger by countercurrent chromatography. *Journal of Liquid Chromatography*, 13(5), 941-950.

Fleming, S. A., Dyer, C. W., Eggington, J. (1999). A convenient one-step gingerol synthesis. *Synthetic Communications*, 29(11), 1933-1939.

Gaikwad, D. D., Shinde, S. K., Kawade, A. V., Jadhav, S. J., Gadhave, M. V. (2017). Isolation and standardization of gingerol from ginger rhizome by using TLC, HPLC, and identification tests. *The Pharma Innovation*, 6(2, Part C), 179-182.

Haque, N., Salma, U., Nurunnabi, T. R., Uddin, M. J., Jahangir, M. F., Islam, S. M., Kamruzzaman, M. (2011). Management of type 2 diabetes mellitus by lifestyle, diet and medicinal plants. *Pakistan Journal of Biological Sciences*, 14(1), 13-24.

Hiserodt, R. D., Franzblau, S. G., Rosen, R. T. (1998). Isolation of 6-, 8-, and 10-Gingerol from Ginger Rhizome by HPLC and Preliminary Evaluation of Inhibition of Mycobacterium a vium and Mycobacterium tuberculosis. *Journal of Agricultural and Food Chemistry*, 46(7), 2504-2508.

Hui, H., Zhao, X., Perfetti, R. (2005). Structure and function studies of glucagon-like peptide-1 (GLP-1): the designing of a novel pharmacological agent for the treatment of diabetes. *Diabetes/Metabolism Research and Reviews*, 21(4), 313-331.

Iranloye, B. O., Arikawe, A. P., Rotimi, G., Sogbade, A. O. (2011). Anti-diabetic and anti-oxidant effects of Zingiber officinale on alloxan-induced and insulin-resistant diabetic male rats. *Nigerian Journal of Physiological Sciences*, 26(1), 89-96.

Isa, Y., Miyakawa, Y., Yanagisawa, M., Goto, T., Kang, M. S., Kawada, T., Morimitsu, Y., Kubota, K., Tsuda, T. (2008). 6-Shogaol and 6-gingerol, the pungent of ginger, inhibit TNF-α mediated downregulation of adiponectin expression via different mechanisms in 3T3-L1 adipocytes. *Biochemical and Biophysical Research Communications*, 373(3), 429-434.

Ji, K., Fang, L., Zhao, H., Li, Q., Shi, Y., Xu, C., Wang, Y., Du, L., Wang, J., Liu, Q. (2017). Ginger oleoresin alleviated γ-ray irradiation-induced reactive oxygen species via the Nrf2 protective response in human mesenchymal stem cells. *Oxidative Medicine and Cellular Longevity*, 2017, 1480294.

Jung, M. Y., Lee, M. K., Park, H. J., Oh, E. B., Shin, J. Y., Park, J. S., Jung, S. Y., Oh, J. H., Choi, D. S. (2018). Heat-induced conversion of gingerols to shogaols in ginger as affected by heat type (dry or moist heat), sample type (fresh or dried), temperature and time. *Food Science and Biotechnology*, 27, 687-693.

Kim, Y. H., Nguyen, H. T., Ding, Y., Park, S. H., Choi, E. M. (2007). Effect of [6]-gingerol, a pungent ingredient of ginger, on osteoblast response to extracellular reducing sugar. *Food Science and Biotechnology*, 16(5), 807-811.

Kooti, W., Farokhipour, M., Asadzadeh, Z., Ashtary-Larky, D., Asadi-Samani, M. (2016). The role of medicinal plants in the treatment of diabetes: a systematic review. *Electronic Physician*, 8(1), 1832.

Kubra, I. R., Mohan Rao, L. J. (2012). Microwave drying of ginger (Z ingiber officinale R oscoe) and its effects on polyphenolic content and antioxidant activity. *International Journal of Food Science & Technology*, 47(11), 2311-2317.

Kumar, N. V., Srinivas, P., Bettadaiah, B. K. (2012). New scalable and eco-friendly synthesis of gingerols. *Tetrahedron Letters*, 53(24), 2993-2995.

Lamuchi-Deli, N., Aberomand, M., Babaahmadi-Rezaei, H., Mohammadzadeh, G. (2017). Effects of the hydroalcoholic extract of Zingiber officinale on arginase I activity and expression in the retina of streptozotocin-induced diabetic rats. *International Journal of Endocrinology and Metabolism*, 15(2), e42161.

Lee, J. O., Kim, N., Lee, H. J., Moon, J. W., Lee, S. K., Kim, S. J., Kim, J. K., Park, S. H., Kim, H. S. (2015). [6]-Gingerol Affects Glucose Metabolism by Dual Regulation via the AMPKα2-Mediated AS160–Rab5 Pathway and AMPK-Mediated Insulin Sensitizing Effects. *Journal of Cellular Biochemistry*, 116(7), 1401-1410.

Li, Y., Tran, V. H., Duke, C. C., Roufogalis, B. D. (2012). Gingerols of Zingiber officinale enhance glucose uptake by increasing cell surface GLUT4 in cultured L6 myotubes. *Planta Medica*, 78(14), 1549-1555.

Li, Y., Tran, V. H., Kota, B. P., Nammi, S., Duke, C. C., Roufogalis, B. D. (2014). Preventative effect of Zingiber officinale on insulin resistance in a high-fat high-carbohydrate diet-fed rat model and its mechanism of action. *Basic & Clinical Pharmacology & Toxicology*, 115(2), 209-215.

Ma, R. H., Ni, Z. J., Zhu, Y. Y., Thakur, K., Zhang, F., Zhang, Y. Y., Wei, Z. J. (2021). A recent update on the multifaceted health benefits associated with ginger and its bioactive components. *Food & Function*, 12(2), 519-542.

Ma, S., Zhang, S., Duan, W., Wang, W. (2009). An enantioselective synthesis of (+)-(S)-[n]-gingerols via the l-proline-catalyzed aldol reaction. *Bioorganic & Medicinal Chemistry Letters*, 19(14), 3909-3911.

Mahluji, S., Attari, V. E., Mobasseri, M., Payahoo, L., Ostadrahimi, A., Golzari, S. E. (2013). Effects of ginger (Zingiber officinale) on plasma glucose level, HbA1c and insulin sensitivity in type 2 diabetic patients. *International Journal of Food Sciences and Nutrition*, 64(6), 682-686.

Mao, Q. Q., Xu, X. Y., Cao, S. Y., Gan, R. Y., Corke, H., Beta, T., Li, H. B. (2019). Bioactive compounds and bioactivities of ginger (Zingiber officinale Roscoe). *Foods*, 8(6), 185.

Masuda, Y., Kikuzaki, H., Hisamoto, M., Nakatani, N. (2004). Antioxidant properties of gingerol related compounds from ginger. *Biofactors*, 21(1-4), 293-296.

Namekata, I., Hamaguchi, S., Wakasugi, Y., Ohhara, M., Hirota, Y., Tanaka, H. (2013). Ellagic acid and gingerol, activators of the sarco-endoplasmic reticulum Ca2+-ATPase, ameliorate diabetes mellitus-induced diastolic dysfunction in isolated murine ventricular myocardia. *European Journal of Pharmacology*, 706(1-3), 48-55.

Nammi, S., Sreemantula, S., Roufogalis, B. D. (2009). Protective effects of ethanolic extract of Zingiber officinale rhizome on the development of metabolic syndrome in high-fat diet-fed rats. *Basic & Clinical Pharmacology & Toxicology*, 104(5), 366-373.

Ogurtsova, K., da Rocha Fernandes, J. D., Huang, Y., Linnenkamp, U., Guariguata, L., Cho, N. H., Cavan, D., Shaw, J. E., Makaroff, L. E. (2017). IDF Diabetes Atlas: Global estimates for the prevalence of diabetes for 2015 and 2040. *Diabetes Research and Clinical Practice*, 128, 40-50.

Oludoyin, A. P., Adegoke, S. R. (2014). Effect of ginger (Zingiber officinale) extracts on blood glucose in normal and streptozotocin-induced diabetic rats. *International Journal of Clinical Nutrition*, 2(2), 32-35.

Otunola, G. A., Afolayan, A. J. (2015). Antidiabetic effect of combined spices of Allium sativum, Zingiber officinale and Capsicum frutescens in alloxan-induced diabetic rats. *Frontiers in Life Science*, 8(4), 314-323.

Packer, L., Wachtel-Galor, S., Ong, C. N., Halliwell, B. (Eds.). (2004). *Herbal and Traditional Medicine: Biomolecular and Clinical Aspects*. CRC Press.

Pajvani, U. B., Accili, D. (2015). The new biology of diabetes. *Diabetologia*, 58, 2459-2468.

Prasad, S., Tyagi, A. K. (2015). Ginger and its constituents: role in prevention and treatment of gastrointestinal cancer. *Gastroenterology Research and Practice*, 2015, 142979.

Priya Rani, M., Padmakumari, K. P., Sankarikutty, B., Lijo Cherian, O., Nisha, V. M., Raghu, K. G. (2011). Inhibitory potential of ginger extracts against enzymes linked to type 2 diabetes, inflammation and induced oxidative stress. *International Journal of Food Sciences and Nutrition*, 62(2), 106-110.

Rani, M. P., Krishna, M. S., Padmakumari, K. P., Raghu, K. G., Sundaresan, A. (2012). Zingiber officinale extract exhibits antidiabetic potential via modulating glucose uptake, protein glycation and inhibiting adipocyte differentiation: an in vitro study. *Journal of the Science of Food and Agriculture*, 92(9), 1948-1955.

Salihu, M., Ajayi, B. O., Adedara, I. A., De Souza, D., Rocha, J. B. T., Farombi, E. O. (2017). 6-Gingerol-rich fraction from Zingiber officinale ameliorates carbendazim-induced endocrine disruption and toxicity in testes and epididymis of rats. *Andrologia*, 49(5), e12658.

Samad, M. B., Mohsin, M. N. A. B., Razu, B. A., Hossain, M. T., Mahzabeen, S., Unnoor, N., Muna, I. A., Akhter, F., Kabir, A. U., Hannan, J. M. A. (2017). [6]-Gingerol, from Zingiber officinale, potentiates GLP-1 mediated glucose-stimulated insulin secretion pathway in pancreatic β-cells and increases RAB8/RAB10-regulated membrane presentation of GLUT4 transporters in skeletal muscle to improve hyperglycemia in Leprdb/db type 2 diabetic mice. *BMC Complementary and Alternative Medicine*, 17(1), 1-13.

Sampath, C., Rashid, M. R., Sang, S., Ahmedna, M. (2017). Specific bioactive compounds in ginger and apple alleviate hyperglycemia in mice with high fat diet-induced obesity via Nrf2 mediated pathway. *Food Chemistry*, 226, 79-88.

Saraswat, M., Suryanarayana, P., Reddy, P. Y., Patil, M. A., Balakrishna, N., Reddy, G. B. (2010). Antiglycating potential of Zingiber officinalis and delay of diabetic cataract in rats. *Molecular Vision*, 16, 1525.

Sattar, N. A., Hussain, F., Iqbal, T., Sheikh, M. A. (2012). Determination of in vitro antidiabetic effects of Zingiber officinale Roscoe. *Brazilian Journal of Pharmaceutical Sciences*, 48, 601-607.

Schadich, E., Hlaváč, J., Volná, T., Varanasi, L., Hajdúch, M., Džubák, P. (2016). Effects of ginger phenylpropanoids and quercetin on Nrf2-ARE pathway in human BJ fibroblasts and HaCaT keratinocytes. *BioMed Research International*, 2016, 2173275.

Schwertner, H. A., Rios, D. C. (2007). High-performance liquid chromatographic analysis of 6-gingerol, 8-gingerol, 10-gingerol, and 6-shogaol in ginger-containing dietary supplements, spices, teas, and beverages. *Journal of Chromatography B*, 856(1-2), 41-47.

Semwal, R. B., Semwal, D. K., Combrinck, S., Viljoen, A. M. (2015). Gingerols and shogaols: important nutraceutical principles from ginger. *Phytochemistry Letters*, 117, 554-568.

Sharma, S., Shukla, M. K., Sharma, K. C., Tirath, Kumar, L., Anal, J. M. H., Upadhyay, S. K., Bhattacharyya, S., Kumar, D. (2022). Revisiting the therapeutic potential of gingerols against different pharmacological activities. *Naunyn-Schmiedeberg's Archives of Pharmacology*, 396(4), 633-647.

Singh, A. B., Akanksha, S. N., Maurya, R., Srivastava, A. K. (2009). Anti-hyperglycaemic, lipid lowering and anti-oxidant properties of [6]-gingerol in db/db mice. *International Journal of Medical Sciences*, 1(12), 536-544.

Son, M. J., Miura, Y., Yagasaki, K. (2015). Mechanisms for antidiabetic effect of gingerol in cultured cells and obese diabetic model mice. *Cytotechnology*, 67, 641-652.

Wang, S., Zhang, C., Yang, G., Yang, Y. (2014). Biological properties of 6-gingerol: a brief review. *Natural Product Communications*, 9(7), 1934578X1400900736.

Wang, Z., Thurmond, D. C. (2009). Mechanisms of biphasic insulin-granule exocytosis–roles of the cytoskeleton, small GTPases and SNARE proteins. *Journal of Cell Science*, 122(7), 893-903.

Yadav, A. K., Garg, A. (2019). Antidiabetic effects of [10]-gingerol in streptozotocin-and high-fat diet-induced diabetic rats. *Asian Journal of Pharmaceutical and Clinical Research*, 12, 77-80.

Yatoo, M. I., Saxena, A., Gopalakris, A., Alagawany, M., Dhama, K. (2017). Promising antidiabetic drugs, medicinal plants and herbs: An update. *International Journal of Pharmacology*, 13(7), 732-745.

Yeh, H. Y., Chuang, C. H., Chen, H. C., Wan, C. J., Chen, T. L., Lin, L. Y. (2014). Bioactive components analysis of two various gingers (Zingiber officinale Roscoe) and antioxidant effect of ginger extracts. *LWT-Food Science and Technology*, 55(1), 329-334.

Zhu, Y., Zhao, Y., Wang, P., Ahmedna, M., Sang, S. (2015). Bioactive ginger constituents alleviate protein glycation by trapping methylglyoxal. *Chemical Research in Toxicology*, 28(9), 1842-1849.

Chapter 12

Organo-Sulphur Compounds for the Management of Diabetes Mellitus

Ritika Singh*
and Neha Singh
Galgotias College of Pharmacy, Galgotias University, Greater Noida, Uttar Pradesh, India

Abstract

Diabetes mellitus is a chronic metabolic disorder characterized by elevated blood glucose levels due to inadequate insulin production or utilization. This condition affects a substantial global population, with its prevalence on the rise. In recent times, natural products have garnered increasing attention as potential alternative treatments for diabetes mellitus. Among these, organo-sulphur compounds stand out as a promising class that holds potential for managing this condition. Numerous studies have showcased the efficacy of organo-sulphur compounds in lowering blood glucose levels, enhancing insulin sensitivity, and preventing diabetes-associated complications. These compounds are naturally present in various sources, including garlic, onions, and cruciferous vegetables. Mechanistic insights suggest that their mode of action involves stimulating insulin secretion, amplifying insulin sensitivity, and improving glucose metabolism. Organo-sulphur compounds offer several distinct advantages as a supplementary therapy for diabetes mellitus. Notably, they boast attributes such as minimal toxicity, cost-effectiveness, and the potential for synergistic use alongside established anti-diabetic medications. However, in order to fully comprehend their mechanism of action and unlock their therapeutic potential, further in-depth research is imperative.

* Corresponding Author's Email: ritika.singh.rs18@gmail.com.

In: Naturally Occurring Chemicals …
Editors: A. Singh Grewal, G. Deswal, A. Kumar Dhingra et al.
ISBN: 979-8-89113-491-1

Keywords: organo-sulphur compounds, diabetes mellitus, natural products, insulin sensitivity, glucose metabolism

Abbreviations

AITC	Allyl isothiocyanate
Akt	Ak strain transforming
AMP	Adenosine monophosphate
AMPK	Adenosine monophosphate-activated protein kinase
DM	Diabetes mellitus
DMSO	Dimethyl sulfoxide
DPP-4	Dipeptidyl peptidase-4
GLP-1	Glucagon-like peptide-1
GLUT	Glucose transporter
GSK-3	Glycogen synthase kinase-3
HbA1c	*Haemoglobin A1C*
IDDM	Insulin-dependent diabetic mellitus
IRS	Insulin receptor substrate
NIDDM	Non-insulin dependent diabetic mellitus
Nrf2	Nuclear factor erythroid 2-related factor 2
PI3K	Phosphatidylinositol-3-kinase
PPAR	Peroxisome proliferator-activated receptor
SAC	S-allyl cysteine
SGLT-2	Sodium-glucose cotransporter-2
SOD	Superoxide dismutase.

Introduction

Diabetes mellitus (DM) is a chronic metabolic disorder characterized by hyperglycemia resulting from defects in insulin secretion, insulin action, or both. It has emerged as a significant health challenge worldwide, affecting populations in developed and developing countries alike. DM is commonly classified into two main types: insulin-dependent diabetes mellitus (IDDM) and non-insulin-dependent diabetes mellitus (NIDDM). Its global impact is substantial, with an estimated 463 million adults affected in 2019, a number projected to surge to 700 million by 2045 (International Diabetes Federation, 2019). The present therapeutic approaches for diabetes encompass lifestyle modifications, oral hypoglycemic agents, injectable medications, and insulin treatment (American Diabetes Association, 2021). Nevertheless, these treatments have inherent limitations, including side effects, cost implications, and challenges related to sustained efficacy (Sharma et al., 2021). Consequently, there is a pressing need for alternative therapies that are not only safe and efficacious but also economically viable. Currently, treatment strategies for diabetes comprise lifestyle adjustments and pharmacological interventions. Lifestyle modifications encompass dietary changes, physical activity, and weight management, all aimed at enhancing insulin sensitivity, reducing insulin resistance, and stabilizing blood glucose levels (American Diabetes Association, 2021). However, the adoption of these changes necessitates significant behavioral shifts, and adherence can be problematic for some individuals. Oral hypoglycemic agents, a category of medications with diverse mechanisms of action, serve to lower blood glucose levels. They achieve this by stimulating insulin secretion, curtailing glucose production by the liver, and bolstering insulin sensitivity (American Diabetes Association, 2021). This group includes sulfonylureas, biguanides, alpha-glucosidase inhibitors, DPP-4 inhibitors, GLP-1 receptor agonists, and SGLT-2 inhibitors. Injectable medications involve GLP-1 receptor agonists and amylin mimetics, which are administered subcutaneously (American Diabetes Association, 2021). For patients with type 1 diabetes or advanced type 2 diabetes unresponsive to other treatments, insulin therapy is employed. This approach seeks to replicate physiological insulin secretion to maintain glucose homeostasis (American Diabetes Association, 2021). Despite the array of options available, the drawbacks associated with current treatments, such as side effects, costs, and limited long-term effectiveness, underscore the necessity for alternative therapeutic avenues (Sharma et al., 2021). Diverse alternative treatments have been explored in the realm of diabetes management, including herbal remedies, probiotics, and organosulfur compounds. Among these, organosulfur compounds have garnered attention for their potential impact. These naturally occurring compounds are found in various foods, including garlic, onions, and cruciferous vegetables (Sharma et al., 2021). Known for their multifaceted health benefits, including anti-inflammatory, antioxidant, and anticancer properties (Kumar et al., 2013), organosulfur compounds have recently emerged as potential contributors to diabetes management. Specific compounds like allyl sulfides, diallyl disulfide, and diallyl trisulfide have shown promise in improving glucose homeostasis, augmenting insulin secretion, and mitigating insulin resistance (Sharma et al., 2021). These compounds exert their effects through modulation of key signaling pathways integral to glucose metabolism, including the AMP-activated protein kinase (AMPK) pathway, peroxisome proliferator-activated receptor (PPAR) pathway, and nuclear factor erythroid 2-related factor 2 (Nrf2) pathway (Sharma et al., 2021).

Organo-Sulphur Compounds

Organosulfur compounds comprise a diverse array of molecules, both natural and synthetic, characterized by the presence of at least one sulfur atom bound to a carbon atom. These compounds are ubiquitously distributed in the natural world and can be sourced from a wide spectrum of foods, including fruits, garlic, onions, cruciferous vegetables, spices, and select grains (Akash et al., 2014). Beyond their culinary significance, these compounds have also found utility in the synthesis of pharmaceuticals, agrochemicals, and various industrial products (Sharma et al., 2021). Of late, organosulfur compounds have garnered escalating attention for their potential health-promoting properties, particularly in the realm of diabetes mellitus management.

Sources of Organo-Sulphur Compounds

Organo-sulfur compounds constitute a substantial and diverse assemblage of molecules that can be categorized based on their distinctive chemical structures. This group encompasses various classes of compounds, including thioethers, thioesters, thioketones, thioamides, sulphides, sulfoxides, and sulfones. These compounds are widespread in the natural world and are present in a range of organisms, spanning plants, animals, and microorganisms (Gruhlke et al., 2020). Their existence spans both natural and synthetic domains, with certain natural sources standing out prominently. Notably, garlic, onions, and cruciferous vegetables like broccoli and cabbage are recognized reservoirs of organo-sulfur compounds, the most notable among them being allicin, diallyl disulfide, and S-allyl cysteine (Jaiswal et al., 2015). These compounds emerge when the vegetables undergo crushing or chopping, thus contributing to the distinct aroma and flavor characterizing these edible items (Sharma et al., 2021). Moreover, they wield substantial influence over a multitude of physiological processes, encompassing the regulation of redox equilibrium, enzyme activities, and gene expression (Akash et al., 2014).

Chemical Properties and Structures

The chemical characteristics of organo-sulfur compounds are primarily dictated by the inherent attributes of the sulfur atom and the functional groups that are affixed to it. For instance, thioethers like methanethiol are characterized by a distinct and somewhat unpleasant odor, whereas the sulfoxide dimethyl sulfoxide (DMSO) is frequently employed as a solvent due to its pronounced polarity and remarkable capacity to dissolve a broad spectrum of both organic and inorganic substances (Sharma et al., 2021). This class of compounds showcases a diverse array of chemical architectures, spanning from elementary entities like hydrogen sulfide (H_2S) to more intricate entities like thiosulfates, thiocyanates, and sulfoxides (Jaiswal et al., 2015). The sulfur atom within these compounds exhibits an aptitude for forming covalent bonds with an array of other elements, encompassing carbon, hydrogen, oxygen, and nitrogen, thus giving rise to an assortment of distinct chemical properties and configurations (Gruhlke et al., 2020). The configurations of organo-sulfur compounds can fluctuate significantly, encompassing straightforward linear chains to intricate cyclic arrangements. Among the most renowned organo-sulfur compounds is allicin, sourced from garlic, and it has been evidenced to exert a diverse spectrum of biological effects, ranging from antibacterial and antifungal attributes to antitumor properties (Kumar et al., 2013).

Bioavailability and Metabolism

The bioavailability and metabolism of organo-sulfur compounds exhibit significant variability contingent on the particular compound and the mode of administration. While certain compounds, like DMSO, boast high bioavailability and are promptly assimilated by the body, others, such as sulforaphane, necessitate specific enzymes for activation and are subject to swift degradation within the body (Sharma et al., 2021). The liver chiefly orchestrates the metabolic fate of organo-sulfur compounds, entailing a sequence of chemical transformations that may yield reactive intermediates like sulfenic acids and thiyl radicals. These reactive entities subsequently engage with other molecules in the body, giving rise to a range of diverse biological consequences (Kumar et al., 2013). Following absorption, enzymes in the liver shepherd the metabolism of organo-sulfur compounds, catalyzing their conversion into an assortment of metabolites endowed with distinct biological functionalities (Akash et al., 2014). Subsequently, these metabolites can be excreted via urine or bile pathways.

Effects of Organo-Sulphur Compounds on Insulin Secretion and Sensitivity

Organo-sulfur compounds have exhibited insulinotropic and insulin-mimetic effects, underscoring their potential as therapeutic agents for diabetes. Numerous studies have highlighted the capacity of organo-sulfur compounds, abundant in sources like garlic, onions, and other Allium vegetables, to bolster insulin release from pancreatic β-cells and enhance insulin sensitivity in peripheral tissues. Likewise, allyl isothiocyanate (AITC), present in cruciferous vegetables, has demonstrated the ability to amplify insulin sensitivity in animal models of diabetes (Liu et al., 2016). Additional organo-sulfur compounds, such as sulforaphane and S-allyl cysteine (SAC), have shown the propensity to influence the activity of enzymes integral to glucose metabolism. Sulforaphane, present in cruciferous vegetables, has been identified as a promoter of gene expression related to glucose uptake and utilization in human liver cells (Bahadoran et al., 2019). In a similar vein, SAC, sourced from garlic, has exhibited the capacity to augment the activity of glucose metabolism-associated enzymes, both in vitro and in animal models (Sharma et al., 2014).

Role of Organo-Sulphur Compounds in Glucose Metabolism

Organo-sulfur compounds found in Allium vegetables have been documented to modulate glucose metabolism through diverse mechanisms. For instance, sulforaphane has demonstrated the ability to enhance glucose metabolism by elevating the activity of the antioxidant enzyme superoxide dismutase (SOD) in animal models of diabetes (Bahadoran et al., 2019). These compounds exhibit the capacity to activate the insulin signaling pathway, thereby augmenting cellular glucose uptake. Moreover, they are observed to impede gluconeogenesis, the hepatic process responsible for generating glucose from non-carbohydrate sources. Furthermore, organo-sulfur compounds have been noted for their antioxidative and anti-inflammatory effects, which serve to amplify their favorable impacts on glucose metabolism. Antioxidants function by neutralizing free radicals and mitigating oxidative stress, a factor implicated in the development of insulin resistance and type 2 diabetes. Meanwhile, anti-inflammatory agents have the potential to alleviate chronic low-grade inflammation, another factor associated with insulin resistance. In sum, the mechanisms underpinning the efficacy of organo-sulfur compounds in diabetes mellitus management are intricate, encompassing the modulation of insulin secretion, insulin sensitivity, glucose metabolism, oxidative stress, and inflammation.

Evidence from Preclinical Studies

Preclinical investigations have yielded valuable insights into the potential therapeutic properties of organo-sulfur compounds in relation to diabetes mellitus. In vitro findings have substantiated the insulin-mimetic and insulinotropic effects of these compounds. For instance, diallyl disulfide, a constituent of garlic, has been documented to stimulate insulin secretion from pancreatic β-cells by activating voltage-gated K+ channels (Kim et al., 2011). Likewise, S-allyl cysteine, another compound derived from garlic, has been observed to enhance insulin sensitivity by activating the AMP-activated protein kinase (AMPK) pathway (Kim et al., 2011). In vivo studies have further corroborated the anti-diabetic potential of organo-sulfur compounds. For instance, a study by Khan et al., (2019) revealed that the administration of garlic extract to streptozotocin-induced diabetic rats resulted in improved glucose homeostasis, reduced insulin resistance, and diminished oxidative stress. Another study conducted by Ali et al., (2017) reported that oral administration of onion extract to diabetic rats led to enhanced glucose uptake, decreased insulin resistance, and lowered inflammation.

Synergistic Effects of Organo-Sulphur Compounds and Anti-Diabetic Drugs

Studies have also explored the potential synergistic effects of organo-sulfur compounds when used in conjunction with anti-diabetic drugs. Ashraf et al., (2019) demonstrated that the co-administration of metformin, a commonly prescribed anti-diabetic medication, along with garlic extract led to improved glucose homeostasis and reduced insulin resistance in diabetic rats. Similarly, Ali et al., (2020) conducted a study showing that combining glibenclamide, another anti-diabetic drug, with onion extract resulted in enhanced glucose metabolism and decreased insulin resistance in diabetic rats. These preclinical investigations offer compelling evidence for the potential therapeutic benefits of organo-sulfur compounds in the context of diabetes mellitus. However, further research is needed to determine the optimal dosage, duration, and method of administration of these compounds in human subjects.

Evidence from Clinical Studies

Clinical studies provide valuable information about the protection and effectiveness of organo-sulphur compounds in managing DM. The following section will discuss the results of some of the clinical trials conducted to date.

Clinical Trials Evaluating the Safety and Efficacy of Organo-Sulphur Compounds in Managing DM

Several clinical trials have explored the impact of organo-sulfur compounds on diabetes mellitus. For instance, a randomized, double-blind, placebo-controlled study aimed to assess the effects of garlic extract on glycemic control among patients with type 2 diabetes (Ashraf et al., 2013). This study involved 60 participants who were randomly assigned to either receive garlic extract or a placebo for a duration of 12 weeks. The results revealed that garlic extract significantly reduced fasting blood glucose levels and HbA1c levels compared to the placebo. Another experimental trial investigated the effects of onion extract on glycemic control in individuals with type 1 diabetes (Mollazadeh et al., 2018). The trial included 30 participants who were randomly divided into two groups, one receiving onion extract and the other receiving a placebo for an 8-week period. The findings demonstrated that onion extract led to a significant reduction in fasting blood glucose levels and HbA1c levels compared to the placebo. Likewise, a randomized, double-blind, placebo-controlled study was conducted to examine the impact of black seed (Nigella sativa) on glycemic control in patients with type 2 diabetes (Ahmad et al., 2013). In this trial, 94 participants were randomly assigned to either the black seed group or the placebo group for a duration of 3 months. The results indicated that black seed extract significantly lowered fasting blood glucose levels and HbA1c levels compared to the placebo.

Limitations and Challenges of Clinical Studies

In spite of the promising outcomes observed in these clinical trials, there exist certain limitations and challenges inherent in conducting studies involving organo-sulfur compounds. One of the primary challenges revolves around ensuring the consistency and standardization of the preparations utilized in these investigations. This task is particularly crucial due to the fact that the chemical composition and effectiveness of organo-sulfur compounds can vary based on the source and method of preparation. Additionally, a notable challenge arises from the relatively small sample sizes often encountered in clinical trials conducted thus far. This limitation restricts the extent to which the findings can be extrapolated to broader populations. Collectively, while the evidence gleaned from clinical studies remains somewhat constrained, the results do indicate the potential utility of organo-sulfur compounds as a supplementary approach to managing diabetes mellitus. Subsequent research is imperative to comprehensively assess both the safety and effectiveness of these compounds, while also addressing the intrinsic limitations and challenges that accompany clinical investigations involving them.

Future Research Directions

Organo-sulphur compounds have emerged as promising candidates in both preclinical and clinical studies, suggesting their potential as valuable adjunctive treatments for diabetes mellitus. While further investigation is needed to thoroughly elucidate their mechanisms of action and determine optimal dosing strategies, an accumulating body of evidence suggests that these compounds could yield substantial advantages in diabetes management. Future research avenues might encompass exploring potential synergies between organo-sulphur compounds and existing anti-diabetic medications, as well as investigating their compatibility with lifestyle interventions such as dietary modifications and physical activity regimens. Furthermore, in-depth studies may be warranted to ascertain the most effective formulations and dosages of organo-sulphur compounds for diabetes management, alongside a comprehensive assessment of their long-term safety and efficacy. Overall, the prospective benefits that organo-sulphur compounds could confer in diabetes management hold significant implications for clinical practice. While current diabetes treatments often yield positive outcomes, they can also introduce notable side effects and may not be universally suitable. The integration of organo-sulphur compounds as complementary therapeutic options could present a safe and efficacious alternative, particularly for patients who cannot tolerate or find relief from conventional treatments.

Conclusion

Diabetes mellitus is an enduring global health challenge that affects a substantial number of individuals worldwide, with its prevalence escalating in both developed and developing nations. Despite considerable strides in comprehending its underlying mechanisms and devising treatment strategies, diabetes mellitus persists as a significant concern. Effectively managing this condition demands a multifaceted strategy involving lifestyle adaptations, pharmaceutical interventions, and consistent monitoring and follow-up. While conventional therapies like insulin and oral hypoglycaemic agents remain fundamental, there's a mounting fascination with alternative and complementary remedies in the domain of diabetes management. In this chapter, we've delved into the potential of organo-sulphur compounds as a supplementary avenue for addressing diabetes mellitus. These naturally occurring compounds, abundant in foods like garlic and onions, have demonstrated a diverse array of effects beneficial to insulin secretion, insulin sensitivity, glucose uptake, and oxidative stress mitigation. Organo-sulphur compounds stand as an auspicious realm of investigation in the realm of diabetes mellitus management. Though further research is warranted to completely fathom their potential benefits and constraints in diabetes management, the prevailing evidence strongly indicates that these compounds hold substantial promise as adjunctive therapies. As our comprehension of their mechanisms of action and optimal dosages advances, healthcare practitioners could potentially proffer safer and more efficacious treatment alternatives to individuals grappling with diabetes. In this light, organo-sulphur compounds may emerge as valuable complementary modalities for diabetes treatment, constituting a crucial component of a comprehensive approach to managing this multifaceted condition.

References

Ahmad, A., Husain, A., Mujeeb, M., Khan, S. A., Najmi, A. K., Siddique, N. A., Damanhouri, Z. A., Anwar, F. (2013). A review on therapeutic potential of Nigella sativa: A miracle herb. *Asian Pacific Journal of Tropical Biomedicine*, 3(5), 337-352.

Akash, M. S., Rehman, K., Chen, S. (2014). Role of sulphur-containing compounds in the prevention and management of diabetes mellitus. *Nutrition & Diabetes*, 4(8), e125.

Ali, M. M., Ahmed, S. A., Ahmed, A. S., Ahmed, O. M., El-Shehawi, A. M. (2017). Onion extract improves blood glucose and lipid profiles, antioxidative capacity, and cecal microflora in streptozotocin-induced diabetic rats. *International Journal of Biological Macromolecules*, 104, 1272-1282.

Ali, M. M., Ahmed, S. A., El-Shehawi, A. M., Ahmed, O. M. (2020). Onion extract exerts synergistic effects with glibenclamide on glucose metabolism and insulin resistance in diabetic rats. *Biomedicine & Pharmacotherapy*, 124, 109890.

Ali, M. M., El-Shehawi, A. M., Ahmed, O. M. (2018). Onion extract improves glycaemic control and lipid profile in patients with type 1 diabetes: A randomized placebo-controlled clinical trial. *Journal of Medicinal Food*, 21(5), 469-476.

American Diabetes Association. (2021). Standards of medical care in diabetes 2021. *Diabetes Care*, 44(Suppl 1), S1-S232.

Ashraf, H., Mahboob, T., Sultana, S. (2019). Antidiabetic and synergistic effects of metformin and Allium cepa extract on streptozotocin-induced diabetic rats. *Journal of Food Biochemistry*, 43(8), e12963.

Ashraf, R., Aamir, K., Shaikh, A. R., Ahmed, T. (2013). Effects of garlic on dyslipidaemia and glucose control in type 2 diabetes mellitus: A randomized controlled trial. *Journal of Ayub Medical College Abbottabad*, 25(1-2), 16-19.

Ashraf, R., Khan, R. A., Ashraf, I., Qureshi, A. A. (2013). Effects of Allium sativum (garlic) on systolic and diastolic blood pressure in patients with essential hypertension. *Pakistan Journal of Pharmaceutical Sciences*, 26(5), 859–863.

Bahadoran, Z., Mirmiran, P., Hosseinpanah, F., Hedayati, M., Hosseinpour-Niazi, S., Azizi, F. (2019). Broccoli sprouts powder improves hepatic glucose metabolism in type 2 diabetes mellitus: A randomized double-blind placebo-controlled clinical trial. *Journal of Functional Foods*, 54, 10-17.

Gruhlke, M. C., Schäfer, H., Jacobsen, I. D. (2020). Organo-sulphur compounds in food and medicine. *Journal of Molecular Sciences*, 25(23), 5526.

Huang, T., Li, X., Xie, Z., Cao, J. (2015). Garlic for treating hypercholesterolemia. A meta-analysis of randomized clinical trials. *Annals of Family Medicine*, 13(6), 555-563.

International Diabetes Federation. (2019). IDF Diabetes Atlas, 9th edn. *International Diabetes Federation*. https://www.diabetesatlas.org.

Jaiswal, N., Kumar, S., Sharma, B. (2015). Anti-diabetic potential of sulphur-containing compounds. *Journal of Diabetes and Metabolic Disorders*, 14(1), 58.

Khan, M. S., Jahan, N., Ahmad, I. (2019). Antidiabetic effect of garlic (Allium sativum L.) extract in streptozotocin-induced diabetic rats. *Pakistan Journal of Pharmaceutical Sciences*, 32(2), 739-744.

Kim, J. Y., Kwon, O., Jung, H. A. (2011). S-allyl cysteine isolated from garlic attenuates diabetic nephropathy by improving oxidative stress and renal inflammatory cytokines in mice. *Food and Chemical Toxicology*, 49(3), 590-597.

Kong, K. W., Khoo, H. E., Prasad, K. N., Ismail, A., Tan, C. P., Rajab, N. F. (2010). Revealing the power of the natural red pigment lycopene. *Molecules*, 15(10), 959-987.

Kumar, R., Sasmal, D., Mazumder, K. (2013). Garlic: A review on potential therapeutic benefits as an adjunct to conventional therapy for diabetes, obesity, and related disorders. *Food & Function*, 4(3), 375-383.

Liu, Y., Li, Y., Liu, X., Zhao, X., Zhong, W. (2016). Allyl isothiocyanate improves insulin sensitivity and glucose metabolism in high-fat-diet-induced obese mice. *Journal of Agricultural and Food Chemistry*, 64(16), 3333-3340.

Mollazadeh, H., Hosseinzadeh, H., Mehri, S. (2018). Effects of garlic extract and its constituents on blood glucose and lipid levels in diabetic and diabetic rats. *Journal of Traditional and Complementary Medicine*, 8(3), 432–437.

Sharma, A. K., Mithal, A., Majumdar, A. (2021). Organosulfur compounds for the management of diabetes mellitus: A comprehensive review. *Journal of Diabetes and Metabolic Disorders*, 20(1), 1-18.

Chapter 13

Steroidal Derivatives in the Management of Diabetes Mellitus

Neha Singh[1,*]
Ananya Pandey[2]
Saumya Das[2]
and Avijit Mazumder[2]
[1]Galgotias College of Pharmacy, Galgotias University, Greater Noida, Uttar Pradesh, India
[2]Noida Institute of Engineering and Technology (Pharmacy Institute), Greater Noida, Uttar Pradesh, India

Abstract

Diabetes mellitus (DM) is a persistent metabolic disorder marked by elevated blood glucose levels stemming from either insufficient insulin production or resistance to its effects. Despite the array of available treatment options, DM remains a significant global health issue, with a surging prevalence and the accompanying complications. The exploration of steroidal derivatives as potential therapeutic interventions for DM management has gained momentum due to their multifaceted pharmacological attributes, encompassing anti-inflammatory, immunomodulatory, and metabolic properties. This chapter offers a synopsis of recent strides in utilizing steroidal derivatives for DM treatment, encompassing glucocorticoids, mineralocorticoids, and sex hormones. Furthermore, we spotlight the hurdles and limitations tied to employing steroidal derivatives in DM management, encompassing their adverse effects and possible

* Corresponding Author's Email: singh21neha24@gmail.com.

In: Naturally Occurring Chemicals …
Editors: A. Singh Grewal, G. Deswal, A. Kumar Dhingra et al.
ISBN: 979-8-89113-491-1

interactions with concurrent medications. Nonetheless, burgeoning evidence points to the potential of steroidal derivatives as adjunctive or alternative strategies for DM therapy, particularly among patients dealing with insulin resistance or concurrent medical conditions. Further exploration is imperative to discern the optimal dosing, duration, and safety profiles of these compounds in real-world clinical scenarios. As the understanding of their potential benefits and drawbacks grows, steroidal derivatives could usher in a novel dimension of diabetes management, catering to a diverse range of patients' needs.

Keywords: steroidal derivatives, diabetes mellitus, glucocorticoids, mineralocorticoids, glucose homeostasis

Abbreviations

DHEA	Dehydroepiandrosterone
DM	Diabetes mellitus
PPARs	Peroxisome proliferator-activated receptor
T2DM	Type 2 diabetes mellitus.

Introduction

Diabetes mellitus (DM), a persistent metabolic condition, is characterized by elevated blood glucose levels resulting from faulty insulin secretion, insulin activity, or both. In 2019, the global count of adults afflicted with DM reached approximately 463 million, with its prevalence growing at a concerning pace (International Diabetes Federation, 2019). Despite the array of available treatment options, effectively managing DM remains a formidable challenge. As a result, alternative therapeutic avenues are being explored, including the potential of steroidal derivatives (Chaudhary et al., 2020). The rationale behind investigating steroidal derivatives as a therapeutic approach for DM stems from their demonstrated antidiabetic properties (Yu et al., 2019). This can be attributed to their capacity to modulate diverse metabolic pathways implicated in maintaining glucose homeostasis. Specifically, these compounds can bolster insulin sensitivity, promote glucose uptake, and impede gluconeogenesis (Jafarpour et al., 2019). Additionally, steroidal derivatives harbor anti-inflammatory and antioxidant attributes that assume a pivotal role in DM pathogenesis. The anti-inflammatory effects help counter insulin resistance, while their antioxidant prowess guards against oxidative stress, a hallmark of DM development (Das et al., 2021). Ursolic acid emerges as a compelling example of a steroidal derivative with promising antidiabetic potential. Research indicates that ursolic acid can enhance insulin sensitivity, augment glucose uptake, and curtail hepatic glucose release (Jafarpour et al., 2019). The compound's anti-inflammatory and antioxidant attributes further contribute to its antidiabetic efficacy. Spironolactone, a synthetic aldosterone antagonist primarily employed for hypertension and edema management, also demonstrates promise in DM control. Studies suggest that spironolactone can enhance glycemic regulation by heightening insulin sensitivity, mitigating insulin resistance, and reducing hepatic glucose production (Singh et al., 2020). Beyond ursolic acid and spironolactone, other steroidal derivatives like dehydroepiandrosterone (DHEA), pregnenolone, and vitamin D exhibit antidiabetic properties (García-Sánchez et al., 2021). DHEA, produced by the adrenal glands, has displayed efficacy in enhancing glucose tolerance, amplifying insulin sensitivity, and quelling inflammation (Falahi et al., 2020). Pregnenolone, a neurosteroid lauded for its anti-inflammatory attributes, has demonstrated the ability to heighten insulin sensitivity and facilitate glucose uptake (Das et al., 2021). Furthermore, vitamin D, a steroid hormone pivotal for bone health and calcium metabolism, has been linked to improved glycemic control and reduced insulin resistance through research (Teegarden & Donkin, 2009).

Glucocorticoids in DM Management

Glucocorticoids constitute a category of steroid hormones synthesized within the adrenal glands. They play a pivotal role in governing diverse physiological functions, encompassing glucose metabolism, immune response, and stress management (Liu et al., 2021). Endogenous glucocorticoids, such as cortisol, are inherently produced by the body. In contrast, synthetic counterparts like prednisone and dexamethasone, endowed with anti-inflammatory and immunosuppressive attributes, find application in addressing an array of conditions, including diabetes mellitus (DM) (Guo et al., 2019).

Mechanisms of Action in Glucose Homeostasis and Insulin Sensitivity

Glucocorticoids play a vital role in upholding glucose homeostasis and insulin sensitivity. They orchestrate glucose metabolism by elevating hepatic glucose production, curtailing glucose uptake in peripheral tissues, and promoting gluconeogenesis (Rizza & Mandarino, 2013). Additionally, glucocorticoids dampen insulin signaling by diminishing insulin receptor expression and compromising insulin receptor efficacy. Consequently, this leads to diminished glucose uptake and utilization by peripheral tissues, culminating in hyperglycemia (Joshi & Bhatt, 2019).

Clinical Evidence and Potential Benefits and Risks

The utilization of glucocorticoids in the management of DM remains a subject of debate. While glucocorticoids possess robust anti-inflammatory and immunosuppressive attributes, their impact on glucose metabolism and insulin sensitivity can exacerbate glycemic control in individuals with DM. Studies indicate that even brief utilization of glucocorticoids can result in noteworthy elevations in blood glucose levels (Guo et al., 2019). Consequently, concerns have arisen regarding the potential hazards linked to glucocorticoid usage in DM patients. However, counterbalancing this, mounting evidence suggests potential benefits of glucocorticoids in DM treatment. For instance, investigations have unveiled that administering glucocorticoids in low doses can amplify insulin sensitivity and diminish insulin resistance among DM patients (Joshi & Bhatt, 2019). Furthermore, glucocorticoids might harbor anti-inflammatory effects capable of mitigating the risk of DM-associated complications, like cardiovascular diseases and nephropathy (Guo et al., 2019).

Mineralocorticoids in DM Management

Mineralocorticoids constitute a class of steroid hormones synthesized within the adrenal glands. Apart from their role in glucose metabolism, these hormones significantly contribute to the regulation of electrolyte equilibrium, particularly with regards to sodium and potassium levels, and the maintenance of blood pressure (Goldberg & Jessup, 2019). The principal endogenous mineralocorticoid is aldosterone, which primarily acts on the kidneys, stimulating the reabsorption of sodium and the excretion of potassium. Synthetic mineralocorticoids, like fludrocortisone, are employed for their capacity to retain salt and are utilized in treating diverse conditions such as adrenal insufficiency and orthostatic hypotension (Lifton & Geller, 2017).

Role in Sodium and Water Balance and Blood Pressure Regulation

Mineralocorticoids, exemplified by aldosterone, play a pivotal role in maintaining sodium and water equilibrium and regulating blood pressure (Wang et al., 2021). Aldosterone specifically acts on the distal tubules and collecting ducts within the kidneys, prompting the reabsorption of sodium and the excretion of potassium. This process culminates in an increase in extracellular fluid volume and subsequently elevates blood pressure. This mechanism holds paramount importance in upholding normal blood pressure levels and safeguarding against dehydration (Lifton & Geller, 2017).

Effects on Glucose Metabolism and Insulin Sensitivity

While the precise impact of mineralocorticoids on glucose metabolism and insulin sensitivity remains somewhat elusive, certain studies have hinted at aldosterone's potential role in insulin resistance, potentially through the hindrance of glucose uptake and utilization in peripheral tissues (Hanslik et al., 2017). On the contrary, other investigations have proposed that aldosterone might yield favorable consequences on glucose metabolism. This could involve the stimulation of insulin secretion and the enhancement of pancreatic beta-cell functionality (Luther & Brown, 2018). However, the exact mechanisms underpinning these effects are not yet fully elucidated and call for further scrutiny (Luther & Brown, 2018).

Clinical Evidence and Potential Benefits and Risks

The exact role of mineralocorticoids in DM management remains uncertain. While certain studies propose that aldosterone might play a role in insulin resistance and disrupted glucose metabolism in DM, other investigations suggest its potential benefits in enhancing pancreatic beta-cell function and insulin secretion. However, the utilization of exogenous mineralocorticoids like fludrocortisone for DM management is not recommended. This is due to their salt-retaining characteristics, which can trigger hypertension and fluid retention (Hanslik et al., 2017).

Sex Hormones in DM Management

Androgens are primarily synthesized in the testes in males and the adrenal glands in females. They play a role in regulating glucose homeostasis and insulin sensitivity. On the other hand, estrogens are predominantly produced in the ovaries in females and have shown both insulin-sensitizing and glucose-lowering effects. Progestins, synthesized mainly in the ovaries in females, have demonstrated both insulin-sensitizing and insulin-resistant effects, contingent upon the dosage and duration of treatment (Liu et al., 2018; Ferrannini et al., 2021).

Effects of Sex Hormones on Glucose Homeostasis and Insulin Sensitivity

The effects of sex hormones, specifically androgens, on glucose homeostasis and insulin sensitivity are intricate and influenced by multiple factors, including hormone type, dosage, treatment duration, and individual sex and hormonal status. Androgens have been demonstrated to negatively impact glucose metabolism and insulin sensitivity in both men and women (Pitteloud et al., 2005). In contrast, estrogens have been found to enhance insulin sensitivity and improve glucose metabolism in individuals of both sexes (Sowers et al., 2008). Meanwhile, progestins have displayed varying effects on insulin sensitivity, being either insulin-sensitizing or insulin-resistant, contingent upon the administered dose and treatment duration (Liu et al., 2018).

Clinical Evidence and Potential Benefits and Risks

The use of sex hormones in the management of DM remains a subject of ongoing investigation, and their potential advantages and risks are not yet firmly established. Studies have produced conflicting outcomes regarding the impact of androgen deprivation therapy in men with prostate cancer on the risk of developing DM (Smith, 2008). While certain studies suggest an increased risk, others propose that testosterone replacement therapy in hypogonadal men might enhance insulin sensitivity and glucose metabolism (Snyder et al., 2016). For postmenopausal women, estrogen utilization has been associated with a reduced risk of DM development; however, determining the optimal treatment dose and duration remains elusive (Sowers et al., 2008). In the case of progestins, like medroxyprogesterone acetate, high doses and prolonged treatment durations have been demonstrated to hinder glucose metabolism and insulin sensitivity (Liu et al., 2018).

Mechanisms of Action of Steroidal Derivatives in DM Management

When insulin binds to its receptor on the surface of target cells, it initiates a intricate signaling cascade that eventually results in the uptake of glucose into cells and the suppression of glucose production in the liver (Saltiel et al., 2021). Other hormones and signaling pathways, including glucagon, adiponectin, leptin, and peroxisome proliferator-activated receptors (PPARs), also play a role in regulating glucose metabolism and insulin sensitivity (Stolarczyk et al., 2021). Insulin resistance develops when insulin fails to efficiently stimulate glucose uptake and utilization in target tissues like muscle, liver, and adipose tissue. Consequently, the pancreas produces more insulin to counterbalance the reduced sensitivity of target tissues, leading to hyperinsulinemia. Over time, this can cause beta-cell dysfunction and impaired insulin secretion, ultimately resulting in the onset of type 2 diabetes (Kahn et al., 2014). Steroidal derivatives, such as glucocorticoids, have the potential to impact various pathways involved in glucose metabolism and insulin sensitivity. Specifically, glucocorticoids have been demonstrated to increase glucose production in the liver while concurrently inhibiting glucose uptake in peripheral tissues. These actions can contribute to the development of hyperglycemia and insulin resistance (Majithia et al., 2018). Mineralocorticoids, on the other hand, not only play a role in regulating sodium and water balance but also influence glucose metabolism and insulin sensitivity. The primary mineralocorticoid, aldosterone, may elevate insulin resistance and impede glucose uptake in peripheral tissues through the activation of the renin-angiotensin-aldosterone system (Goodfriend et al., 2011). Nonetheless, certain studies propose that mineralocorticoid antagonists like spironolactone and eplerenone might benefit glycemic control and insulin sensitivity in individuals with type 2 diabetes due to their anti-inflammatory and vasodilatory properties (Struthers et al., 2014). Sex hormones, encompassing androgens, estrogens, and progestins, also play a role in regulating glucose metabolism and insulin sensitivity. Androgens like testosterone have been linked to reduced insulin sensitivity in certain studies, potentially affecting adipose tissue and muscle metabolism (Pasquali et al., 2011). Estrogens, on the other hand, have been associated with improved insulin sensitivity and glycemic control in certain studies, possibly through their effects on adipose tissue and the PPAR signaling pathway (Gomez-Sanchez et al., 2016). However, the role of progestins in glucose metabolism and insulin sensitivity remains not fully elucidated, warranting further research to understand their impact on the management of diabetes (De Leo et al., 2011).

Challenges and Limitations

Adverse Effects and Safety Concerns

While steroidal derivatives might offer potential benefits for managing DM, their utilization comes with associated risks. For example, glucocorticoids have been linked to adverse metabolic effects, including weight gain, hypertension, dyslipidemia, and glucose intolerance, particularly with prolonged usage (Saunders et al., 2016). Conversely, mineralocorticoids may contribute to issues like sodium and water retention, electrolyte imbalances, and hypertension, which could further exacerbate existing cardiovascular risk factors in individuals with DM (Khan et al., 2019). Furthermore, the utilization of sex hormones in DM management could potentially heighten the likelihood of thromboembolic events, especially among older women with pre-existing cardiovascular conditions (de Candia et al., 2018). As such, it is imperative to meticulously balance the potential benefits and risks associated with employing steroidal derivatives in DM management and to closely monitor patients for any adverse effects.

Interactions with Other Medications and Potential Drug-Drug Interactions

Steroidal derivatives have the potential to interact with other medications frequently employed in DM management, possibly resulting in undesirable outcomes or modified therapeutic outcomes. For instance, glucocorticoids could heighten the chances of hypoglycemia in individuals using insulin or other hypoglycemic agents, and might also diminish the efficacy of certain antihyperglycemic drugs like metformin (Majithia et al., 2018). Moreover, mineralocorticoid antagonists might similarly interact with particular antihyperglycemic agents.

Patient Selection and Individualized Therapy

Given the diverse nature of DM, it holds significance to identify patients who are likely to derive the most benefit from steroidal derivative therapy. For instance, glucocorticoids might show greater effectiveness in individuals with type 2 DM who also contend with inflammatory conditions like rheumatoid arthritis or lupus (Saunders et al., 2016). Mineralocorticoids could be considered for patients having both DM and hypertension as comorbidities (Khan et al., 2019). Moreover, personalized treatment strategies are pivotal to enhance treatment outcomes while mitigating the risk of adverse effects. This could involve customizing the dosage and treatment duration based on the patient's requirements, routinely monitoring blood glucose levels and other pertinent biomarkers, and making therapy adjustments as deemed necessary (Khan et al., 2019).

Cost-Effectiveness and Access to Treatment

The expense associated with steroidal derivative therapy could present a barrier to accessibility for certain patients, especially those lacking insurance coverage or facing financial constraints. Additionally, the cost-effectiveness of these therapies in comparison to other treatments for DM remains uncertain and warrants further investigation (Khan et al., 2019). Initiatives aimed at enhancing access to steroidal derivative therapy and promoting its cost-effective utilization might encompass negotiating reduced drug costs, expanding insurance coverage, and formulating guidelines for appropriate utilization. Thoughtful consideration of individual patient factors, vigilant monitoring of potential adverse effects, and endeavors to enhance treatment accessibility can collectively contribute to optimizing the potential advantages of these therapies for individuals with DM (Khan et al., 2019).

Conclusion

While steroidal derivatives hold promise for the management of DM, their utilization is not devoid of limitations and challenges. It's important to closely monitor adverse effects, such as weight gain and hypertension, in patients undergoing glucocorticoid and mineralocorticoid therapies. The intricacies of how steroidal derivatives influence glucose metabolism and insulin sensitivity are intricate and warrant further investigation. Subsequent studies should strive to elucidate the underlying molecular and cellular pathways at play, as well as potential mechanisms of action. Clinicians must exercise caution regarding potential adverse effects and interactions with other medications when contemplating the use of steroidal derivatives in DM patients. The future direction of research in this field should focus on shedding light on mechanisms of action and exploring potential combination therapies to enhance the management of DM.

References

Chaudhary, P., Chaudhary, P. (2020). Steroidal derivatives as therapeutic agents in the management of diabetes mellitus: a review. *Steroids*, 163, 108697.

De Fronzo, R. A., Tripathy, D. (2009). Skeletal muscle insulin resistance is the primary defect in type 2 diabetes. *Diabetes Care*, 32(Supplement 2), S157-S163.

Ferrannini, E., Natali, A., Bellastella, G. (2021). Androgens and glucose metabolism in men and women. *Endocrine Reviews*, 42(3), 401-438.

García-Sánchez, J. R., García-Sánchez, E., García-González, J. J., García-González, A. (2021). Steroids beyond ursolic acid and spironolactone: Dehydroepiandrosterone, pregnenolone, and vitamin D as new antidiabetic agents. *Molecules*, 26(5), 1445.

Guo, L., Meng, R., Tang, J. (2019). Glucocorticoids in the treatment of diabetes mellitus. *International Journal of Endocrinology*, 2019, 1-11.

Hanslik, G., Wallaschofski, H., Dietz, A., Rettig, R., Baumeister, S. E., Völzke, H. (2017). Aldosterone and glucose metabolism: A review of the evidence. *Hormone and Metabolic Research*, 49(10), 757-763.

Joshi, S. R., Bhatt, H. (2019). Glucocorticoid use in diabetes mellitus: Is there still a role? *Indian Journal of Endocrinology and Metabolism*, 23(6), 610-614.

Kahn, S. E., Cooper, M. E., Del Prato, S. (2014). Pathophysiology and treatment of type 2 diabetes: perspectives on the past, present, and future. *Lancet*, 383(9922), 1068-1083.

Khan, M. H., Khan, S., Rahman, A. A., Islam, M. T., Islam, M. T. (2019). Steroidal derivatives: An emerging class of therapeutics for the management of diabetes mellitus. *Frontiers in Pharmacology*, 10, 380.

Lifton, R. P., Geller, D. S. (2017). Molecular mechanisms of human hypertension. *Cell*, 171(3), 557-571.

Liu, H., Yao, Y., Wang, W., Fu, C., Meng, L. (2018). Progestins and insulin resistance. *Endocrine, Metabolic & Immune Disorders-Drug Targets*, 18(2), 168-175.

Liu, J. J., Ching, A. L. S. (2021). Steroidal derivatives: potential modulators of glucose metabolism and insulin sensitivity. *European Journal of Medicinal Chemistry*, 211, 113070.

Liu, Y., Liu, Y., Cao, X., Ji, B. (2021). Glucocorticoids in physiological and pathological conditions: new insights and therapeutic implications. *Frontiers in Endocrinology*, 12, 652619.

Luther, J. M., Brown, N. J. (2018). The renin-angiotensin-aldosterone system and glucose homeostasis. *Trends in Pharmacological Sciences*, 39(7), 624-633.

Pitteloud, N., Hardin, M., Dwyer, A. A., Valassi, E., Yialamas, M., Elahi, D. (2005). Increasing insulin resistance is associated with a decrease in Leydig cell testosterone secretion in men. T*he Journal of Clinical Endocrinology & Metabolism*, 90(5), 2636-2641.

Rizza, R. A., Mandarino, L. J. (2013). Cortisol-induced insulin resistance in man: Impaired suppression of glucose production and stimulation of glucose utilization due to a postreceptor detect of insulin action. *Journal of Clinical Endocrinology and Metabolism*, 75(1), 131-138.

Saltiel, A. R., Kahn, C. R. (2021). Insulin signaling and the regulation of glucose and lipid metabolism. *Nature*, 414(6865), 799-806.

Saunders, E. A., Oliver, T. F., Wahid, S. T. (2016). Glucocorticoids and type 2 diabetes: from physiology to pathology. *Journal of Diabetes & Metabolic Disorders*, 15(1), 1-11.

Smith, M. R. (2008). Androgen deprivation therapy and risk for diabetes and cardiovascular disease in prostate cancer survivors. *Current Urology Reports*, 9(3), 197-202.

Snyder, P. J., Bhasin, S., Cunningham, G. R., Matsumoto, A. M., Stephens-Shields, de Candia, P., Prattichizzo, F., Garavelli, S., De Rosa, V., Galgani, M., Di Rella, F., Ceriello, A., Matarese, G. (2018). Hormonal and metabolic interplay in the regulation of immunity and inflammation. *Reviews in Endocrine & Metabolic Disorders*, 19(3), 235-254.

Stolarczyk, E. (2021). Hormonal regulation of glucose homeostasis. *International Journal of Molecular Sciences*, 22(9), 4567.

Teegarden, D., Donkin, S. S. (2009). Vitamin D: emerging new roles in insulin sensitivity. *Nutrition Research Reviews*, 22(1), 82-92.

Wang, W., Gomez-Sanchez, C. E. (2021). Mineralocorticoid receptor antagonists: Their current use and future prospects. *International Journal of Molecular Sciences*, 22(13), 6702.

Yu, L., Zhang, W., Jin, Y., Yang, H. (2019). Recent advances in steroidal anti-diabetic agents. *Steroids*, 149, 108411.

Chapter 14

Saponins as Potential Therapeutic Agents for Diabetes Mellitus Management

Deepshi Arora[1,*]
Manish Kumar[2]
Yugam Taneja[3]
Anjali Sharma[1]
Aakriti Saini[1]
Diksha Gulati[1]
and Sharad Visht[4]
[1]Guru Gobind Singh College of Pharmacy, Yamuna Nagar, Haryana, India
[2]School of Pharmaceutical Sciences, C. T. University, Ludhiana, Punjab, India
[3]Zeon Lifesciences Ltd, Paonta Sahib, Himachal Pradesh, India
[4]Tishk International University, Erbil, Kurdistan Region, Iraq

Abstract

Diabetes mellitus (DM) is a major global public health concern, marked by chronic hyperglycemia due to insufficient insulin secretion or activity. The World Health Organization (WHO) predicts that by 2025, over 300 million people worldwide will have diabetes, particularly in low- and middle-income countries where healthcare access is limited. The current synthetic drugs and insulin used for treatment are expensive, hard to access in remote areas, and carry significant side effects. Thus, exploring alternative methods like phytochemicals from medicinal plants, which possess hypoglycemic properties, is crucial.

---

* Corresponding Author's Email: aroradeepshi1992@gmail.com.

In: Naturally Occurring Chemicals …
Editors: A. Singh Grewal, G. Deswal, A. Kumar Dhingra et al.
ISBN: 979-8-89113-491-1

Saponins, a group of phytochemicals with diverse structural and metabolic functions, hold promise as anti-diabetic agents. This chapter delves into saponins, their sources in various plants, and their potential benefits in treating diabetes. Adipokine secretion dysregulation has been linked to type 2 diabetes and insulin resistance. It's imperative to investigate these natural compounds to provide effective, accessible, and safer treatments for diabetes.

Keywords: saponins, diabetes, insulin, phytochemicals, adipokines, hyperglycemia, anti-diabetic

Abbreviations

AMPK	AMP-activated protein kinase
ASP	Acylation stimulating protein
DM	Diabetes mellitus
GSK	Glycogen synthase kinase
JAK-STAT	Janus kinase-signal transducer and activator of transcription
MAPK	Mitogen-activated protein kinase
mRNA	Messenger ribonucleic acid
p-STAT3	Phosphorylated signal transducer and activator of transcription-3
STZ	Streptozotocin
TNF	Tumour necrosis factor
WHO	World health organization.

Introduction

Diabetes mellitus (DM) is a chronic metabolic disorder arising from reduced insulin levels or insulin resistance, causing elevated blood glucose levels (LeRoith et al., 2019). It ranks as the fifth fastest-growing global ailment, with an estimated 300 million individuals presently affected and a projected prevalence of 5.4% by 2025 (El Ghoul et al., 2012). In response to costly and adverse chemically derived medications, approximately 80% of people worldwide are turning to plant-based treatments containing phytoconstituents for diabetes management (Srinivasan, 2005). This underscores the significance of seeking novel plant-derived therapies, as saponins, as an additional metabolite in known anti-diabetic plants, have contributed to their hypoglycemic effects (El Barky et al., 2017). Thus, a strategic exploration and assessment of saponins can potentially advance improved diabetes treatments. Saponins, widely distributed in plants and named after their soap-like properties ("sapo" in Latin), have found extensive pharmaceutical use due to their medicinal attributes (Marrelli et al., 2016). Recent studies showcase saponins' various pharmacological potentials, including immune enhancement, antibacterial, antioxidant, anticancer, anti-diabetic, and anti-obesity properties. The use of saponin in the pharmaceutical sector is widespread due to the discovery of its medicinal qualities (Vinarov et al., 2018). Current efforts are focusing on harnessing saponins for more potent phytomedicines to manage type II diabetes effectively. These endeavors highlight saponins' versatile role in advancing medical treatments, especially for diabetes management.

Chemical Nature of Saponins

Saponins are intricate chemical compounds characterized by high-molecular-weight glycosides linked to an aglycone moiety. These glycosides can encompass sugars like xylose, rhamnose, galactose, glucose, or methyl pentose. The aglycone moiety, devoid of sugars, varies chemically from the glycone part and is positioned in proximity (Desai et al., 2009). Saponins fall into two primary groups based on their composition: triterpenoid saponins and steroid saponins. Their aglycone moieties exhibit distinct structures. Triterpenoid saponins feature a triterpene aglycone, comprising six isoprene units, while steroid saponins incorporate a steroid aglycone with a characteristic four-ring structure. This chemical diversity underpins their utility in diverse applications, serving as natural surfactants, foaming agents, and emulsifiers (Faizal & Geelen, 2013). The categorization of saponins into neutral and acidic types hinges on their chemical structure. Neutral saponins encompass a triterpenoid aglycone linked to sugar chains, commonly present in plants like soybeans, ginseng, and licorice. In contrast, acidic saponins possess a steroid backbone with spirostane or furostane side chains, often accompanied by carboxylic acid groups that confer acidity. These acidic saponins are found in animal sources such as fish, sea cucumbers, starfish, and some plants.

Mechanism of Antidiabetic Action of Saponins

Saponins, complex molecules composed of high-molecular-weight glycosides like xylose, rhamnose, galactose, glucose, or methyl pentose, are uniquely structured with chemically distinct aglycone and glycone portions closely linked. In the context of type II diabetes mellitus treatment, saponins show promise by influencing multiple organs including the intestine, liver, pancreas, adipose tissue, and skeletal muscle. Their actions encompass stimulating insulin secretion (Deshpande & Bhalsing, 2014), reducing insulin resistance, suppressing disaccharide activity, enhancing glycogen formation, curtailing glucose production, and modulating hormone synthesis in adipose tissue (Jimenez-Sanchez et al., 2017), collectively leading to decreased insulin levels. Saponins offer a potential therapeutic strategy for diabetes mellitus treatment. They exert their hypoglycemic effects through several mechanisms, including restoring insulin response and refining insulin signaling for improved glucose uptake and metabolism. Saponins elevate plasma insulin levels and prompt pancreatic insulin release, thereby lowering blood glucose. Their inhibition of disaccharide activity lessens glucose absorption, while promoting glycogen synthesis aids glucose storage in liver and muscle tissues. Furthermore, saponins hinder gluconeogenesis and the catalytic activity of α-glucosidase, an enzyme crucial in carbohydrate breakdown. These multifaceted mechanisms underscore saponins' potential as an effective therapeutic avenue for diabetes mellitus management (Guo et al., 2015).

Saponins Effective in the Management of Type II Diabetes

Arjunolic Acid

The plants *Terminalia arjuna, Cochlospermum tinctorium, Cornus capitata,* and *Leandra chaetodon* are notable sources of arjunolic acid, a triterpenoid saponin (Manna & Sil, 2012). This substance exhibits potent anti-diabetic effects by inhibiting α-glycosidase and reducing levels of reactive oxygen species. Furthermore, it has demonstrated the ability to decrease the activation of phospho-P38, NF-KB, and phospho-ERK1/2, while suppressing signal transduction pathways triggered by streptozotocin (STZ). This leads to the alleviation of diabetic symptoms (Manna, 2009).

Astragaloside IV

Astragaloside IV is a triterpenoid saponin with cycloartane characteristics that are obtained from the roots of *Astragalus membranaceus*. It has been identified as a potential diabetes treatment as it promotes insulin production, reduces the formation of free radicals, and inhibits the formation of glycation products (Agyemang et al., 2013). Additionally, it has been found to prevent the development of diabetic renal disease and inhibit peripheral nerve damage in rats induced with STZ-induced diabetes. Administration of Astragaloside IV at doses of 25 and 50 milligrams per kilogram via oral means was observed to significantly reduce blood glucose and lipid levels in diabetic mice. Furthermore, the expression of mRNA and protein was effectively blocked (Lu et al., 2015).

Charantin

Charantin, a steroid saponin extractable from Momordica charantia Linn seeds (Family: Cucurbitaceae), possesses the capacity to enhance insulin secretion, resulting in the effective reduction of blood glucose levels. This attribute positions it as a valuable therapeutic agent for diabetes management (Desai & Tatke, 2015).

Christinin-A

Zizyphus spina-christi L. leaves are employed for the extraction of the phytochemical christinin using a butanolic extraction technique. In animal models induced with STZ, this compound has demonstrated anti-diabetic effects. The anti-diabetic mechanism of christinin entails reducing blood glucose levels and inhibiting phosphorylase activity in the liver. Additionally, research has shown that administering christinin for four weeks leads to increased serum levels of pyruvate and glycogen (Michel, 2011).

Diosgenin

Diosgenin, derived from Dioscorea polygonoides, displays anti-diabetic effects in STZ-induced diabetic rats (Governa, 2018). In a different study, diosgenin isolated from Trigonella foenum-graecum exhibited reduced mRNA expression and inhibited triglyceride levels in HepG2 cells and diabetic obese rats. Furthermore, three weeks of feeding male diabetic rats with a 1% diosgenin-supplemented diet resulted in significantly lower plasma glucose levels, decreased liver glucose synthesis, and increased α-amylase activity in the proximal region of the small intestinal mucosa.

Elatosides G, H and I

In a Wistar rat oral glucose tolerance test, the phytochemicals extracted from the tender shoots and roots of Aralia elata Seem exhibited potent in vivo anti-diabetic activity (Roghani-Dehkordi et al., 2015).

Senegasaponins A, B and C

Senegasaponins A, B, and C, extracted from the tender shoots and roots of Aralia elata Seem (Family: Araliaceae), displayed robust anti-diabetic activity in a Wistar rat oral glucose tolerance test (Roghani-Dehkordi et al., 2015).

Ginsenosides

Ginsenosides, a diverse class of steroid saponins derived from ginseng (*Panax* spp.), exhibit hypoglycemic effects (Gaikwad et al., 2014). The carbohydrate portion of ginseng root extract contains numerous pannaxoides, demonstrating hypoglycemic efficacy in a mouse model of alloxan-induced diabetes (Jia et al., 2017). Isolated Quinquefolans A, B, and C from the roots also demonstrate anti-diabetic effects in mice (Jia et al., 2017). Recent research indicates that ginseng exerts an anti-diabetic impact, potentially due to insulin stimulation from pancreatic cells (Roghani-Dehkordi, 2018).

Gymnemic Acid

Derived from the *Gymnema sylvestre* plant, gymnemic acid, a triterpenoid glycoside, has demonstrated success in a diabetic rat model induced by a high-fat diet and STZ. This compound has exhibited the capacity to enhance insulin signal transduction and activate PI3K/AKT and AMPK-mediated signaling pathways in diabetic rats when administered at doses of 40–80 mg/kg/day. These actions lead to improved glucose uptake and utilization. These findings suggest the potential therapeutic utility of gymnemic acid in diabetes management (Gaikwad et al., 2014).

Momordin Ic

This compound originates from the methanol extract of the fruit of *Kochia scoparia* Linn. They have been observed to effectively reduce blood glucose levels and inhibit ethanol absorption in Wistar rats (Gaikwad et al., 2014).

28-O-Monoglucosides

The triterpenoid saponin sourced from *Gypsophila oldhamiana* Miq. (Caryophyllaceae) roots has demonstrated potent α-glucosidase inhibitory activity (Jia et al., 2017). Additionally, it possesses anti-amylase properties (Luo et al., 2008).

Platyconic Acid

Platyconic acid is a chemical compound obtained from Platycodi radix (Platycodon grandiflorum root). It has been demonstrated to function as a peroxisome proliferator activator in 3T3-L1 adipocytes, enhancing glucose absorption. This compound also elevates glycogen accumulation and reduces triacylglycerol levels in the liver, consequently lowering hepatic insulin levels. Furthermore, platyconic acid has been noted to stimulate adiponectin production in adipose tissue.

Prototinosaponin AIII and Pseudoprototinosaponin

Prototinosaponin AIII and pseudoprototinosaponin were extracted from the rhizomes of Anemarrhena asphodeloides Bunge. When evaluated in KK-Ay mice, these compounds exhibited insulin secretion-mimicking effects and impacted hepatic glycogenolysis and gluconeogenesis, suggesting their potential for enhancing diabetes medication development.

Role of Adipokines in Insulin Resistance and Glucose Metabolism

Obesity significantly elevates the risk of developing insulin resistance and type 2 diabetes, characterized by reduced tissue responsiveness to insulin. Among the responsive tissues, adipose tissue notably contributes to these conditions by storing triglycerides through mechanisms like enhancing lipogenesis and suppressing lipolysis. Insulin signaling initiates when insulin binds to its cell membrane receptor, activating the PI3K-AKT/PKB and Ras-MAPK pathways via IRS protein phosphorylation (Jung et al., 2014). Adipose tissue, a major player in obesity, is pivotal for insulin sensitivity regulation. In adipose tissue, insulin activates two primary pathways: the PI3K-AKT/PKB pathway, predominantly responsible for metabolic actions like glucose uptake via Glut 4 transporter translocation to the plasma membrane, and the MAPK pathway, associated with mitogenic and growth effects rather than metabolic ones (Brown et al., 2012). Adipokines, hormones secreted by adipose tissue, also exert a vital influence on insulin sensitivity. Obesity alters adipokine release. While some, such as resistin and visfatin, link to insulin resistance, others like adiponectin and leptin enhance insulin sensitivity. Inflammatory cytokines like TNF-alpha and IL-6, released from adipose tissue, are linked to insulin resistance and type 2 diabetes onset (Andrade-Oliveira et al., 2015). The disrupted secretion of adipokines due to obesity can contribute to insulin resistance and type 2 diabetes development by affecting pivotal insulin action signaling pathways like JAK2/STAT3, MAPK, PI3K, and AMPK. Identifying therapeutic agents capable of modulating adipokine secretion and function is crucial to enhance insulin sensitivity and prevent or treat type 2 diabetes. Saponins derived from various plant sources exhibit promise in adjusting insulin signaling and boosting insulin sensitivity. For instance, saponins from Panax notoginseng have demonstrated the ability to lower fasting blood glucose levels and enhance glucose homeostasis in KK-Ay mice. Saponin-rich extracts from Panax odoratum have ameliorated diabetes symptoms in STZ-induced diabetic rats, concurrently elevating superoxide dismutase activity. Additionally, these extracts exhibited inhibitory activity against α-glycosidase, a crucial enzyme in carbohydrate digestion and absorption

(Frühbeck et al., 2008). Thus, saponins hold potential therapeutic value for preventing and treating type 2 diabetes by modulating insulin signaling pathways and adipokine secretion (Uzayisenga et al., 2014).

Saponin' s Effect on Leptin

Saponins possess the ability to regulate energy metabolism by activating AMPK and influencing multiple signaling pathways also impacted by leptin, including JAK2/STAT3, MAPK, PI3K, and AMPK (Andrade-Oliveira et al., 2015). Notably, Panax notoginseng saponins have demonstrated the potential to enhance insulin and leptin sensitivity, yielding anti-hyperglycemic and anti-obesity effects. Similarly, the administration of tea saponins has been associated with reduced inflammation in adipose tissue, the liver, and the hypothalamus. Saponins present in tea and Yucca schidigera plants have showcased anti-obesity and anti-diabetic capabilities by enhancing the anorexigenic effects of central leptin administration and restoring leptin-phosphorylated signal transducer and activator of transcription-3 (p-STAT3) signaling in the arcuate nucleus. These saponins elevate insulin sensitivity, regulate energy balance, and control fat metabolism through AMP-activated protein kinase (AMPK) and PI3K signaling activation. Consequently, these findings suggest that saponins could serve as valuable anti-obesity medications by ameliorating insulin resistance and augmenting insulin sensitivity (Kucukkurt et al., 2015). Adiponectin, a protein hormone originating from adipocytes, holds a vital role in regulating metabolic processes such as blood sugar control and fatty acid oxidation. Its insufficiency has been associated with atherosclerosis and insulin resistance development, particularly among obese individuals and those with type 2 diabetes. Research indicates that administering adiponectin can lower blood glucose levels and heighten insulin sensitivity. However, further investigation is imperative to evaluate its safety and effectiveness in treating metabolic disorders. Animal studies propose that adiponectin deficiency triggers insulin resistance through reduced expression of AdipoR1 and AdipoR2, distinct receptors largely found in skeletal muscle. The diminished expression of AdipoR1 and AdipoR2 in obesity-related insulin resistance is believed to underlie adiponectin's anti-diabetic metabolic impacts (Kucukkurt et al., 2015; Al-Braich et al., 2014).

Effect of Saponins on Adiponectin

A study conducted on diabetic mice revealed that Chikusetsu saponin elevated adiponectin levels and improved the expression of neuronal AdipoR1 along with downstream molecules like AMPK and GSK-3 in a concentration-dependent manner. Platyconic acid, a saponin present in Platycodi radix, has been demonstrated to enhance insulin signaling and stimulate adiponectin expression in adipose tissue. The ASP system, which governs adipocyte triglyceride metabolism by facilitating glucose transport and triglyceride synthesis, might also contribute to this mechanism (Yadav et al., 2013; Bhavsar et al., 2009).

Recent research highlights an accumulating body of evidence from literature suggesting that saponin therapy holds the potential to elevate adiponectin levels, thereby potentially playing a crucial role in enhancing insulin sensitivity (Coelho et al., 2013). In a study involving diabetic mice, Chikusetsu saponin was discovered to elevate adiponectin levels and enhance the expression of neuronal AdipoR1, as well as downstream molecules like AMPK and GSK-3, in a concentration-dependent manner. Platyconic acid, a saponin derived from Platycodi radix, has demonstrated the ability to augment insulin signaling and stimulate adiponectin expression within adipose tissue. The ASP system, which governs adipocyte triglyceride metabolism by facilitating glucose transport and triglyceride synthesis, might also play a role in this context (Kwon et al., 2012). Adipsin, implicated in obesity and diabetes models, exhibits dysregulation. It is associated with the complement pathway and can enhance insulin secretion by generating the peptide complement 3a (C3a) through catalyzing the formation of C3 convertase via the alternative complement pathway. Adipsin achieves this by cleaving complement factor B, initiating the production of C3 convertase and generating various complement fragments, including C3a (Lo et al., 2014).

Saponin's Effect on Adipsin

Bhavsar et al.'s study reveals a significant increase in adipsin expression due to Helicteres isora saponins when compared to control db/db mice (Bhavsar et al., 2009). The association between Panax notoginseng saponins and complement factor 3 (C3) has also been investigated (Zhang et al., 2007). The positive influence of saponins on reducing hyperglycemia and improving insulin sensitivity is underscored by their ability to stimulate adipsin and C3 (Zhang et al., 2007).

Visfatin and Insulin Sensitivity

Research indicates that Helicteres isora and Panax notoginseng saponins have the potential to enhance the expression of adipsin and C3, resulting in decreased hyperglycemia and enhanced insulin sensitivity. Visfatin, which exhibits affinity for insulin receptors akin to insulin but binds at a distinct site, can trigger diverse signaling pathways, regulating insulin secretion and signaling within pancreatic beta cells. Furthermore, visfatin has been associated with TNFα-mediated insulin resistance through the NAD+/Sirt1/PTP1B pathway in adipocytes (Brown et al., 2008).

Saponin's Effect on Visfatin

Saponins have the capacity to activate the insulin transduction pathway by stimulating PI3K, protein kinase B (AKT), and MAPK, similar to visfatin. Macrostemonoside A, a steroidal saponin derived from the Allium genus, has been shown to enhance visfatin production and release, along with elevating mRNA levels in 3T3-L1 adipocytes in a dose- and time-dependent manner (Sobolewska et al., 2016).

Apelin and Insulin Sensitivity

Apelin, a 36-amino acid peptide, functions as an endogenous ligand for the G-protein-coupled receptor APJ, which is found in various human organs (Turer et al., 2012). Apelin and APJ play roles in regulating energy metabolism, fluid balance, cardiovascular function, and angiogenesis. Serum apelin levels exhibit an inverse relationship with insulin resistance and liver cirrhosis, while oxidative stress and inflammation elevate plasma apelin levels (Hurt et al., 2014). Beyond its involvement in insulin secretion, apelin influences glucose metabolism and insulin sensitivity. Research has demonstrated that apelin can lower fasting glucose levels and enhance glucose tolerance in in vivo mouse models. Apelin's impact on insulin sensitivity may extend beyond its role in glucose metabolism, requiring further investigation for a comprehensive understanding of the underlying mechanisms and potential therapeutic applications. In vitro studies utilizing C2C12 muscle cells have indicated that apelin can enhance glucose transport through the AMPK pathway. Moreover, ex vivo and in vitro studies have revealed that apelin contributes to increased Akt phosphorylation in muscle. These effects may contribute to apelin's potential to enhance insulin sensitivity and facilitate glucose uptake in the muscles of insulin-resistant and obese animals (Bertrand et al., 2015).

Conclusion

The potential of saponins as an anti-diabetic agent is indeed promising. With their historical use in various medicinal traditions and growing scientific interest, saponins have garnered attention for their diverse biological activities. Their hypoglycemic and antioxidant properties position them as a viable therapeutic avenue for diabetes management and prevention of related complications. Notably, saponins' hypocholesterolemic and hypotriglyceridemic effects hold potential for mitigating atherosclerosis risk in diabetic individuals. Additionally, their capacity to reduce body fat without inducing weight gain offers a favorable trait in an anti-diabetic agent. However, as outlined in the review, comprehensive research is necessary to assess the toxicological profile of saponins and potential adverse effects. Identifying specific saponin types and their mechanisms of action will be crucial for optimizing their therapeutic utility. In sum, saponins show substantial promise as an anti-diabetic agent, and further exploration may yield improved strategies for diabetes management and complication prevention.

References

Agyemang, K., Han, L., Liu, E., Zhang, Y., Wang, T., Gao, X. (2013). Recent advances in Astragalus membranaceus anti-diabetic research: pharmacological effects of its phytochemical constituents. *Evidence-Based Complementary and Alternative Medicine*, 2013, 654643.

Al-Braich, M. S., Al-Husaini, N. K., Saleh, S. H. (2014). Effect of adiponectin level in type II diabetic postmenopausal women compared to healthy women. *European Journal of Medicine*, 2014(1), 4-7.

Andrade-Oliveira, V., Câmara, N. O., Moraes-Vieira, P. M. (2015). Adipokines as drug targets in diabetes and underlying disturbances. *Journal of Diabetes Research*, 2015, 681612.

Bertrand, C., Valet, P., Castan-Laurell, I. (2015). Apelin and energy metabolism. *Frontiers in Physiology*, 6, 115.

Bhavsar, S. K., Singh, S., Giri, S., Jain, M. R., Santani, D. D. (2009). Effect of saponins from Helicteresisora on lipid and glucose metabolism regulating genes expression. *Journal of Ethnopharmacology*, 124(3), 426-433.

Blanco-Montenegro, I., De Ritis, R., Chiappini, M. (2007). Imaging and modelling the subsurface structure of volcanic calderas with high-resolution aeromagnetic data at Vulcano (Aeolian Islands, Italy). *Bulletin of Volcanology*, 69, 643-659.

Brown, J. E., Onyango, D. J., Ramanjaneya, M., Conner, A. C., Patel, S. T., Dunmore, S. J., Randeva, H. S. (2010). Visfatin regulates insulin secretion, insulin receptor signalling and mRNA expression of diabetes-related genes in mouse pancreatic β-cells. *Journal of Molecular Endocrinology*, 44(3), 171-178.

Brown, J. E. (2012). Dysregulated adipokines in the pathogenesis of type 2 diabetes and vascular disease. *British Journal of Diabetes & Vascular Disease*, 12(5), 249-254.

Cheok, C. Y., Salman, H. A. K., Sulaiman, R. (2014). Extraction and quantification of saponins: A review. *Food Research International*, 59, 16-40.

Coelho, M., Oliveira, T., Fernandes, R. (2013). Biochemistry of adipose tissue: an endocrine organ. *Archives of Medical Science*, 9(2), 191-200.

Desai, S. D., Desai, D. G., Kaur, H. (2009). Saponins and their biological activities. *Pharma Times*, 41(3), 13-16.

Desai, S., Tatke, P. (2015). Charantin: An important lead compound from Momordica charantia for the treatment of diabetes. *Journal of Pharmacognosy and Phytochemistry*, 3(6), 163-166.

El Barky, A. R., Hussein, S. A., Alm-Eldeen, A. E., Hafez, Y. A., Mohamed, T. M. (2017). Saponins and their potential role in diabetes mellitus. *Diabetes Management*, 7(1), 148-58.

El Ghoul, J., Smiri, M., Ghrab, S., Boughattas, N. A., Ben-Attia, M. (2012). Antihyperglycemic, antihyperlipidemic and antioxidant activities of traditional aqueous extract of Zygophyllum album in streptozotocin diabetic mice. *Pathophysiology*, 19(1), 35-42.

Faizal, A., Geelen, D. (2013). Saponins and their role in biological processes in plants. *Phytochemistry Reviews*, 12, 877-893.

Frühbeck, G. (2006). Intracellular signalling pathways activated by leptin. *Biochemical Journal*, 393(1), 7-20.

Gaikwad, S. B., Krishna Mohan, G., Sandhya Rani, M. (2014). Phytochemicals for diabetes management. *Pharmaceutical Crops*, 5, 11-28.

Governa, P., Baini, G., Borgonetti, V., Cettolin, G., Giachetti, D., Magnano, A. R., Miraldi, E., Biagi, M. (2018). Phytotherapy in the management of diabetes: a review. *Molecules*, 23(1), 105.

Hurt, R. T., EdakkanambethVarayil, J., Ebbert, J. O. (2014). New pharmacological treatments for the management of obesity. *Current Gastroenterology Reports*, 16, 1-8.

Jia, S., Shen, M., Zhang, F., Xie, J. (2017). Recent advances in Momordica charantia: functional components and biological activities. *International Journal of Molecular Sciences*, 18(12), 2555.

Jung, U. J., Choi, M. S. (2014). Obesity and its metabolic complications: the role of adipokines and the relationship between obesity, inflammation, insulin resistance, dyslipidemia and nonalcoholic fatty liver disease. *International Journal of Molecular Sciences*, 15(4), 6184-6223.

Kucukkurt, I., Dundar, Y. (2013). Effects of dietary Yucca schidigera supplementation on plasma leptin, insulin, iodated thyroid hormones and some biochemical parameters in rats. *Revue de Medecine Veterinaire*, 164(7), 362-367.

Kwon, D. Y., Kim, Y. S., Ryu, S. Y., Choi, Y. H., Cha, M. R., Yang, H. J., Park, S. (2012). Platyconic acid, a saponin from Platycodi radix, improves glucose homeostasis by enhancing insulin sensitivity in vitro and in vivo. *European Journal of Nutrition*, 51, 529-540.

Le Roith, D., Biessels, G. J., Braithwaite, S. S., Casanueva, F. F., Draznin, B., Halter, J. B., Sinclair, A. J. (2019). Treatment of diabetes in older adults: an Endocrine Society clinical practice guideline. *Journal of Clinical Endocrinology & Metabolism*, 104(5), 1520-1574.

Lo, J. C., Ljubicic, S., Leibiger, B., Kern, M., Leibiger, I. B., Moede, T., Kelly, M. E., Bhowmick, D. C., Murano, I., Cohen, P., Banks, A. S. (2014). Adipsin is an adipokine that improves β cell function in diabetes. *Cell*, 158(1), 41-53.

Lu, W. S., Li, S., Guo, W. W., Chen, L. L., Li, Y. S. (2015). Effects of Astragaloside IV on diabetic nephropathy in rats. *Genetics and Molecular Research*, 14(2), 5427-5434.

Luo, J. G., Ma, L., Kong, L. Y. (2008). New triterpenoid saponins with strong α-glucosidase inhibitory activity from the roots of Gypsophila oldhamiana. *Bioorganic & Medicinal Chemistry*, 16(6), 2912-2920.

Manna, P., Sil, P. C. (2012). Arjunolic acid: beneficial role in type 1 diabetes and its associated organ pathophysiology. *Free Radical Research*, 46(7): 815-30.

Manna, P., Sinha, M., Sil, P. C. (2009). Prophylactic role of arjunolic acid in response to streptozotocin mediated diabetic renal injury: activation of polyol pathway and oxidative stress responsive signaling cascades. *Chemico-Biological Interactions*, 181(3), 297-308.

Marrelli, M., Conforti, F., Araniti, F., Statti, G. A. (2016). Effects of saponins on lipid metabolism: A review of potential health benefits in the treatment of obesity. *Molecules*, 21(10), 1404.

Michel, C. G., Nesseem, D. I., Ismail, M. F. (2011). Anti-diabetic activity and stability study of the formulated leaf extract of Zizyphus spina-christi (L.) Willd with the influence of seasonal variation. *Journal of Ethnopharmacology*, 133(1), 53-62.

Roghani-Dehkordi, F., Roghani, M., Baluchnejadmojarad, T. (2015). Diosgenin mitigates streptozotocin diabetes-induced vascular dysfunction of the rat aorta: the involved mechanisms. *Journal of Cardiovascular Pharmacology*, 66(6), 584-592.

Sobolewska, D., Michalska, K., Podolak, I., Grabowska, K. (2016). Steroidal saponins from the genus Allium. *Phytochemistry Reviews*, 15, 1-35.

Srinivasan, K. (2005). Plant foods in the management of diabetes mellitus: spices as beneficial anti-diabetic food adjuncts. *International Journal of Food Sciences and Nutrition*, 56 (6), 399-414.

Turer, A. T., Scherer, P. E. (2012). Adiponectin: mechanistic insights and clinical implications. *Diabetologia*, 55, 2319-2326.

Vinarov, Z., Radeva, D., Katev, V., Tcholakova, S., Denkov, N. (2018). Solubilisation of hydrophobic drugs by saponins. *Indian Journal of Pharmaceutical Sciences*, 80(4), 709-718.

Yadav, A., Kataria, M. A., Saini, V., Yadav, A. (2013). Role of leptin and adiponectin in insulin resistance. *Clinica Chimica Acta*, 417, 80-84.

Zhang, J. H., Wang, J. P., Wang, H. J. (2007). Clinical study on effect of total panax notoginseng saponins on immune-related inner environment imbalance in rheumatoid arthritis patients. *Chinese Journal of Integrated Traditional and Western Medicine*, 27(7), 589-592.

Chapter 15

The Role of Catechins in Diabetes and Its Complications

Surbhi Gupta[1]
Prabhat Singh[2,*]
Vaishali Negi[2]
and Bhupesh Sharma[3]
[1]Department of Pharmacology, School of Pharmacy, Bharat Institute of Technology, Meerut, Uttar Pradesh, India
[2]Faculty of Pharmacy, Swami Vivekanand Subharti University, Meerut, Uttar Pradesh, India
[3]Department of Pharmacology, Amity Institute of Pharmacy, Amity University, Noida, Uttar Pradesh, India

Abstract

Diabetes mellitus, characterized by prolonged hyperglycemia, is a complex metabolic disorder affecting nearly 4% of the global population. Chronic elevated blood glucose levels can lead to organ damage and failure in various body systems, including the nervous system, kidneys, gastrointestinal tract, eyes, blood vessels, and heart. Managing diabetes is challenging due to its multifaceted emotional and physical implications, often complicating effective control strategies. Current pharmacological therapies pose cardiovascular risks and mortality concerns, underscoring the need for safer, non-toxic nutritional alternatives. Catechins, natural polyphenols belonging to the flavonoid family, are prevalent in vegetables, fruits, and plant-derived beverages. High concentrations are found in fresh tea leaves, red wine,

* Corresponding Author's Email: prabhatsingh509@gmail.com.

In: Naturally Occurring Chemicals …
Editors: A. Singh Grewal, G. Deswal, A. Kumar Dhingra et al.
ISBN: 979-8-89113-491-1

strawberries, black grapes, and apricots. Catechins exhibit anti-diabetic, antioxidant, anti-inflammatory, and anti-obesity properties. They counter alloxan-induced diabetes through their free radical scavenging ability, and they ameliorate oxidative stress, endoplasmic reticulum stress, insulin resistance, hyperglycemia, and intestinal dysfunction. By inhibiting α-amylase and α-glucosidase enzymes, catechins lower lipid metabolites, blood sugar, and albuminuria. These diverse pharmacological effects position catechins as a promising therapeutic option for diabetes management and associated complications, warranting further exploration.

Keywords: epigalocatechin, hyperglycemia, endoplasmic stress, oxidative insult, anti-inflammatory, diabetes

Abbreviations

AMPK	AMP-activated protein kinase
ATP	Adenosine triphosphate
CKK	Cholecystokinin
DM	Diabetes mellitus
EC	Epicatechin
ECG	Epicatechin gallate
EGC	Epigallocatechin
EGCG	Epigallocatechin gallate
ETC	Electron transport chain
g	Gram
G-6-Pase	Glucose-6-phosphatase
GLP	Glucagon-like peptide
GLUT	Glucose transporter
GSK	Glycogen synthase-kinase
H_2O_2	Hydrogen peroxide
IGF	Insulin-like growth factor
IL	Interleukin
IR	Insulin resistance
IRS	Insulin receptor substrate
IST	Insulin signal transduction
JNK	Janus-kinase pathways
mg	Miligran
NADPH	Nicotinamide adenine dinucleotide phosphate

NF-κB	Nuclear factor kappa B
PI3K	Phosphatidylinositol-3-kinase
ROS	Reactive oxygen species
TNF-α	Tumor necrosis factor-alpha
UCP-3	Uncoupling protein-3.

Introduction

Flavonoids are the most prevalent polyphenolic secondary metabolites known for their health-promoting properties in both plants and foods. In the food industry, the supplementation of aglycones is essential to enhance serum concentrations and absorption rates. Within plants, flavonoids play a pivotal role in determining the quality, color, antioxidants, and nutritional value of fruits (Zhu et al., 2023). Naturally occurring flavonoids such as catechins, epigallocatechin, alpinetin, hesperetin, diosmetin, rutin, quercetin, and luteolin exhibit extensive therapeutic effects, including antioxidative and anti-inflammatory properties (Ye & Zhou, 2023). Catechins are a type of flavonoid found among polyphenolic compounds, naturally sourced from plants and various vegetable sources. The term "catechu" is derived from a boiled extract of Mimosa catechu, reflecting its relationship to catechins. Catechins are widely distributed in a diverse range of foods and herbs, including apples, broad beans, apricots, pears, strawberries, red wine, cocoa products, and black grapes (Cabrera & Giménez, 2006; Isemura, 2019). Green tea leaves, particularly those of the non-fermented variety, stand out as a significant dietary source of catechins, containing more of these compounds compared to black tea. Reports from the European Food Safety Agency confirm that every 100 ml of green tea typically contains around 126 mg of catechins (Sheng et al., 2023). Fresh leaves undergo a drying and steaming process to create green tea, which effectively preserves the majority of catechins by inactivating the polyphenol-oxidase enzyme (Bartoszek et al., 2018). Products derived from cocoa, such as chocolate, also contain substantial quantities of catechin and epicatechin. Strawberries, cherries, and apples are rich sources of catechins, with content ranging from 2-50 mg, 5–22 mg, and 10-43 mg per 100 g of these fruits, respectively. Recently, catechins have garnered increased attention due to their notable positive impact on health.

Chemistry of Catechins

Catechins, represented by the chemical formula C15H14O6, constitute a crucial subgroup of flavonoids. They are characterized by possessing two or more aromatic rings (A and B), each bearing at least one aromatic hydroxyl group linked to a carbon atom, as well as a dihydropyran heterocyclic C ring with an attached OH group (Braicu et al., 2013). Catechins are classified into four primary classes based on variations in their carbon ring structures: epicatechin gallate (ECG), epicatechin (EC), epigallocatechin gallate (EGCG), and epigallocatechin (EGC) (Peluso & Serafini, 2017). In EC, there are OH groups at the 4′ and 3′ positions of ring B, along with an OH group at the 3rd position of the C ring. The sole structural distinction between EC and EGC is the presence of an additional OH group at the 5′ position of ring B in EGC. EGCG and ECG are ester derivatives of EGC and EC, respectively, formed through esterification with gallate at three OH positions of ring C (Braicu et al., 2013). Notably, the pyrogallol ring in ECG lacks an OH group, and the galloyl group is substituted with a hydrogen atom (Peluso & Serafini, et al., 2017) (Figure 1).

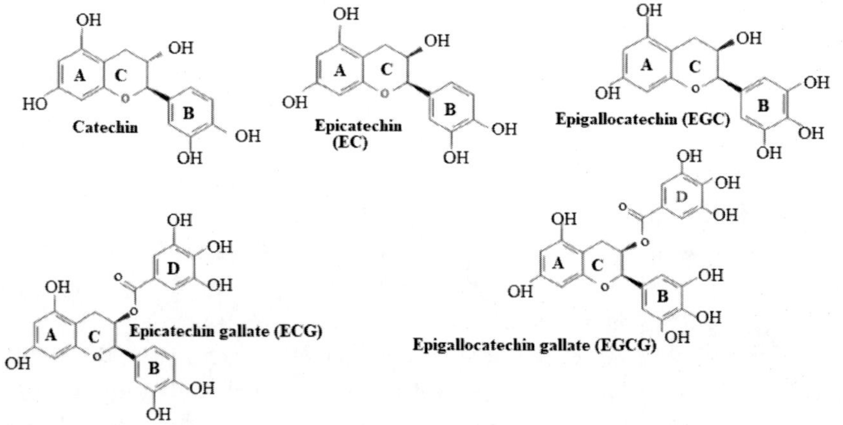

Figure 1. Catechins chemical structures.

Mechanism of Action of Catechins

Studies have revealed that catechins exhibit higher stability within the pH range of 4 to 6, and they are notably less stable below pH 3. Extensive research has been conducted to explore the therapeutic potential of catechins in both human and animal models. While many of the activities associated with catechins are recognized, their underlying mechanisms remain incompletely understood. Notably, their biological effects are largely attributed to their capacity for scavenging free radicals and their antioxidant properties (Bernatoniene & Kopustinskiene, 2018). Based on the current body of evidence, catechins have been identified to possess a range of beneficial properties, including anticancer, anti-allergic, anti-inflammatory, antioxidant (Fan et al., 2017), antidiabetic, anti-obesity, antiviral, antimicrobial, and hypotensive activities (Bernatoniene & Kopustinskiene, 2018). Catechins also offer neuroprotection by inhibiting the phosphorylation of tau proteins, curbing amyloid-β protein aggregation, and suppressing the release of apoptotic proteins (Özduran et al., 2021). Catechins are also known for their ability to form chelates with heavy metals such as copper and iron, effectively preventing metal toxicity. This chelation of transition metals is likely facilitated by the presence of di/tri-hydroxy groups within the catechins' ring structure (Botten et al., 2015). Furthermore, catechins play a role in regulating intracellular nitro-oxidative stress, which contributes to their anticancer activity. These compounds also exhibit antiapoptotic effects by modulating the expressions of both antiapoptotic and proapoptotic genes. As the body of evidence continues to grow, the diverse impacts of catechins on various cellular pathways have garnered significant attention. Catechins offer therapeutic potential owing to their antioxidant, anti-apoptotic, anti-inflammatory, and free-radical scavenging properties. These characteristics make them promising candidates for the prevention and treatment of conditions such as cancer, neurodegeneration, cardiovascular disorders, and various metabolic disorders (Özduran et al., 2021). Recognizing their beneficial effects, catechins are currently under investigation in a range of approaches and are finding their way into pharmaceutical, cosmetic, and medicinal products.

Role of Catechins in Diabetes Mellitus (DM)

Glucose is an essential component for sustaining life. However, when glucose levels exceed the upper limit, it leads to a condition called hyperglycemia. One of the major contributors to hyperglycemia is insulin resistance (IR). Prolonged hyperglycemia can trigger various complications, including diabetes, nephropathy, neurodegenerative disorders, cardiovascular diseases, and other metabolic conditions. Catechins and epigallocatechin, as highlighted in numerous studies, have been identified for their potential to provide protection against diabetes (Wen et al., 2022). They may play a role in mitigating diabetes by reducing oxidative stress, addressing insulin resistance, modulating mitochondrial and intestinal functions, and exerting anti-inflammatory effects (Xu et al., 2019). Moreover, catechins have shown the ability to inhibit enzymes involved in carbohydrate metabolism, such as α-amylase and α-glucosidase, leading to reduced fasting glucose levels in individuals with diabetes (Nazir et al., 2020). This chapter offers a comprehensive overview of the potential mechanistic pathways through which catechins can contribute to diabetes management. It aims to provide a scientific foundation for further investigations into the effectiveness of catechins in ameliorating diabetes (Figure 2).

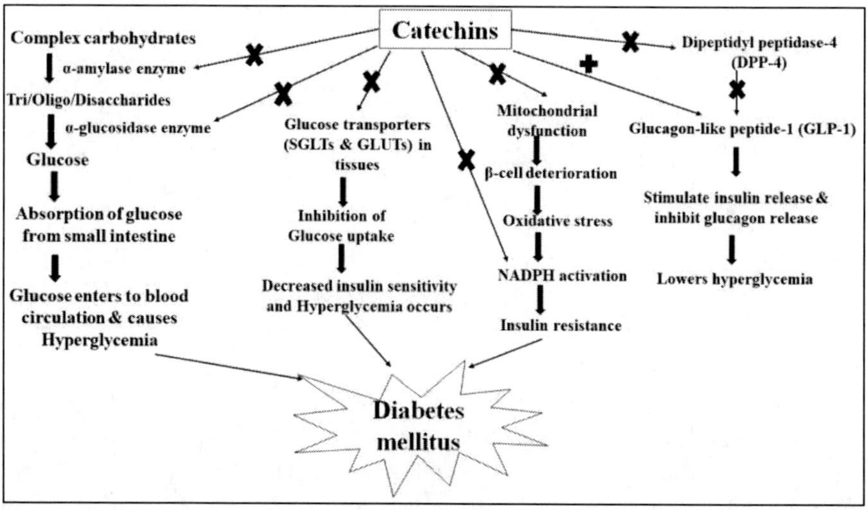

Figure 2. Antidiabetic mechanism of catechins.

Catechins: Recuperate Oxidative Stressand Diabetes

Chronic hyperglycemia triggers oxidative damage primarily due to the excessive generation of reactive oxygen species (ROS), commonly known as free radicals. This phenomenon results from processes such as glucose auto-oxidation, alterations in glutathione levels, antioxidant dysfunction, and lipid peroxidation (Samarghandian et al., 2017). The impact of ROS is extensive, causing chemical modifications in various cellular components and specifically contributing to lipid peroxidation. Lipid peroxidation is directly implicated in initiating oxidative stress, a significant factor in the development of diabetes. Elevated blood glucose levels lead to increased production of hydrogen peroxide (H2O2) and the suppression of catalase gene expression. In cases where there's a deficiency in catalase, pancreatic β-cells are particularly vulnerable to oxidative damage caused by the excessive ROS generated by mitochondria. This oxidative damage impairs the functions of β-cells, ultimately contributing to the onset of diabetes (Asmat et al., 2016). Furthermore, oxidative insults disrupt insulin signaling, decrease insulin sensitivity, and elevate the risk of diabetes. Catechins play a pivotal role in alleviating oxidative stress in diabetes by modulating various pathways. They act as scavengers of free radicals and enhance antioxidant levels, contributing to the mitigation of oxidative damage and its associated complications (Wen et al., 2022). Catechins exhibit anti-hyperglycemic and antioxidant effects by donating hydrogen ions and restoring the activity of various antioxidant enzymes such as catalase, superoxide dismutase, and glutathione in diabetes (Samarghandian et al., 2017). In cases of diabetes, oxidative stress can elevate the production of pro-inflammatory cytokines, which may contribute to apoptosis of pancreatic cells and subsequent decline in insulin secretion (Alipour et al., 2018). Oxidative stress resulting from hyperglycemia can activate nuclear factor kappa-B (NFκB), a protein complex that stimulates the production of inflammatory chemokines (Beckman et al., 2002). In this context, epicatechins (ECs) and epigallocatechin gallate (EGCG) have been found to potentially reduce NFκB activation induced by hyperglycemia, leading to a reduction in cytokine production and subsequently inhibiting vascular inflammation associated with diabetes (Babu et al., 2012). Furthermore, oxidative stress can be triggered by the activation of nicotinamide adenine dinucleotide phosphate (NADPH), a key source of intracellular hydrogen peroxide (H2O2) and superoxide. Epicatechins have demonstrated the ability to decrease NADPH oxidase activity by modulating Janus-kinase (JNK) pathways, thereby enhancing insulin sensitivity (Janus-kinase) pathways, and consequently improving insulin sensitivity (Cremonini & Oteiza, 2018).

Catechins: Improve Mitochondrial Performance

Mitochondria play a crucial role in regulating both oxidative phosphorylation and insulin release from pancreatic β-cells. When glucose levels increase, β-cells sense this change and stimulate oxidative phosphorylation, leading to the production of adenosine triphosphate (ATP) within the mitochondria. This ATP generation subsequently triggers the release of insulin (Kaufman et al., 2015). Mitochondrial dysfunction is closely associated with metabolic disorders such as obesity, cardiac issues, diabetes, and insulin resistance (IR), contributing to the deterioration of β-cell function and IR (Wen et al., 2022). Ample evidence supports the notion that proper mitochondrial activity is crucial for regulating insulin release in response to glucose in diabetes. In the context of diabetes, mitochondria are a primary source of oxidative stress. Impaired mitochondria can lead to the accumulation of a toxic substance called ceramide, along with oxidative damage, which in turn can promote insulin resistance (Chen et al., 2022). Additionally, mitochondria function as a redox sink and play a pivotal role in controlling the activity of NADPH oxidase, which is essential for maintaining the cellular redox balance (Wen et al., 2022). Catechins, particularly ECG and EGCG, possess the ability to safeguard mitochondria and their genetic material, including mitochondrial DNA, from the detrimental effects of reactive oxygen species (ROS) and oxidative stress (Chen et al., 2022). In the context of diabetes (DM), proinflammatory cytokines like IL-1β and TNF-α contribute to the destruction of pancreatic β-cells and impair insulin secretion. Emerging research has consistently demonstrated that EGCG can preserve impaired β-cell function through mitochondrial signaling pathways (Zhang et al., 2011). The mitochondrial electron transport chain (ETC) plays a significant role in regulating insulin release triggered by glucose. Catechins, such as epicatechin, have been shown to protect and restore the integrity of pancreatic β-cells, leading to improved insulin secretion. Additionally, catechins facilitate the replication of mitochondrial DNA and support the regeneration of β-cells. By upregulating the activity of the mitochondrial ETC, catechins enhance ATP generation and insulin secretion from β-cells in the context of DM (Rowley et al., 2017). Uncoupling Protein-3 (UCP-3), a mitochondrial transporter located on the mitochondrial membrane of pancreatic cells, governs processes like ATP production, glucose oxidation, and the initiation of insulin release (Mailloux & Harper, 2011). In DM, proinflammatory cytokines, particularly IL-1β, trigger apoptosis and mitochondrial damage through the UCP-3 signaling cascade.

EGCG has shown evidence of protecting against UCP-3 mediated mitochondrial damage and apoptosis, which may in turn enhance insulin secretion (Jia et al., 2020).

Catechins: Mitigate Insulin Resistance

The fundamental mechanism that maintains blood glucose homeostasis revolves around insulin signal transduction (IST), which governs processes like glycogen synthesis in the liver and glucose uptake by adipose tissues and muscles (Yaribeygi et al., 2019). Insulin, along with insulin-like growth factors IGF-1 and IGF-2, initiates the activation of insulin receptors or binding sites. Subsequently, these insulin receptors induce autophosphorylation of insulin receptor substrate IRS-1. This activation triggers insulin-dependent kinases such as glycogen synthase kinase GSK-3, AMP-activated protein kinase AMPK, and insulin-inducible kinase (AKT, PKC), initiating downstream signaling pathways. In an indirect manner, IRS-1 can activate the AKT pathway, which has been demonstrated to upregulate glucose transporter GLUT4. This transporter facilitates the uptake of glucose, thereby helping to regulate body glucose levels (Ho et al., 2016). Insulin resistance (IR) or insulin insensitivity refers to the reduced responsiveness of insulin-targeted tissues to insulin's effects. This condition contributes to the progression of various health issues such as atherosclerosis, type-2 diabetes, impaired glucose metabolism, hypertension, and dyslipidemia (Chen et al., 2022). Research has consistently shown that insulin resistance (IR) can lead to impaired mitochondrial function and disrupted glucose metabolism, resulting in increased production of reactive oxygen species (ROS). This oxidative stress and mitochondrial dysfunction have been associated with the progression of insulin resistance and diabetes (Lilja et al., 2020). Continuous consumption of tea catechins has been found to modify lipid metabolism and potentially mitigate disturbances in glucose and lipid metabolism as well as obesity associated with type-2 diabetes (Crespy & Williamson, 2004). Catechins have the capacity to reduce oxidative stress by preserving mitochondrial integrity and decreasing ROS production, thereby counteracting various intracellular signaling processes and insulin resistance (Chen et al., 2022). Catechins play a role in mitigating the detrimental effects of insulin resistance by promoting insulin signal transduction (IST), which encourages glycogen synthesis and enhances glucose uptake through GLUT4. Among these catechins, epigallocatechin gallate (EGCG) is particularly recognized for its ability to prevent diabetes due to its insulin-mimetic action and its promotion of GLUT4 translocation to the cellular membrane. This effect might be mediated through the PI3K/AKT signaling pathway, leading to increased glucose uptake (Xu et al., 2019). Therefore, catechins have the potential to significantly improve insulin resistance and reduce the risk of developing diabetes.

Catechins: Enhance Gastrointestinal Function

The gastrointestinal tract plays a direct role in human health, particularly in the context of metabolic conditions like type-2 diabetes and obesity. Gut hormones have significant roles in controlling intestinal function, food intake, insulin release, and nutrient absorption (Gribble & Reimann, 2019). For instance, GLP-1 regulates insulin secretion and glucose homeostasis, while GLP-2 is involved in energy regulation and maintaining the integrity of intestinal barriers, which in turn has implications for controlling diabetes (Baldassano et al., 2016). Catechin metabolites in the stomach offer potential benefits for diabetes treatment. Epicatechins and EGCG have been shown to enhance the release of GLP-1 from the ileum and increase CCK from the duodenum. Additionally, they reduce the activity of dipeptidyl-peptidase-IV, which plays a role in controlling insulin secretion and glucose homeostasis (Cremonini et al., 2021). Green tea catechins also support the growth of beneficial gut bacteria like Lactobacillus, functioning as probiotics that may help maintain glucose levels (Wen et al., 2022). Catechins have the ability to improve intestinal function and regulate diabetes through mechanisms such as enhancing intestinal barriers, influencing microbial composition, and increasing the production of gut hormones.

Catechins: α-Glucosidase and α-Amylase Activity

One of the primary ways blood glucose levels are raised is through the digestion and absorption of carbohydrates, facilitated by enzymes like α-glucosidase and α-amylase (Xu et al., 2019). Another mechanism involves gluconeogenesis, which employs enzymes such as fructose 1,6-bisphosphatase and glucose-6-phosphatase (Wang & Dong, 2019). Interventions that inhibit α-glucosidase and α-amylase have been shown to mitigate the postprandial rise in blood sugar levels in diabetes. Among catechins, EGCG stands out as a potent α-glucosidase inhibitor due to its unique gallic acyl group and the presence of an OH group in its chemical structure (Liu et al., 2016). EGCG's ability to inhibit α-glucosidase contributes to its effectiveness in managing diabetes. It achieves this by modulating the PI3K/AKT signaling pathway in muscle cells, promoting glucose uptake. Furthermore, EGCG helps maintain glucose homeostasis by reducing glucose production in hepatocytes through the attenuation of PKA signaling, which regulates insulin and glucagon signaling (Xu et al., 2019). In essence, catechins play a significant role in managing diabetes by curbing the availability of glucose.

Nano-Formulations of Catechins

Bioactive compounds like catechins are often encapsulated to achieve several objectives, such as improving stability, masking undesirable odors or flavors, converting from liquid to powder forms, and enhancing bioavailability. In the realm of food applications, safe and generally recognized materials are commonly employed for the development of delivery techniques to optimize catechin delivery. Nanoparticles are a popular choice for encapsulating catechins, aiming to enhance their effectiveness (Gomez-Mascaraque et al., 2016). The functionality and size of nanoparticles are influenced by formulation development and processing methods. Nanoparticles typically fall within the size range of 10-100 nm. Various properties of nanoparticles include their size, encapsulation efficiency, zeta potential, stability, loading capacity, and the release behavior of the encapsulated core material. Previous studies have revealed that formulations involving catechin nanoparticles can enhance various factors, such as gastrointestinal absorption, stability, oral bioavailability, bioformulation, and overall therapeutic effectiveness (Cai et al., 2018; Sistanipour et al., 2018). Incorporating catechin into inulin-embedded and chitosan-embedded nanoparticles has been shown to exhibit antidiabetic properties by enhancing the activity of α-amylase and α-glucosidase enzymes, surpassing the effects of free acarbose and catechins alone (Liu et al., 2014). Moreover, chitosan-embedded catechin nanoparticles have demonstrated enhanced antioxidant capabilities compared to natural catechins (Zhu et al., 2014). The development of nano-formulated lipid carriers and solid-lipid nanoparticles has aimed to enhance the stability, solubility, cellular compatibility, and sustained release properties of EGCG (Frias et al., 2016). Utilizing chitosan peptide nanoparticles to deliver epigallocatechin-3-gallate (EGCG) has shown improved antioxidant status and cellular uptake compared to the free form of the drug (Hu et al., 2013). Cationic lipid nanoparticles loaded with EGCG have shown promising results in mitigating oxidative damage and ocular inflammatory responses, highlighting the potential efficacy of EGCG in diabetes and its complications (Fangueiro et al., 2016). Additionally, epigallocatechin gallate-loaded self-assembled gelatin nanoparticles have been found to inhibit angiogenesis in the eyes through targeted action on integrin αvβ3 (Chang et al., 2017). These findings collectively suggest that catechin in the form of nano-formulations holds therapeutic potential for managing diabetes and its associated complications. However, further research is needed to develop novel catechin nano-formulations that can offer enhanced therapeutic benefits in diabetes management.

Conclusion

Numerous past research studies have extensively explored the antidiabetic, antioxidant, anti-inflammatory, cardio-protective, antihyperlipidemic, anti-cancer, and neuroprotective potentials of catechins. The findings from these studies collectively support the beneficial effects of catechins in addressing hyperglycemia and related conditions associated with diabetes. Catechins contribute to the improvement of hyperglycemia by mitigating oxidative stress, enhancing mitochondrial function, promoting glycogen synthesis, facilitating glucose uptake, and addressing insulin resistance. Moreover, even nano-formulations of catechins have demonstrated favorable outcomes in managing diabetes and its associated complications by enhancing the physicochemical properties of catechins. To establish a comprehensive understanding of the therapeutic benefits and potential limitations of catechins for diabetes management, well-designed future investigations are essential. Further research is warranted to validate and expand upon the positive impacts of catechins, thus paving the way for more effective strategies in utilizing catechins for the management of diabetes.

References

Alipour, M., Malihi, R., Hosseini, S. A., Abbasnezhad, A., Ghavami, A., Shahmohammadi, H. A., Ghanavati, M. (2018). The effects of catechins on related risk factors with type 2 diabetes: a review. *Progress in Nutrition*, 20(1), 12-20.

Asmat, U., Abad, K., Ismail, K. (2016). Diabetes mellitus and oxidative stress—A concise review. *Saudi Pharmaceutical Journal*, 24(5), 547-553.

Babu, P. V. A., Si, H., Liu, D. (2012). Epigallocatechin gallate reduces vascular inflammation in db/db mice possibly through an NF-κ B-mediated mechanism. *Molecular Nutrition & Food Research*, 56(9), 1424-1432.

Baldassano, S., Amato, A., Mulè, F. (2016). Influence of glucagon-like peptide 2 on energy homeostasis. *Peptides*, 86, 1-5.

Bartoszek, M., Polak, J., Chorążewski, M. (2018). Comparison of antioxidant capacities of different types of tea using the spectroscopy methods and semi-empirical mathematical model. *European Food Research and Technology*, 244, 595-601.

Beckman, J. A., Creager, M. A., Libby, P. (2002). Diabetes and atherosclerosis: epidemiology, pathophysiology, and management. *JAMA*, 287(19), 2570-2581.

Bernatoniene, J., Kopustinskiene, D. M. (2018). The role of catechins in cellular responses to oxidative stress. *Molecules*, 23(4), 965.

Botten, D., Fugallo, G., Fraternali, F., Molteni, C. (2015). Structural properties of green tea catechins. *The Journal of Physical Chemistry B*, 119(40), 12860-12867.

Braicu, C., Ladomery, M. R., Chedea, V. S., Irimie, A., Berindan-Neagoe, I. (2013). The relationship between the structure and biological actions of green tea catechins. *Food Chemistry*, 141(3), 3282-3289.

Cabrera, C., Artacho, R., Giménez, R. (2006). Beneficial effects of green tea—a review. *Journal of the American College of Nutrition*, 25(2), 79-99.

Cai, Z. Y., Li, X. M., Liang, J. P., Xiang, L. P., Wang, K. R., Shi, Y. L., Liang, Y. R. (2018). Bioavailability of tea catechins and its improvement. *Molecules*, 23(9), 2346.

Chang, C. Y., Wang, M. C., Miyagawa, T., Chen, Z. Y., Lin, F. H., Chen, K. H., Tseng, C. L. (2017). Preparation of arginine–glycine–aspartic acid-modified biopolymeric nanoparticles containing epigalloccatechin-3-gallate for targeting vascular endothelial cells to inhibit corneal neovascularization. *International Journal of Nanomedicine*, 12, 279.

Chen, B., Zhang, W., Lin, C., Zhang, L. (2022). A comprehensive review on beneficial effects of catechins on secondary mitochondrial diseases. *International Journal of Molecular Sciences*, 23(19), 11569.

Cremonini, E., Oteiza, P. I. (2018). (-)-Epicatechin and its metabolites prevent palmitate-induced NADPH oxidase upregulation, oxidative stress and insulin resistance in HepG2 cells. *Archives of Biochemistry and Biophysics*, 646, 55-63.

Cremonini, E., Daveri, E., Mastaloudis, A., Oteiza, P. I. (2021). (–)-Epicatechin and anthocyanins modulate GLP-1 metabolism: Evidence from C57BL/6J mice and GLUTag cells. *The Journal of Nutrition*, 151(6), 1497-1506.

Crespy, V., Williamson, G. (2004). A review of the health effects of green tea catechins in in vivo animal models. *The Journal of Nutrition*, 134(12), 3431S-3440S.

Fan, F. Y., Sang, L. X., Jiang, M. (2017). Catechins and their therapeutic benefits to inflammatory bowel disease. *Molecules*, 22(3), 484.

Fangueiro, J. F., Calpena, A. C., Clares, B., Andreani, T., Egea, M. A., Veiga, F. J., Souto, E. B. (2016). Biopharmaceutical evaluation of epigallocatechin gallate-loaded cationic lipid nanoparticles (EGCG-LNs): In vivo, in vitro and ex vivo studies. *International Journal of Pharmaceutics*, 502(1-2), 161-169.

Frias, I., Neves, A. R., Pinheiro, M., Reis, S. (2016). Design, development, and characterization of lipid nanocarriers-based epigallocatechin gallate delivery system for preventive and therapeutic supplementation. *Drug Design, Development and Therapy*, 3519-3528.

Gómez-Mascaraque, L. G., Soler, C., Lopez-Rubio, A. (2016). Stability and bioaccessibility of EGCG within edible micro-hydrogels. Chitosan vs. gelatin, a comparative study. *Food Hydrocolloids*, 61, 128-138.

Gribble, F. M., Reimann, F. (2019). Function and mechanisms of enteroendocrine cells and gut hormones in metabolism. *Nature Reviews Endocrinology*, 15(4), 226-237.

Ho, C. K., Sriram, G., Dipple, K. M. (2016). Insulin sensitivity predictions in individuals with obesity and type II diabetes mellitus using mathematical model of the insulin signal transduction pathway. *Molecular Genetics and Metabolism*, 119(3), 288-292.

Hu, B., Ting, Y., Zeng, X., Huang, Q. (2013). Bioactive peptides/chitosan nanoparticles enhance cellular antioxidant activity of (−)-epigallocatechin-3-gallate. *Journal of Agricultural and Food Chemistry*, 61(4), 875-881.

Isemura, M. (2019). Catechin in human health and disease. *Molecules*, 24(3), 528.

Jia, X., Luo, Z., Gao, Y., Liu, H., Liu, X., Mai, W., Zheng, Q. (2020). EGCG Upregulates UCP3 Levels to Protect MIN6 Pancreatic Islet Cells from Interleukin-1β-Induced Apoptosis. *Drug Design, Development and Therapy*, 4251-4261.

Kaufman, B. A., Li, C., Soleimanpour, S. A. (2015). Mitochondrial regulation of β-cell function: maintaining the momentum for insulin release. *Molecular Aspects of Medicine*, 42, 91-104.

Lilja, S., Oldenburg, J., Pointner, A., Dewald, L., Lerch, M., Hippe, B., Haslberger, A. (2020). Epigallocatechin gallate effectively affects senescence and anti-SASP via SIRT3 in 3T3-L1 preadipocytes in comparison with other bioactive substances. *Oxidative Medicine and Cellular Longevity*, 2020, 4793125.

Liu, J., Ding, H., Yan, C., He, Z., Zhu, H., Ma, K. Y. (2023). Effect of tea catechins on gut microbiota in high fat diet-induced obese mice. *Journal of the Science of Food and Agriculture*, 103(5), 2436-2445.

Liu, J., Lu, J. F., Kan, J., Wen, X. Y., Jin, C. H. (2014). Synthesis, characterization and in vitro anti-diabetic activity of catechin grafted inulin. *International Journal of Biological Macromolecules*, 64, 76-83.

Liu, S., Yu, Z., Zhu, H., Zhang, W., Chen, Y. (2016). In vitro α-glucosidase inhibitory activity of isolated fractions from water extract of Qingzhuan dark tea. *BMC Complementary and Alternative Medicine*, 16(1), 1-8.

Mailloux, R. J., Harper, M. E. (2011). Uncoupling proteins and the control of mitochondrial reactive oxygen species production. *Free Radical Biology and Medicine*, 51(6), 1106-1115.

Nazir, N., Zahoor, M., Ullah, R., Ezzeldin, E., Mostafa, G. A. (2020). Curative effect of catechin isolated from Elaeagnus umbellata Thunb. berries for diabetes and related complications in streptozotocin-induced diabetic rats model. *Molecules*, 26(1), 137.

Özduran, G., Becer, E., Vatansever, H. S. (2023). The role and mechanisms of action of catechins in neurodegenerative diseases. *Journal of the American Nutrition Association*, 42(1), 67-74.

Peluso, I., Serafini, M. (2017). Antioxidants from black and green tea: From dietary modulation of oxidative stress to pharmacological mechanisms. *British Journal of Pharmacology*, 174(11), 1195-1208.

Rowley, T. J. 4th, Bitner, B. F., Ray, J. D., Lathen, D. R., Smithson, A. T., Dallon, B. W., Plowman, C. J., Bikman, B. T., Hansen, J. M., Dorenkott, M. R., Goodrich, K. M., Ye, L., O'Keefe, S. F., Neilson, A. P., Tessem, J. S. (2017). Monomeric cocoa catechins enhance β-cell function by increasing mitochondrial respiration. *The Journal of Nutritional Biochemistry*, 49, 30-41.

Samarghandian, S., Azimi-Nezhad, M., Farkhondeh, T. (2017). Catechin treatment ameliorates diabetes and its complications in streptozotocin-induced diabetic rats. *Dose-Response*, 15(1), 1559325817691158.

Sheng, Y., Sun, Y., Tang, Y., Yu, Y., Wang, J., Zheng, F., Sun, Y. (2023). Catechins: Protective mechanism of antioxidant stress in atherosclerosis. *Frontiers in Pharmacology*, 14, 1144878.

Sistanipour, E., Meshkini, A., Oveisi, H. (2018). Catechin-conjugated mesoporous hydroxyapatite nanoparticle: A novel nano-antioxidant with enhanced osteogenic property. *Colloids and Surfaces B: Biointerfaces*, 169, 329-339.

Wang, Z., Dong, C. (2019). Gluconeogenesis in cancer: function and regulation of PEPCK, FBPase, and G6Pase. *Trends in Cancer*, 5(1), 30-45.

Wen, L., Wu, D., Tan, X., Zhong, M., Xing, J., Li, W., Cao, F. (2022). The role of catechins in regulating diabetes: an update review. *Nutrients*, 14(21), 4681.

Xu, L., Li, W., Chen, Z., Guo, Q., Wang, C., Santhanam, R. K., Chen, H. (2019). Inhibitory effect of epigallocatechin-3-O-gallate on α-glucosidase and its hypoglycemic effect via targeting PI3K/AKT signaling pathway in L6 skeletal muscle cells. *International Journal of Biological Macromolecules*, 125, 605-611.

Yaribeygi, H., Farrokhi, F. R., Butler, A. E., Sahebkar, A. (2019). Insulin resistance: Review of the underlying molecular mechanisms. *Journal of Cellular Physiology*, 234(6), 8152-8161.

Ye, Y., Zhou, J. (2023). The protective activity of natural flavonoids against osteoarthritis by targeting NF-κB signaling pathway. *Frontiers in Endocrinology*, 14, 1117489.

Zhang, Z., Ding, Y., Dai, X., Wang, J., Li, Y. (2011). Epigallocatechin-3-gallate protects pro-inflammatory cytokine induced injuries in insulin-producing cells through the mitochondrial pathway. E*uropean Journal of Pharmacology*, 670(1), 311-316.

Zhu, W., Zhang, Z. (2014). Preparation and characterization of catechin-grafted chitosan with antioxidant and antidiabetic potential. *International Journal of Biological Macromolecules*, 70, 150-155.

Zhu, W., Wu, H., Yang, C., Shi, B., Zheng, B., Ma, X., Qian, M. (2023). Postharvest light-induced flavonoids accumulation in mango (Mangifera indica L.) peel is associated with the up-regulation of flavonoids-related and light signal pathway genes. *Frontiers in Plant Science*, 14, 1136281.

Chapter 16

Allicin in the Management of Diabetes Mellitus

Diksha Gulati*
Aakriti Saini
Deepshi Arora
and Ashwani K. Dhingra
Guru Gobind Singh College of Pharmacy, Yamuna Nagar, Haryana, India

Abstract

Elevated blood sugar levels are a characteristic of diabetes mellitus, a complex condition wherein the body's insulin production falls short of meeting its needs. Urgent attention is needed globally to address this issue with effective, affordable, and easily accessible treatments that carry minimal or no side effects. Given the adverse effects associated with synthetic hypoglycemic drugs, the spotlight has turned towards traditional herbal remedies for the management and prevention of diabetes mellitus. Among these, garlic (*Allium sativum* L.) and other Allium species contain the protective organosulfur compound known as allicin. The health benefits of allicin have been studied throughout human history, and its distinct aroma is easily recognizable. When garlic is crushed and macerated, the enzyme allinase transforms it into allicin. Allicin has demonstrated antioxidant, antibacterial, antihypertensive, antidiabetic, immunomodulatory, and cardioprotective properties. The anti-diabetic effects of garlic stem from its ability to enhance glucose utilization, reduce intestinal glucose absorption, and stimulate insulin release from existing cells or insulin-bound reserves within the pancreas. In addition to its role in diabetes management,

* Corresponding Author's Email: dikshagulatir@gmail.com.

In: Naturally Occurring Chemicals …
Editors: A. Singh Grewal, G. Deswal, A. Kumar Dhingra et al.
ISBN: 979-8-89113-491-1

allicin's positive impact extends to other related conditions like diabetic nephropathy and diabetic hypertension. As diabetes often coexists with various other ailments, allicin's potential benefits can extend to addressing these interconnected health issues.

Keywords: diabetes mellitus, allicin, insulin, diabetic nephropathy, diabetic hypertension

Abbreviations

CRDH	Cohen-rosenthal diabetic hypertensive
CTGF	Connective tissue growth factor
DM	Diabetes mellitus
HDL	High density lipoprotein
LDL	Low density lipoprotein
STZ	Streptozotocin
TGF	Transforming growth factor.

Introduction

Diabetes is characterized by a disruption in the body's ability to produce sufficient insulin, produce inadequate insulin, or develop decreased sensitivity to insulin's actions (Barar, 2002). Its prevalence is rapidly increasing, with a global prevalence of around 5% among the general population (Torben, 2002). In India alone, there are already 30 million individuals affected by diabetes mellitus (DM), and this number continues to rise rapidly (Shankar & Sundraka, 2001). Additionally, diabetes cases are widespread in many regions. Over the next 25 years, diabetes is projected to become a leading cause of mortality and disability worldwide (Edwin et al., 2006). There has been a global demand for plant-based products for a considerable time. Various herbal remedies have shown promise in alleviating symptoms and mitigating the potential side effects associated with diabetes. Certain herbs have demonstrated the ability to support the renewal of ß-cells and reduce insulin resistance. Additionally, several herbs are believed to possess antioxidant and cholesterol-lowering properties, helping to maintain healthy blood sugar levels. To manage type 2 diabetes (NIDDM), medications that lower blood sugar levels and increase liver glycogen levels can be used (Shrabana et al., 2003). Apart from white garlic (*Allium sativum* L.), other members of the Allium species include elephant garlic (*Allium ampeloprasum* L.), wild garlic (*Allium ursinum* L.), field garlic (*Allium vineale* L.), and alpine leek (*Allium victorialis* L.). All these species of Allium contain the sulfur-containing volatile compound allicin. Allicin is considered one of the primary bioactive organosulfur compounds in Allium species, contributing to their distinctive strong flavor and aroma. Among the thiosulfinate compounds found in fresh garlic, allicin is the most prevalent, typically constituting about 70% (w/w) of all thiosulfinates or approximately 0.4% of the fresh mass (Rybak et al., 2004). When garlic cloves are crushed or mashed, the enzyme alliinase (also known as alliin lyase, EC 4.4.1.4), found in Allium spp., catalyzes the production of allicin. Allicin is a colorless oil with limited solubility in water, and its formation naturally leads to the release of pyruvate, ammonia, and the non-protein amino acid alliin, which serves as its precursor (Marchese et al., 2016). A garlic clove contains distinct compartments housing both alliin and alliinase. When the clove is cut or crushed, allicin is released. Allicin serves as a protective chemical that can trigger inflammation and discomfort in animal predators. This is believed to act as a deterrent by activating excitatory ion channels known as transient receptor potential cation channel subfamily V member 1 (TRPV1) and transient receptor potential ankyrin 1 (TRPA1) on primary sensory neurons within the pain pathway (Okada et al., 2005). The discovery of allicin and its biological properties in garlic can be attributed to Chester John Cavallito and John Hays Bailey, who first reported it in 1944. This pivotal discovery-initiated decades of comprehensive research into the renowned "heart of garlic" (Josling, 2007). Allicin has demonstrated anticancer effects by inducing apoptosis in cancer cells (Chu et al., 2013). Moreover, allicin has shown the ability to eliminate various types of bacteria, encompassing both gram-positive and gram-negative species (Fujisawa et al., 2009). Furthermore, allicin holds significant potential in the treatment of cardiovascular diseases (CVD). It demonstrates the ability to enhance antioxidant status, prevent hyperlipidemia and cardiac hypertrophy, induce vasorelaxation, inhibit angiogenesis, and even reduce platelet aggregation (Chan et al., 2013). Notably, recent research has revealed that pretreatment with allicin notably reduced the biochemical and histological alterations induced by doxorubicin (DOX) in experimental mice. This suggests that allicin might serve as a promising cytoprotective agent against DOX-induced oxidative damage in the hearts of cancer patients (Abdel et al., 2017).

Anti-Diabetic Effects of Allicin

Numerous preclinical and clinical investigations have highlighted garlic's potential to lower blood sugar levels (Padiya & Banerjee, 2013; Wang et al., 2017). Garlic formulations contain a range of metabolites containing sulfur. The antidiabetic properties of allicin were initially discovered in rabbits, where it was found to effectively reduce fasting blood sugar levels in a dose-dependent manner, similar to the action of tolbutamide (Augusti, 1975). Furthermore, allicin has shown promise in mitigating diabetes-associated cardiovascular complications. For instance, studies have demonstrated that allicin effectively hindered the progression of cardiac fibrosis in streptozotocin (STZ)-induced diabetic rats. Mechanistic insights supported this observation, indicating that allicin suppressed the expression of proteins like Bcl-2, Fas, connective tissue growth factor (CTGF), and transforming growth factor 1 (TGF1), thus potentially slowing down the development of diabetes-related cardiac issues (Liu et al., 2012). Bcl-2 and Fas play pivotal roles in determining the fate of a cell, while cardiac fibrosis indicators CTGF and TGF-1 are more indicative of the overall state. In a separate study, allicin demonstrated significant reduction in ventricular arrhythmias induced by Bcl-2 therapy in diabetic rats. Ventricular arrhythmias disrupt the electrical conduction within cardiomyocytes. The balance of electrolytes within these cells is primarily regulated by action potential duration (APD), L-type calcium current (ICa-L), and inward rectifier potassium current (IK1). Electrophysiological findings indicated that allicin reduced APD by inhibiting ICa-L and enhancing IK1. The prophylactic administration of allicin to type 1 diabetic rats led to a reduction in the levels of anti-islet cell antibodies, which are produced during the progression of diabetes. This improvement was associated with increased serum insulin levels from repaired Langerhans islet cells in the diabetic rats after allicin treatment (Osman et al., 2012b). Huang et al. (2017) investigated the impact of allicin on diabetic nephropathy (DN), characterized by elevated blood urea nitrogen and serum creatinine levels along with a reduction in creatinine clearance rate. Allicin administration effectively mitigated the progression of kidney damage in DN rats by preventing diabetes-induced kidney histological changes. This effect might be attributed to allicin's ability to inhibit the TGF-1/p-ERK1/2 downstream signaling pathway (Huang et al., 2017). To enhance its efficacy and stability, allicin was combined with captopril to create S-allyl-mercapto-captopril (CPSSA). Long-term administration of CPSSA to Cohen-rosenthal diabetic hypertensive (CRDH) rats not only prevented weight gain but also mitigated blood pressure elevation and reduced blood glucose levels. These findings underscore allicin's potential role in mitigating the risk of cardiometabolic disorders like type II diabetes, hypertension, and obesity (Younis et al., 2010).

Effects of Garlic on DM Complications

Glycemic control, a crucial aspect of managing diabetes, has shown promising enhancements through the use of garlic. Research indicates that garlic extracts may enhance insulin production, increase insulin sensitivity, and reduce insulin resistance (Ashraf et al., 2005). These findings contribute to improved glucose control, potentially aiding individuals with diabetes in maintaining stable blood sugar levels. Diabetes patients often face an increased risk of dyslipidemia, a condition characterized by abnormal lipid levels. Garlic possesses lipid-lowering properties, including the reduction of triglyceride, LDL ("bad" cholesterol), and total cholesterol levels, while simultaneously increasing HDL ("good" cholesterol) levels (Reinhart et al., 2008). These effects can potentially contribute to the reduction of cardiovascular risks and improved management of dyslipidemia associated with diabetes. Increased oxidative stress in diabetes is linked to the development of complications such as diabetic neuropathy, nephropathy, and retinopathy. Garlic's robust antioxidant capabilities, thanks to sulfur-containing compounds like allicin and allyl cysteine, can help mitigate this oxidative stress (Rahman K, 2001). Diabetes and its related complications are often associated with chronic inflammation. Garlic has demonstrated anti-inflammatory benefits by reducing pro-inflammatory cytokines and inhibiting the activation of inflammatory pathways (Iciek, Kwiecien & Wlodek, 2009). By mitigating inflammation, garlic may offer potential relief from some of the challenges associated with diabetes. Figure 1 provides a comprehensive overview of the potential role of garlic in diabetes prevention and addressing its associated complications.

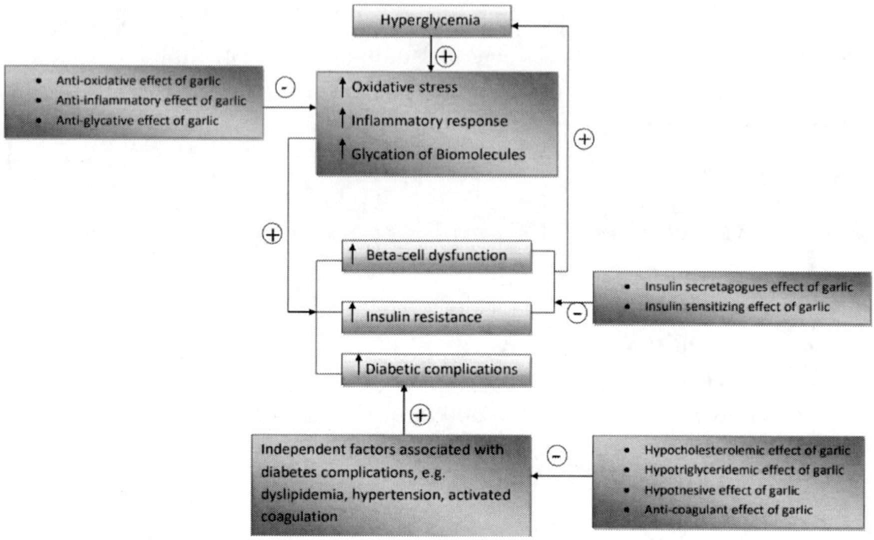

Figure 1. Role of garlic in diabetes and its complication.

Effects of Garlic on Diabetic Hypertension

Both diabetes and hypertension involve ATP-sensitive potassium (KATP) channels and often coexist as common comorbidities. Drugs targeting these channels can influence the performance of the cardiovascular system and insulin secretion (Nichols, 2006). Garlic, a herbal remedy, has been utilized to address both diabetes and hypertension due to its vasodilator properties and potential effects on glucose metabolism (Ried et al., 2008). Garlic acts as a vasodilator by hyperpolarizing vascular smooth muscle cells through the opening action of K+ channels (Reiter and Brandt, 1991). Studies have found that the vasodilator effect of garlic is diminished by the K+ channel blocker glibenclamide (Hosseini & Shafiee-Nick, 2008). Furthermore, garlic reduces intestinal glucose absorption, enhances glucose utilization, and may enhance insulin release (Ried et al., 2008). The antioxidant qualities of garlic (Ashraf et al., 2005) and its potential role in producing nitric oxide, possibly through endothelial function (Kiesewetter et al., 1991), may contribute to the relaxation of vascular smooth muscle, potentially mediated by nitric oxide production. Moreover, garlic extract has shown promise as an ACE inhibitor, contributing to its antihypertensive effects by lowering blood pressure. The antioxidative and anti-diabetic properties of garlic may underlie its ability to lower blood pressure, considering that oxidative stress plays a role in hypertension development among diabetic individuals (Durak et al., 2004).

Effects of Garlic on Diabetic Nephropathy

Research has explored the potential benefits of garlic for diabetic nephropathy (DN), a kidney condition triggered by diabetes. Garlic's impact on oxidative stress, inflammation, and fibrosis, three key contributors to the development and advancement of DN, has been studied. It is suggested that garlic's antioxidant properties could aid in mitigating oxidative stress, a significant factor in DN. In animal diabetes models, garlic extract has shown the ability to decrease markers of oxidative stress and enhance the activity of antioxidant enzymes (Asmat et al., 2016; Fiorentino et al., 2013). These findings could potentially provide protection against kidney injury induced by reactive oxygen species. Additionally, garlic's anti-inflammatory properties have been demonstrated, which could be advantageous in the context of diabetic nephropathy. Studies on animal diabetes models have indicated that garlic extract has the ability to inhibit the synthesis of pro-inflammatory molecules, leading to a reduction in inflammation (Gioscia Ryan et al., 2014; Al Waili et al., 2017). By modulating the inflammatory response, garlic might help alleviate kidney inflammation associated with diabetic nephropathy. Furthermore, garlic's potential to mitigate fibrosis, a common feature of diabetic nephropathy, has also been investigated. Fibrosis, characterized by an excessive accumulation of extracellular matrix proteins in the kidney, compromises kidney function. Garlic extract may counteract fibrosis by reducing collagen deposition and the expression of fibrotic markers in animal models of diabetic nephropathy (Qiu et al., 2020; Fine et al., 2000). These findings suggest that garlic could potentially prevent the development of renal fibrosis in the context of diabetic nephropathy. In summary, garlic's anti-inflammatory, anti-fibrotic, and antioxidant properties hold promise for potential therapeutic benefits in the management of diabetic nephropathy. However, further clinical research is necessary to validate these findings and establish the optimal dosage and duration of garlic supplementation for individuals with diabetic nephropathy.

Effects of Garlic on Diabetic Macroangiopathy

Indeed, garlic's vasodilatory properties, as demonstrated by studies (Ried et al., 2008), could potentially enhance blood flow and mitigate the risk of vascular complications associated with diabetes. Moreover, garlic has been shown to possess antiplatelet and anticoagulant characteristics (Rahman, 2007), which might aid in the prevention of blood clot formation and subsequently reduce the likelihood of cardiovascular events. Furthermore, garlic's antioxidant attributes may hold significance in diminishing oxidative stress and inflammation, both of which contribute to the development and progression of macrovascular complications in diabetes. The role of oxidative stress in the formation of atherosclerotic plaque and endothelial dysfunction is well-established. While the potential mechanisms are suggestive, more extensive research is necessary to precisely elucidate how garlic may impact cardiovascular health and potentially mitigate the risk of macrovascular complications in individuals with diabetes, particularly diabetic macroangiopathy. In summary, the various potential mechanisms associated with garlic, such as its vasodilatory, antiplatelet, anticoagulant, and antioxidant properties, suggest that it could hold some beneficial effects in conditions related to cardiovascular health and macrovascular complications in diabetes. However, further rigorous investigations are needed to better understand and validate these effects.

Interactions of Allicin and Anti-Diabetic Drugs

Garlic's extensive range of medicinal benefits is widely recognized. Its composition is primarily comprised of allicin and various sulfur compounds, some of which are considered bioactive (Lawson and Cardner, 2005). Garlic's potential as an anti-diabetic agent has been suggested and explored. The interaction between garlic and anti-diabetic medications has been the subject of numerous experimental and clinical investigations. In a rat model, the impact of garlic on the pharmacokinetics of metformin, a common anti-diabetic drug, was examined. The study revealed that garlic led to an increase in both the area under the curve (AUC) and peak plasma concentration (Cmax) of metformin. These findings indicate the importance of adjusting the dosage of the medication when administered concurrently with garlic. This highlights the need for careful consideration of potential drug interactions when incorporating garlic into a treatment regimen for diabetes or other medical conditions (Shikha et al., 2011). In another study, a rat model of streptozocin-induced diabetes was utilized to investigate the combined therapy of garlic extract (at doses of 50 or 100 mg/kg) and metformin over a 28-day period. It was observed that garlic extract, both alone and in combination with metformin, led to an increase in body weight. However, the combined therapy proved to be more effective in reducing blood glucose levels. This suggests that garlic extract enhances the hypoglycemic effects of metformin (Poonam et al., 2013). Moreover, both garlic juice and metformin have demonstrated potential therapeutic benefits by mitigating the tubular toxicity induced by gentamicin (Tavafi, 2013). In a clinical trial involving 60 patients with diabetes, the participants were randomly divided into two groups. One group received a combination of placebo and metformin (500 mg twice a day), while the other group received garlic tablets (300 mg three times daily), over a period of 24 weeks. The group receiving the combined treatment of garlic and metformin exhibited a significant drop in blood glucose levels (3-12%) compared to the groups treated with metformin alone or placebo, indicating an enhanced effect of garlic on glucose control (Asraf et al., 2011).

Conclusion

Allicin, a compound found in garlic, has shown promising outcomes in the treatment of diabetes and its associated complications. Evidence suggests that allicin can lower blood sugar levels, improve insulin sensitivity, and prevent the development of both microvascular and macrovascular problems. Furthermore, allicin's antioxidant and cholesterol-lowering properties contribute to its positive effects on diabetes management. The findings from numerous studies investigating allicin's therapeutic potential in diabetes and related disorders are encouraging. However, further research is necessary to fully understand the precise mechanisms through which allicin exerts its effects, as well as to determine the optimal dosage and treatment duration. The discovery of allicin's potential in mitigating the consequences of diabetes offers the possibility of developing more effective and safe treatments for this condition. With the increasing global prevalence of diabetes, there is a growing need for accessible and affordable medications that can effectively manage the disease and its complications. As such, allicin presents a promising avenue for addressing this urgent health challenge.

References

Abdel-Daim, M. M., Kilany, O. E., Khalifa, H. A., Ahmed, A. A. M. (2017). Allicin-ameliorates doxorubicin-induced cardiotoxicity in rats via suppression of oxidative stress, inflammation and apoptosis. *Cancer Chemotherapy and Pharmacology*, 80, 745-753.

Al-Waili, N. S., Saloom, K. S., Al-Waili, T. N., Al-Waili, A. N. (2017). The safety and efficacy of a mixture of honey, olive oil, and beeswax for the management of hemorrhoids and anal fissure: A pilot study. *Scientific World Journal*, 6, 1998-2005.

Ashraf, R., Aamir, K., Shaikh, A. R., Ahmed, T. (2005). Effects of garlic on dyslipidemia in patients with type 2 diabetes mellitus. *Journal of Ayub Medical College*, 17(3), 60-64.

Ashraf, R., Khan, R. A., Ashraf, I. (2011). Garlic (Allium sativum) supplementation with standard antidiabetic agent provides better diabetic control in type 2 diabetes patients. *Pakistan Journal of Pharmaceutical Sciences*, 24(4), 565-570.

Asmat, U., Abad, K., Ismail, K. (2016). Diabetes mellitus and oxidative stress—A concise review. *Saudi Pharmaceutical Journal*, 24(5), 547-553.

Augusti, K. T. (1975). Studies on the effect of allicin (diallyl disulphide-oxide) on alloxan diabetes. *Experientia*, 31, 1263-1265.

Barar, F. S. K. (2000). *Essentials of Pharmacotherapeutics* (3rd ed.). S. Chand and Company Ltd: New Delhi.

Chan, J. Y., Yuen, A. C. Y., Chan, R. Y. K., Chan, S. W. (2013). A review of the cardiovascular benefits and antioxidant properties of allicin. *Phytotherapy Research*, 27, 637-646.

Chu, Y. L., Ho, C. T., Chung, J. G., Raghu, R., Lo, Y. C., Sheen, L. Y. (2013). Allicin induces anti-human liver cancer cells through the p53 gene modulating apoptosis and autophagy. *Journal of Agricultural and Food Chemistry*, 61, 9839–9848.

Durak, I., Kavutcu, M., Aytaç, B., Avci, A., Devrim, E., Ozbek, H., Oztürk, H. S. (2004). Effects of garlic extract consumption on blood lipid and oxidant/antioxidant parameters in humans with high blood cholesterol. *Journal of Nutrition and Biochemistry*, 15(6), 373-377.

Fine, L. G., Bandoyopadhay, D., Norman, J. T. (2000). Cellular events in renal tubulointerstitial fibrosis. *Annals of the New York Academy of Sciences*, 928(1), 22-45.

Fiorentino, T. V., Prioletta, A., Zuo, P., Folli, F. (2013). Hyperglycemia-induced oxidative stress and its role in diabetes mellitus related cardiovascular diseases. *Current Pharmaceutical Design*, 19(32), 5695-5703.

Fujisawa, H., Watanabe, K., Suma, K., Origuchi, K., Matsufuji, H., Seki, T., Ariga, T. (2009). Antibacterial potential of garlic-derived allicin and its cancellation by sulfhydryl compounds. *Bioscience Biotechnology and Biochemistry*, 73, 1948-1955.

Gioscia Ryan, R. A., McCullough, M. J., Domaille, D. W. (2014). Garlic-derived organosulfur compounds inhibit inflammation induced by endothelial cells: Potential mechanism(s) of action. *Nutrition Journal*, 13, 5.

Hosseini, M., Shafiee-Nick, R. (2008). Interaction of Glibenclamide with Garlic in Control and Diabetic Rats. *Indian Journal of Biochemistry & Biophysics*, 45(5), 316-320.

Huang, H., Jiang, Y., Mao, G., Yuan, F., Zheng, H., Ruan, Y., Wu, T. (2017). Protective effects of allicin on streptozotocin-induced diabetic nephropathy in rats. *Journal of the Science of Food and Agriculture*, 97, 1359-1366.

Iciek, M., Kwiecien, I., Wlodek, L. (2009). Biological properties of garlic and garlic-derived organosulfur compounds. *Environmental and Molecular Mutagenesis*, 50(3), 247-265.

Josling, P. (2007). *Allicin—the heart of garlic*. Callahan Florida, FL, USA: NWI Publishing.

Kiesewetter, H., Jung, F., Pindur, G., Jung, E. M., Mrowietz, C., Wenzel, E. (1991). Effect of garlic on thrombocyte aggregation, microcirculation, and other risk factors. *International Journal of Clinical Pharmacology, Therapy, and Toxicology*, 29(4), 151-155.

Lawson, L. D., Cardner, C. D. (2005). Composition, stability and bioavailability of garlic products being used in a clinical trial. *Journal of Agricultural and Food Chemistry*, 53, 6254-6261.

Liu, Y., Qi, H., Wang, Y., Wu, M., Cao, Y., Huang, W., Li, L., Ji, Z., Sun, H. (2012). Allicin protects against myocardial apoptosis and fibrosis in streptozotocin-induced diabetic rats. *Phytomedicine*, 19, 693-698.

Marchese, A., Barbieri, R., Sanches-Silva, A., Daglia, M., Nabavi, S. F., Jafari, N. J., Izadi, M., Ajami, M., Nabavi, S. M. (2016). Antifungal and antibacterial activities of allicin: A review. *Trends in Food Science & Technology*, 52, 49-56.

Nichols, C. G. (2006). KATP Channels as Molecular Sensors of Cellular Metabolism. *Nature*, 440 (7083), 470-476.

Okada, Y., Tanaka, K., Fujita, I., Sato, E., Okajima, H. (2005). Antioxidant activity of thiosulfinates derived from garlic. *Redox Report*, 10, 96-102.

Osman, M., Adnan, A., Salmah Bakar, N., Alashkham, F. (2012). Allicin has significant effect on autoimmune anti-islet cell antibodies in type 1 diabetic rats. *Polish Journal of Pathology*, 63, 248-254.

Padiya, R., Banerjee, S. (2013). Garlic as an anti-diabetic agent: Recent progress and patent reviews. *Recent Patents on Food, Nutrition & Agriculture*, 5, 105-127.

Poonam, T., Prakash, G. P., Kumar, L. V. (2013). Effect of co-administration of Allium sativum extract and Metformin on Blood glucose of Streptozotocin induced diabetic rats. *Journal of Intercultural Ethnopharmacology*, 2, 81-84.

Qiu, Y., Huang, J., He, J. (2020). HIF-1α and its role in the pathogenesis of diabetic nephropathy. *Frontiers in Medicine*, 7, 570890.

Rahman, K. (2001). Historical perspective on garlic and cardiovascular disease. *Journal of Nutrition*, 131(3s), 977S-979S.

Rahman, K. (2007). Effects of garlic on platelet biochemistry and physiology. *Molecular Nutrition & Food Research*, 51(11), 1335-1344.

Reinhart, K. M., Coleman, C. I., Teevan, C., Vachhani, P., White, C. M. (2008). Effects of garlic on blood pressure in patients with and without systolic hypertension: A meta-analysis. *Annals of Pharmacotherapy*, 42(12), 1766-1771.

Reiter, M., Brandt, W. (1991). Relaxant Effects on Tracheal and Ileal Smooth Muscles of the Guinea Pig. *Arzneimittelforschung*, 41(4), 387-391

Ried, K., Frank, O. R., Stocks, N. P., Fakler, P., Sullivan, T. (2008). Effect of Garlic on Blood Pressure: A Systematic Review and Meta-Analysis. *BMC Cardiovascular Disorders*, 8, 13.

Rybak, M. E., Calvey, E. M., Harnly, J. M. (2004). Quantitative determination of allicin in garlic: Supercritical fluid extraction and standard addition of alliin. *Journal of Agricultural and Food Chemistry*, 52, 682-687.

Shankar, P., Sundarka, M. K. (2001). Management of type 2 diabetes: evidence-based approach. *Journal of Indian Academy of Clinical Medicine*, 2, 244-250.

Shikha, C., Tamanna, N., Kumar, S. L. (2011). Effect of Allium sativum on the pharmacokinetic of Metformin in rat plasma: a herb–drug interaction study. *Der Pharmacia Lettre*, 3, 287–291.

Shrabana, C., Tuhin, K. B., Begum, R., Liaquat, A., Mosihuzzaman, M., Nilufer, N., Azad, K. A. K., Biswapati, M. (2003). Advanced studies on the hypoglycemic effect of Caesalpinia bonducella F. in type 1 and 2 diabetes in Long Evans rats. *Journal of Ethnopharmacology*, 84, 41-46.

Tavafi, M. (2013). Protection of renal tubules against gentamicin induced nephrotoxicity. *Journal of Renal Injury Prevention*, 2(1), 5–6.

Torben, H. (2002). Genetics of type 2 diabetes. *Current Science*, 83, 1477-1482.

Wang, J., Zhang, X., Lan, H., Wang, W. (2017). Effect of garlic supplement in the management of type 2 diabetes mellitus (T2DM): A meta-analysis of randomized controlled trials. *Food & Nutrition Research*, 61, 1377571.

Younis, F., Mirelman, D., Rabinkov, A., Rosenthal, T. (2010). S-Allyl-Mercapto-Captopril: A novel compound in the treatment of cohen-rosenthal diabetic hypertensive rats. *Journal of Clinical Hypertension*, 12, 451-455.

Chapter 17

Arginine in the Management of Diabetes Mellitus

Neha Singh[*]
Kartikey Panday
Ashish Tiwari
and Pratibha Dwivedi
Krishnarpit Institute of Pharmacy, Prayagraj, Uttar Pradesh, India

Abstract

Diabetes mellitus (DM) is a chronic metabolic disorder characterized by high blood glucose levels. It affects a significant number of individuals worldwide and is associated with various complications such as cardiovascular disease, neuropathy, and nephropathy. As researchers continue to search for effective treatments for DM, arginine has emerged as a promising avenue. Arginine, an amino acid, has shown potential benefits in the management of DM. Studies have demonstrated that arginine supplementation can improve insulin sensitivity and glucose metabolism in patients with DM. By enhancing insulin sensitivity, arginine aids in the regulation of blood sugar levels and improves the body's ability to utilize glucose effectively. Arginine's antioxidant properties help protect against oxidative stress, potentially reducing the risk of complications associated with DM. Furthermore, arginine has been shown to improve endothelial function, which is often impaired in individuals with DM. By promoting better endothelial function, arginine may help reduce the risk of cardiovascular complications, which are prevalent in DM patients. In conclusion,

[*] Corresponding Author's Email: nehasinghkip657@gmail.com.

In: Naturally Occurring Chemicals ...
Editors: A. Singh Grewal, G. Deswal, A. Kumar Dhingra et al.
ISBN: 979-8-89113-491-1

arginine holds promise as a potential treatment for DM. It has been shown to improve insulin sensitivity, glucose metabolism, and endothelial function while providing antioxidant protection. However, further research is required before arginine can be recommended as a standard treatment for DM.

Keywords: arginine, diabetes mellitus, insulin sensitivity, glucose metabolism, endothelial function

Abbreviations

CVD	Cardiovascular disease
DM	Diabetes mellitus
DPP-4	Dipeptidyl peptidase-4
GLP-1	Glucagon-like peptide-1
NO	Nitric oxide
RCT	Randomized controlled trial
T1DM	Type 1 diabetes mellitus
T2DM	Type 2 diabetes mellitus.

Introduction

Diabetes mellitus (DM) is an enduring metabolic disorder marked by elevated blood glucose levels. This condition emerges from either inadequate insulin production or ineffective insulin utilization—a hormone pivotal in regulating blood sugar levels. Globally prevalent, this ailment demands vigilant management to avert severe complications. It encompasses three primary types: type 1, type 2, and gestational diabetes. Type 1 diabetes, referred to as insulin-dependent diabetes, manifests when the pancreas' insulin-producing cells are destroyed, leading to insufficient insulin creation. Conversely, type 2 diabetes arises due to insulin resistance, where body cells exhibit reduced responsiveness to insulin. Gestational diabetes, occurring during pregnancy, generally subsides post childbirth. Neglecting proper diabetes management can foster diverse complications, such as cardiovascular disease, renal failure, impaired vision, and potential limb amputation necessities. Controlling blood glucose levels and adeptly managing diabetes is crucial for diminishing these risks. Such complications contribute significantly to the condition's associated morbidity and mortality rates (IDF Diabetes Atlas, 2021). Diabetes management entails adopting lifestyle adjustments, employing pharmacological interventions, and implementing insulin therapy (American Diabetes Association, 2022). Incorporating lifestyle modifications stands as a cornerstone of effective diabetes management. These changes typically encompass dietary adjustments, regular physical activity, and weight management, all of which contribute to enhanced glycemic control and reduced complications risk. By embracing these lifestyle modifications, individuals with diabetes can significantly influence their glycemic control, lower complications risk, and improve overall well-being. However, it's imperative to collaborate closely with healthcare professionals to tailor these adjustments according to individual needs and circumstances (Evert et al., 2021). Pharmacological therapy involves the use of oral hypoglycemic agents and injectable medications that either enhance insulin sensitivity or stimulate insulin secretion (Inzucchi et al., 2018). According to the American Diabetes Association (2022), insulin treatment is advised for patients with type 1 diabetes and for those with type 2 diabetes who grapple with severe hyperglycemia or fail to achieve glycemic targets through other treatments. The primary objective of diabetes treatment remains to maintain blood sugar levels within a normal range to prevent complications. The choice of treatment options hinges on the type and severity of diabetes.

Overview of Arginine as an Amino Acid and Its Potential Benefits in DM

Arginine, an indispensable amino acid, plays a pivotal role in a multitude of metabolic pathways within the body. While dietary sources like meat, poultry, fish, dairy products, and legumes provide arginine, supplementation might be necessary when dietary intake falls short or specific therapeutic objectives are pursued (Wu et al., 2019). It stands as a critical foundational component for synthesizing essential molecules, including proteins, nitric oxide (NO), urea, creatine, and polyamines. Arginine's involvement extends to the regulation of immune function, hormone secretion, and wound healing processes. It additionally contributes to the cardiovascular system's normal operation by fostering vasodilation and sustaining healthy blood pressure levels. Moreover, arginine's potential benefits span various realms, from conditions like erectile dysfunction and sports performance to certain medical disorders. Notably, arginine showcases a favorable impact on insulin secretion and glucose uptake in skeletal muscles. It triggers insulin secretion from pancreatic beta cells and stimulates glucose uptake by skeletal muscle cells. The potential of arginine in managing diabetes mellitus (DM) has captured considerable attention among researchers. Multiple studies have investigated the impact of arginine supplementation on glucose metabolism, insulin sensitivity, and glycemic control in individuals with diabetes. While the results have been promising, additional research is needed to fully understand the potential advantages and identify optimal arginine dosages for effective DM management. Arginine, a semi-essential amino acid, plays a pivotal role in various physiological processes like nitric oxide synthesis, protein synthesis, and immune function. Studies have showcased arginine's ability to enhance insulin sensitivity, stimulate glucose uptake in skeletal muscle, and alleviate insulin resistance in both animal and human trials (Li et al., 2018; Jobgen et al., 2006). Given its favorable effects on glucose metabolism and insulin sensitivity, arginine supplementation has emerged as a potential therapeutic avenue for diabetes mellitus (DM). Numerous clinical trials have aimed to investigate the impact of arginine supplementation on glycemic control in individuals with diabetes. However, the results have displayed inconsistency, with some studies noting enhancements in glycemic control while others report no substantial effects (Wu et al., 2019). Research efforts have extensively explored arginine's potential role in diabetes management. An influential study highlighted arginine supplementation's role in elevating insulin sensitivity and diminishing fasting blood glucose levels among individuals with type 2 diabetes. Moreover, another study indicated that arginine supplementation increased glucose uptake in skeletal muscle cells, suggesting potential improvements in insulin sensitivity (Tang et al., 2013). Beyond its influence on insulin sensitivity, arginine might confer supplementary advantages for those with diabetes (Wu et al., 2009). Significantly, arginine has demonstrated the ability to restore endothelial function, often compromised in individuals with diabetes. This restoration could potentially mitigate the risk of cardiovascular complications, commonly encountered by individuals with diabetes (Cortese-Krott et al., 2014). A noteworthy randomized controlled trial conducted by Jobgen et al., (2006) provided evidence that arginine supplementation enhanced insulin sensitivity and glucose uptake in both healthy individuals and those with type 2 DM. Li et al., (2018) conducted another study that highlighted how arginine supplementation elicited enhancements in glucose metabolism and insulin sensitivity specifically within patients with type 2 DM. An additional potential advantage of arginine in diabetes management lies in its capacity to mitigate oxidative stress. Oxidative stress arises when an imbalance occurs between free radicals and antioxidants in the body, leading to cellular damage and inflammation. Wu et al.,'s study in 2019 showcased that arginine supplementation reduced markers of oxidative stress among patients with Type 2 DM. Numerous other studies have also underscored arginine's potential to diminish oxidative stress in individuals with diabetes. This attribute might serve as a preventive measure against the emergence of diabetic complications, such as cardiovascular disease and neuropathy, as implied by Vallianou et al., in 2017. Furthermore, arginine supplementation has demonstrated the ability to enhance endothelial function in patients with diabetes mellitus. Endothelial dysfunction, characterized by impaired blood vessel function, stands as a common complication within diabetes.

Arginine and Glucose Metabolism

Arginine has demonstrated a noteworthy impact on glucose metabolism, evident in both animal and human studies. Animal research reveals that arginine supplementation can elevate glucose tolerance and enhance insulin sensitivity; findings echoed by Kim et al., (2017). Human studies have similarly revealed positive effects of arginine supplementation on glucose metabolism among individuals with Type 2 diabetes. Notably, randomized controlled trials by Piatti et al., (2001) and Lucotti et al., (2002) have provided substantiation for the potential advantages of arginine supplementation in refining glucose metabolism in individuals with Type 2 diabetes and impaired glucose tolerance, respectively. These investigations propose that arginine could amplify insulin-mediated glucose uptake, possibly through mechanisms entailing insulin secretion and nitric oxide production. However, a more comprehensive understanding of the intricate mechanisms, optimal dosages, and enduring effects of arginine supplementation within these specific populations requires further research.

Arginine and Insulin Secretion

Insulin, a critical hormone produced by the pancreas, serves as a pivotal regulator of glucose metabolism in the body. In cases of diabetes, disruptions in insulin production or utilization led to elevated blood glucose levels.

Several studies, conducted in both animal models and human subjects, have highlighted arginine's capacity to facilitate insulin secretion (Jobgen et al., 2006). Numerous animal studies have uncovered arginine supplementation's potential to amplify insulin secretion. Clinical studies involving human participants have similarly demonstrated that intravenous arginine infusion can stimulate insulin secretion in both healthy individuals and those diagnosed with Type 2 diabetes. These compelling findings imply that arginine could potentially offer a beneficial role in diabetes management by bolstering insulin secretion (Cersosimo et al., 1996).

Arginine and Cardiovascular Health

Cardiovascular disease poses a prevalent challenge for individuals dealing with diabetes, significantly elevating morbidity and mortality risks. Arginine's positive influence on cardiovascular health is noteworthy, attributed to its capacity to enhance endothelial function, reduce blood pressure, and alleviate oxidative stress. Endothelial dysfunction is a hallmark of diabetes, marked by compromised nitric oxide (NO) production and diminished vasodilation. Arginine serves as a precursor for nitric oxide (NO) synthesis, consistently been shown to enhance endothelial function in both human and animal studies (Boger, 2006). The efficacy of arginine supplementation in managing blood pressure, especially among hypertensive individuals, is evident (Dong et al., 2011). Additionally, arginine has proven to mitigate oxidative stress in people with diabetes, a primary driver of cardiovascular disease development (Sena et al., 2011).

Arginine and Diabetic Nephropathy

Diabetic nephropathy is a common complication of diabetes and is acknowledged as a prominent contributor to end-stage kidney disease (ESKD). This condition is marked by proteinuria, hypertension, and renal impairment. Arginine has demonstrated a beneficial impact on the management of diabetic nephropathy (Mori et al., 2018).

Role of Arginine in Nitric Oxide Production

One of the most prominent mechanisms of arginine is its involvement in the synthesis of nitric oxide (NO). Nitric oxide serves as a potent vasodilator and possesses anti-inflammatory properties (Jobgen et al., 2006). It plays a pivotal role in maintaining homeostasis and ensuring the proper functionality of diverse physiological processes within the human body. Arginine serves as a precursor for the generation of NO, and existing evidence indicates that supplementation with arginine could heighten the production of NO (Wu et al., 2019). Numerous studies have underscored the critical role of nitric oxide (NO) in enhancing insulin sensitivity and refining glucose metabolism in individuals with diabetes mellitus (DM) (Jobgen et al., 2006).

Role of Arginine in Glucose Uptake

Arginine's potential to enhance glucose uptake in DM patients is noteworthy. Jobgen et al., (2006) conducted an analysis indicating that arginine supplementation augmented glucose uptake in both healthy individuals and those with type 2 DM (T2DM). Likewise, Li et al., (2018) showcased in their study that arginine supplementation ameliorated glucose metabolism in T2DM patients. These findings suggest that arginine could enhance glucose uptake and utilization, thus potentially enhancing glycemic control among individuals with DM.

Role of Arginine in Antioxidant Protection

Oxidative stress is a prevalent characteristic of diabetes mellitus (DM) and its associated complications. Emerging evidence indicates that arginine could possess antioxidant properties capable of mitigating oxidative stress in DM patients. A study by Wu et al., (2019) demonstrated that arginine supplementation effectively lowered oxidative stress markers among individuals with Type 2 DM. Furthermore, arginine might fortify the body's antioxidant defense mechanisms, thus providing a shield against oxidative harm, as suggested by Jobgen et al., (2006). Collectively, the diverse mechanisms through which arginine operates propose its potential role in diabetes mellitus management. Its capacity to enhance insulin sensitivity, diminish oxidative stress, and ameliorate endothelial function positions it as an appealing therapeutic agent for addressing DM.

Dosage and Duration of Treatment

Numerous studies have examined the most effective arginine dosage for individuals with DM. Li et al., (2018) conducted a randomized, double-blind, placebo-controlled trial indicating that a daily 9-gram arginine dose over 12 weeks enhanced glucose metabolism in Type 2 DM patients. Conversely, Wu et al., (2019) found that a lower 3-gram daily dose effectively reduced oxidative stress in Type 2 DM patients. The optimal arginine dosage for DM management remains uncertain which may possibly be influenced by variables like age, gender, and concurrent health conditions. The duration of arginine treatment for DM patients also lacks clarity. Most studies analyzing arginine's impact on DM have been short-term, spanning a few weeks to months. Extended treatment durations might be necessary to evaluate potential long-term effects on DM and its complications (Flogel et al., 2007).

Future Directions

Future research efforts should be directed towards conducting larger randomized controlled trials. These trials should specifically delve into determining the optimal dosage and duration of arginine supplementation to effectively manage diabetes mellitus (DM). Furthermore, it is crucial to explore potential interactions between arginine and other medications commonly employed to treat DM, such as antihyperglycemic agents and antihypertensive drugs. In addition, there is a need to investigate the potential of arginine in averting or delaying DM complications, including diabetic neuropathy, nephropathy, and retinopathy. Expanding the scope of research to encompass the benefits of arginine supplementation in patients with related metabolic disorders like metabolic syndrome and obesity would also be valuable. These conditions share close associations with DM and warrant exploration for potential therapeutic advantages offered by arginine.

Conclusion

Diabetes mellitus (DM) is a chronic metabolic disease necessitating ongoing management to prevent complications. Treatment approaches depend on diabetes type and severity, encompassing lifestyle adjustments, medications, insulin therapy, and other interventions. Close collaboration with healthcare professionals is vital for personalized treatment planning based on individual needs. Diabetes management entails diverse aspects: monitoring blood sugar, medication use, dietary changes, physical activity, and lifestyle tweaks. Arginine holds promise as a natural therapeutic for diabetes, potentially enhancing insulin sensitivity, glucose metabolism, and endothelial function, while reducing oxidative stress. Despite promising study outcomes, research on arginine's role in diabetes is limited. Further exploration is imperative to understand its potential in halting or slowing DM progression. Larger randomized trials are necessary to ascertain optimal arginine dosage, duration, safety, efficacy, and potential interactions with other drugs. In summary, arginine could offer a valuable natural approach for managing diabetes, but more investigation is essential to comprehend its benefits and risks comprehensively.

References

American Diabetes Association. (2022). Standards of medical care in diabetes—2022. *Diabetes Care*, 45(Suppl. 1), S1-S214.

Boger, R. H. (2006). The pharmacodynamics of L-arginine. *Alternative Therapies in Health and Medicine*, 12(6 Suppl 1), S50-S55.

Cersosimo, E., De Fronzo, R. A., Mandarino, L. J. (1996). A role for the nitric oxide pathway in glucose uptake stimulated by insulin in skeletal muscle. *Diabetes*, 45(3), 375-379.

Cortese-Krott, M. M., Kelm, M., Feelisch, M. (2014). The role of nitric oxide in the regulation of cardiovascular health and disease. *Frontiers in Bioscience*, 19(6), 1101-1124.

Dong, J. Y., Qin, L. Q., Zhang, Z. (2011). Effect of oral L-arginine supplementation on blood pressure: a meta-analysis of randomized, double-blind, placebo-controlled trials. *American Heart Journal*, 162(6), 959-965.

Evert, A. B., Dennison Mendoza, C., Tella, S. H. (2021). Lifestyle medicine approaches to glycaemic control. *Endocrinology and Metabolism Clinics of North America*, 50(2), 315-327.

Flögel, U., Ding, Z., Hardung, H., Jander, S., Reichmann, G., Jacoby, C. (2007). In vivo monitoring of EPR-visible nitric oxide formation in an animal model of sepsis: effect of L-arginine infusion on organ blood flow. *British Journal of Pharmacology*, 152(4), 513-519.

International Diabetes Federation. (2019). *IDF Diabetes Atlas* (9th ed.). https://diabetesatlas.org/upload/resources/material/20200302_133351_IDFATLAS9e-final-web.pdf.

Inzucchi, S. E., Bergenstal, R. M., Buse, J. B., Diamant, M., Ferrannini, E., Nauck, M., Peters, A. L., Tsapas, A., Wender, R., Matthews, D. R., Davies, M. J. (2015). Management of hyperglycaemia in type 2 diabetes, 2015: A patient-centered approach. *Diabetes Care*, 38(1), 140-149.

Jobgen, W. S., Fried, S. K., Fu, W. J., Meininger, C. J., Wu, G. (2006). Regulatory role for the arginine-nitric oxide pathway in metabolism of energy substrates. *Journal of Nutritional Biochemistry*, 17(9), 571-588.

Kim, J. Y., Park, J., Kim, Y. J., Lee, K. W., Kim, M. S. (2017). Arginine enhances glucose metabolism and insulin signaling in myocytes. *Molecular and Cellular Endocrinology*, 439, 138-145.

Li, M., Chen, L., Wang, Y., Wang, Y. (2018). Effects of arginine on glucose metabolism in patients with type 2 diabetes: A randomized, double-blind, placebo-controlled clinical trial. *Journal of Diabetes Investigation*, 9(2), 366-374.

Lucotti, P., Setola, E., Monti, L. D., Galluccio, E., Costa, S., Sandoli, E. P., Fermo, I., Rabaiotti, G., Gatti, R., Piatti, P. (2002). Beneficial effects of a long-term oral L-arginine treatment added to a hypocaloric diet and exercise training program in obese, insulin-resistant type 2 diabetic patients. *American Journal of Physiology-Endocrinology and Metabolism*, 303(9), E1177-E1187.

Mori, M. A., Silva, M. A. F., Moraes, C., Sanches, T. R., Corrêa, C. R., Abreu, G. R. (2018). Arginine supplementation in diabetic rats improves the utilization of amino acids and reduces the accumulation of advanced glycation end products in the kidney. *Applied Physiology, Nutrition, and Metabolism*, 43(5), 444-452.

Piatti, P. M., Monti, L. D., Valsecchi, G., Magni, F., Setola, E., Marchesi, F., Galli-Kienle, M., Pozza, G. (2001). Long-term oral L-arginine administration improves peripheral and hepatic insulin sensitivity in type 2 diabetic patients. *Diabetes Care*, 24(5), 875-880.

Santilli, F., Bucciarelli, L., Noto, D., Cefalù, A., Davì, G., Ferrante, E. (2015). Decreased plasma levels of L-arginine in diabetes: a possible link to impaired nitric oxide signaling and endothelial dysfunction. *Journal of Endocrinological Investigation*, 38(12), 1369-1374.

Sena, C. M., Nunes, E., Louro, T., Proença, T., Fernandes, R., Boarder, M. R., Seiça, R., Timoteo, M. A. (2013). Effects of oral l-arginine supplementation on oxidative stress and endothelial function in patients with type 2 diabetes mellitus and resistant hypertension: a randomized, double-blind, placebo-controlled crossover study. *Atherosclerosis,* 231(2), 208-214.

Tang, Q., Li, X., Song, P., Xu, L., Optiz, T., Li, D., Zhu, T. (2013). L-Arginine improves insulin sensitivity and glucose metabolism in mice fed a high-fat diet. *Nutrition Research*, 33(6), 464-471.

Vallianou, N., Evangelopoulos, A., Koutalas, P., Samathrakis, E. (2017). Arginine and its role in nutrition and health. *Journal of the International Society of Sports Nutrition*, 14(1), 1-13.

Wu, G., Bazer, F. W., Davis, T. A., Kim, S. W., Li, P. (2009). Arginine metabolism and nutrition in growth, health and disease. *Amino Acids*, 37(1), 153-168.

Wu, G., Meininger, C. J., Knabe, D. A. (2000). Arginine nutrition and cardiovascular function. *Journal of Nutrition*, 130(11), 2626S-2629S.

Wu, G., Meininger, C. J., Li, X. (2019). Novel roles of arginine in endothelial cell oxidative stress and inflammation. *Frontiers in Bioscience*, 24, 1258-1275.

Chapter 18

Berberine in the Management of Diabetes Mellitus

**Jatin Kumar*
and Neha Kanojia**
Chitkara University School of Pharmacy, Chitkara University, Himachal Pradesh, India

Abstract

Globally, the prevalence of diabetes mellitus (DM) has been on the rise. The International Diabetes Federation (IDF) has reported that there are now 366 million individuals worldwide living with diabetes, resulting in 4.6 million annual fatalities. Among the various types, Type 2 diabetes mellitus (T2DM) is the most widespread. The primary approaches for treating T2DM start with dietary and exercise interventions, followed by oral hypoglycemic medications and possibly subcutaneous insulin injections. Notably, Rhizoma coptidis and its key component, berberine, have been recognized as potent natural agents for lowering blood sugar levels. Berberine's hypoglycemic effects were initially observed when it was prescribed for diabetic patients with diarrhea back in 1988. Since then, Chinese medical practitioners have commonly recommended berberine as an anti-hyperglycemic agent. Over the past three decades, numerous pre-clinical and clinical studies have been discussed in medical literature on this subject. While berberine shows promise in reducing hyperglycemia, a few challenges persist. The availability of multicenter clinical studies to validate its hypoglycemic effects across a broader patient population is currently limited. Additionally, further research is required to substantiate the claim that berberine offers comparable benefits to other established

* Corresponding Author's Email: jatinkashyap4401@gmail.com.

In: Naturally Occurring Chemicals …
Editors: A. Singh Grewal, G. Deswal, A. Kumar Dhingra et al.
ISBN: 979-8-89113-491-1

T2DM therapies. In terms of safety, uncertainties remain about the long-term consumption of berberine, particularly considering the severity of diabetes.

Keywords: berberine, diabetes mellitus, hyperglycemia, *Berberis vulgaris*, T2DM

Abbreviations

AMP	Adenosine monophosphate
AMPK	Activated Protein kinase
ATP	Adenosine triphosphate
BBR	Berberine
COX-2	Cyclooxygenase-2
CVRF	Cardiovascular risk factor
DM	Diabetes mellitus
FBG	Fasting blood sugar
GLP-1	Glucagon-like protein-1
GLUT1	Glucose transporter-1
GTPase	Guanidine triphosphatase
H_2O_2	Hydrogen peroxide
HDL	High-density lipoprotein
HNF-4	Hepatocyte nuclear factor-4
IDF	International Diabetes Federation
IL-1	Interluckine-1
IL-6	Interluckine-6
iNOS	Inducible nitric oxide synthase
InsR	Insulin receptor
LD50	Lethal dose
LDL	Low-density lipoprotein
MAPK	Mitogen-activated protein kinase
MCP-1	Monocyte chemoattractant protein-1
MMP-9	Matrix metallopeptidase-9
mRNA	Messenger ribonucleic acid
NADPH	Nicotinamide di phosphate dehydrogenase
NF-kB	Nuclear factor-kB
PPAR	Peroxisome proliferator-activator receptor
T1DM	Type 2 diabetes mellitus

T2DM	Type 2 diabetes mellitus
TG	Triglycerides
TLR-4	Toll-like receptor 4
TNF-α	Tumour necrosis factor-α.

Introduction

The alkaloid berberine is present in plants such as Coptis chinensis (Chinese goldthread), Hydrastis, Mahonia, Xanthorhiza, and the stems and roots of *Berberis vulgaris* (barberry). Its diverse functions encompass neuroprotection, memory enhancement, cardioprotective properties, cholesterol level reduction, and alleviation of inflammatory diseases. This compound effectively modulates glucose levels by engaging various pathways and mechanisms. It improves insulin sensitivity, activates the 5' adenosine monophosphate-activated protein kinase (AMPK) pathway, boosts glycolysis in peripheral tissues, curtails gluconeogenesis in the liver, enhances the secretion of glucagon-like peptide-1, elevates glucose transporter levels, and regulates intestinal flora. In comparison to sulfonylurea and metformin, berberine demonstrates greater effectiveness (Belwal et al., 2020; Habtemariam, 2020b; Pang et al., 2015; Yin et al., 2012). Berberine (BBR), an isoquinoline alkaloid found in plants, possesses the ability to enhance insulin sensitivity and reduce blood sugar levels. Moreover, BBR's impact extends to supporting improved mitochondrial activity (Cole et al., 2021). This isoquinoline alkaloid, specifically known as a plant-derived quaternary ammonium salt, has a molar mass of 336.36122 g/mol. Its chemical nomenclature is 2,3-methylenedioxy-9,10-dimethoxyprotoberberine chloride (Derosa, Maffioli, & Cicero, 2012). Several plants, such as Coptis chinensis (Goldthread), Berberis aquifolium (Oregon grape), Hydrastis canadensis (Goldenseal), Arcangelisia flava, *Berberis vulgaris* (Barberry), and Berberis aristata (Tree Turmeric), can serve as sources for isolating this compound (I. P. Singh & Mahajan, 2013). Given the challenges associated with berberine's limited intestinal absorption and suboptimal bioavailability, there is a growing emphasis on researching synthetic derivatives. This approach aims to enhance the drug's effectiveness and therapeutic potential (Habtemariam, 2020b). Diabetes mellitus can be categorized into two types: type 1 diabetes mellitus (insulin-dependent) and type 2 diabetes mellitus (insulin-independent). From a clinical perspective, more than 90% of individuals with diabetes have type 2 diabetes mellitus (T2DM). A significant contributing factor for the development of type 2 diabetes mellitus is insulin resistance (IR), a pathological condition where target cells or organs fail to respond appropriately to insulin, impeding its ability to promote glucose elimination. Besides its direct association with T2DM, insulin resistance is also a precursor to the onset of other metabolic disorders, including hypertension, obesity, and atherosclerosis (Rodríguez-Gutiérrez et al., 2018). T2DM, characterized as one of the most prevalent chronic ailments and a complex metabolic disorder, stands as a distinct cardiovascular risk factor (García-Fontana et al., 2016; Gu et al., 2010; Pang et al., 2015). Various clinical, in vivo, and in vitro scientific studies have extensively documented the antidiabetic and hypoglycemic effects of *Berberis vulgaris* (*B. vulgaris*) and berberine (BBR). These investigations have found substantial support for the plant's efficacy in diabetes treatment. For instance, studies involving individuals with newly diagnosed type 2 diabetes mellitus (T2DM) and those with poorly controlled T2DM revealed that administration of 0.5 g of BBR three times a day for three months led to reductions in HbA1c, fasting blood glucose (FBG), postprandial blood glucose (PBG), triglycerides (TG), total cholesterol (TC), and low-density lipoprotein cholesterol (LDL-C). The authors highlighted BBR's potential as a potent oral hypoglycemic agent with favorable impacts on lipid metabolism. Owing to its antibacterial, antiprotozoal, and antidiarrheal properties, berberine has a history of use in traditional Chinese medicine and Ayurvedic medicine for bacterial diarrhea treatment. A multitude of studies have suggested that BBR possesses a broad spectrum of therapeutic effects, making it potentially valuable in addressing various chronic conditions. These include depression, inflammatory diseases, inflammatory diabetes (with antihyperglycemic, antihyperlipidemic, and antihypertensive effects), as well as cancer (demonstrating cytotoxic effects and inhibitory actions against the proliferation and replication of specific tumorigenic microorganisms and viruses). The antihyperglycemic properties of BBR were first observed in 1986 (Chen & Xie, 1986; Singh & Mahajan, 2013; Vuddanda et al., 2010). Berberine (BBR) exerts its regulation on glucose metabolism through a diverse array of mechanisms and signaling pathways. These encompass enhancing insulin sensitivity, activating the AMP-activated protein kinase (AMPK) pathway, influencing gut microbiota composition, inhibiting gluconeogenesis in the liver, encouraging the secretion of intestinal glucagon-like protein-1 (GLP-1), elevating hepatic low-density lipoprotein receptor mRNA expression, and prompting peripheral tissue cells to engage glucose transporters (Derosa et al., 2012; Singh & Mahajan, 2013; Vuddanda et al., 2010; Zhang et al., 2010).

Pharmacokinetic Profile of Berberine

Absorption

Despite its potential therapeutic benefits for various diseases, the clinical application of berberine is hindered by its sluggish oral absorption and limited bioavailability (Habtemariam, 2020a; Khashayar et al., 2021). Clinical investigations have demonstrated that intravenous (IV) administration can elevate the drug's blood concentration, but it can also lead to significant adverse effects. However, in rats, the absolute bioavailability of BBR is only around 1%. Poor absorption after oral administration of berberine is primarily attributed to factors like low permeability, hepatobiliary excretion, P-glycoprotein-mediated efflux, and self-aggregation. Additionally, the combination of low absorption and metabolism by the liver and the human intestine contributes to its low oral bioavailability (Liu et al., 2016). Previous studies have explored multiple strategies to enhance berberine's bioavailability. One approach involves altering the administration method. Another common strategy to boost berberine's efficacy is to modify its chemical structure, particularly through the creation of derivatives with antidiabetic effects (Habtemariam, 2020b).

Distribution

Following oral administration, BBR is predominantly distributed in tissues due to its relatively low plasma concentration. Upon intragastric dosing, berberine rapidly spreads throughout the body, with the liver, lungs, kidneys, pancreas, muscles, brain, heart, and fat showing descending levels of distribution. Notably, the liver stands as the primary organ of distribution. Around four hours after administration, most tissues exhibited BBR concentrations approximately 70 times higher than those found in the plasma. However, in certain tissues such as the liver, muscles, brain, heart, and pancreas, the BBR levels remained relatively stable over time (Liu et al., 2010; Tan et al., 2013).

Metabolism

In vivo, berberine undergoes rapid metabolism, primarily facilitated by the liver and intestinal flora, as indicated by multiple experimental studies. During this process, berberine undergoes extensive fragmentation. Key metabolic routes for berberine involve demethylation, demethylation, reduction, and hydroxylation, leading to the formation of phase I berberine metabolites. Additionally, glucuronidation, methylation, and sulfation are the primary pathways for berberine metabolism within the body (Alolga et al., 2016; Liu et al., 2009; Wang et al., 2017). This metabolic process is closely linked to the liver's cytochrome P450 enzymes. Among these, CYP2D6 and CYP1A2 are pivotal for the biotransformation of berberine in both mice and humans. Various subtypes of CYP450 enzymes participate in the metabolism of berberine (Guo et al., 2011; Li et al., 2011; Wang et al., 2015).

Excretion

Berberine (BBR) is primarily eliminated from the body through the bile and kidneys, manifested as excretion in urine and feces in various animal species. The process of bile excretion is relatively slow due to the presence of hepato-enteric circulation. Notably, different experimental subjects such as humans, rabbits, rats, and mice, as well as variations in BBR delivery methods including gavage, oral administration, and intravenous administration, have been shown to lead to variations in the excretion patterns. These findings are consistent with relevant experimental studies (Feng et al., 2021; Ma et al., 2013).

Mechanisms of Antidiabetic Action of Berberine

Berberine's Effects on Insulin Sensitivity and Secretion

Berberine (BBR) exhibits two distinct protective effects on islet function. First, in individuals with type 2 diabetes mellitus (T2DM) who also display insulin resistance, berberine enhances insulin sensitivity (Chueh & Lin, 2011; Yang et al., 2012). Second, BBR promotes insulin secretion and provides protection to pancreatic islet cells due to its antioxidant properties.

This effect is observed in advanced-stage T2DM with impaired islet function and in type 1 diabetes mellitus (T1DM) (Chueh & Lin, 2011, 2012). In both in vitro and animal experiments, berberine has been shown to elevate the expression of the insulin receptor (InsR), leading to reductions in fasting serum insulin levels and fasting blood sugar levels. This molecular action of berberine serves as a defense against insulin resistance. Researchers have further explored how BBR triggers the promoter of InsR in a protein kinase C dependent manner across various human cell types. This activation enhances the messenger RNA (mRNA) and protein expression of InsR. Several studies conducted on adipose and muscle cells have suggested that BBR might enhance the expression of insulin-sensitizing protein retinol binding protein-4 and GLUT1, respectively (Ko et al., 2005; Zhang et al., 2008). As resistance to insulin progresses, the action of Berberine (BBR) comes into play. BBR increases the activity of AMP-activated protein kinase (AMPK), leading to enhanced insulin sensitivity and stimulation of glycolysis. This effect is achieved by influencing the phosphorylation of insulin receptors (InsR) and the expression of insulin receptor substrate-1 (IRS-1). AMPK is a pivotal protein kinase responsible for energy sensing and signaling. Acting as a cellular "fuel gauge," it monitors energy levels and helps prevent metabolic disorders (Chen et al., 2010; Hwang et al., 2009; Kahn et al., 2005; Lee et al., 2006). BBR significantly raises the phosphorylation of AMPK subunits, which seems to be another critical mechanism in AMPK activation (Kim et al., 2007; Lu et al., 2009). This process involves an increase in intracellular potassium, leading to calcium influx through voltage-dependent calcium channels. The resulting elevation in intracellular Ca2+ facilitates the migration and exocytosis of insulin granules (Derosa et al., 2012). Furthermore, BBR has been demonstrated to enhance Min6 cell proliferation and glucose-stimulated insulin secretion by activating the insulin and insulin-like growth factor-1 signaling cascade (Ko et al., 2005).

Berberine's Effects on the Liver's Metabolism of Glucolipids

The liver plays a pivotal role in glucolipid metabolism, and Berberine (BBR) exerts significant influence over this process by regulating intranuclear transcription factors (Xia et al., 2011). By directly inhibiting hepatic gluconeogenesis, BBR leads to a reduction in blood sugar levels. Hepatocyte nuclear factor 4 (HNF-4), belonging to the hepatic nuclear factor family, holds the ability to suppress gluconeogenesis. Research has indicated that BBR has the potential to elevate HNF-4 mRNA expression, mitigate hepatic steatosis, counteract hepatic gluconeogenesis, and consequently lower blood glucose levels. Furthermore, the expression of fatty acid synthase (FAS) is downregulated (Wang et al., 2008). Through mechanisms such as reducing hepatic glycogen levels and modifying glucolipid metabolism, potentially by upregulating PPAR-α and PPAR-γ protein expression to enhance lipid metabolism, and significantly downregulating PPAR-δ expression in the liver, BBR effectively curbs the progression of liver degeneration. The activation of PPAR-agonists could potentially ameliorate metabolic disorders by enhancing the utilization of fatty acids in skeletal muscle and adipose tissues (Berger & Moller, 2002; Zhou et al., 2008).

Berberine's Effects on the Reduction of Intestinal Absorption of Glucose

Berberine (BBR) effectively reduces blood sugar levels by impeding the activity of α-glucosidase, an intestinal enzyme responsible for enhancing the absorption of glucose from the intestines. This inhibition of α-glucosidase, which catalyzes the breakdown of carbohydrates into monosaccharides, curtails the digestion and subsequent absorption of carbohydrates (Yin et al., 2008). BBR is also believed to potentially suppress the production of intestinal disaccharidases, with the duodenum being particularly affected (Liu et al., 2010). In addition, BBR has been shown to decrease α-glucuronidase in diabetic rats, a response similar to that achieved with the medication acarbose. This effect leads to an improvement in glucose tolerance among rats with diabetes induced by streptozotocin (Liu et al., 2008).

Berberine's Effects on Modulating Gut Microbiota

Berberine (BBR) possesses robust antibacterial properties that could be interconnected with its antidiabetic effects. BBR's influence on stomach microbiota seems to underlie its potential for treating type 2 diabetes mellitus (T2DM). T2DM is linked to alterations in the composition of gut microbiota, triggering an inflammatory cascade through the CD14/toll-like receptor 4 (TLR-4) pathway and lipopolysaccharides (LPS). This, in turn, leads to low-grade inflammation in the body and the onset of T2DM (Cani & Delzenne, 2009; Han et al., 2011; Hotamisligil, 2006). Both probiotic and antibiotic treatments have been shown to be critical in managing type 2 diabetes mellitus. BBR demonstrates substantial antibacterial effectiveness against parasites, worms, and diseases caused by viruses, bacteria, and fungi (Iwazaki et al., 2010; Singh & Mahajan, 2013). Notably, obese individuals exhibit fewer Bacteroidetes compared to lean control counterparts (Ley et al., 2006).

Berberine's Effects on Antioxidant and Anti-Inflammatory Activities

The development of diabetes mellitus (DM) and its subsequent effects are intricately linked with oxidative stress and inflammation (Li et al., 2014; Xie & Du, 2011). Berberine (BBR) is capable of impacting proinflammatory cytokines, antioxidant enzymes, and indicators of oxidative stress, thus contributing to the regulation of glucose homeostasis through the reduction of oxidative stress (Li et al., 2014; Singh & Kakkar, 2009; Zhou & Zhou, 2011). The administration of BBR exhibits the potential to decrease malondialdehyde (MDA) levels while concurrently raising the levels of glutathione (GSH), glutathione peroxidase (GSH-Px), and superoxide dismutase (SOD). These alterations contribute to the scavenging of excessive free radicals and the mitigation of oxidative stress (Bhutada et al., 2011; Zhou & Zhou, 2011). Diabetes, functioning as a metabolic disorder, can induce oxidative stress that disrupts specific pathways and generates radicals like superoxide anion and hydrogen peroxide, ultimately impairing insulin activity. The generated free radicals have the potential to inflict damage on the functionality of the pancreatic islets, thereby reducing insulin secretion. Moreover, reactive oxygen species-induced activation of protein kinase C and NF-κB further aggravates insulin resistance and production, thereby disrupting insulin signaling pathways. Inflammatory processes play a pivotal role in diabetes development. The metabolic disruption caused by diabetes leads to oxidative stress, which interferes with insulin function through the generation of free radicals such as H_2O_2 and superoxide anion, while also disrupting various metabolic pathways. Individuals with diabetes are believed to have an impaired antioxidative system, which is responsible for compromised reduction responses (Lao-ong et al., 2012; Ma et al., 2018). Berberine's anti-inflammatory effects are believed to stem from the inhibition of acute-phase proteins and proinflammatory cytokines.

Experimental treatments involving immune cells, splenic cells, adipocytes, pancreatic cells, and hepatocytes with berberine have shown reductions in concentrations of MMP9, TNF-α, COX-2, iNOS, MCP1, IL-6, IL-1, C-reactive protein, and haptoglobin.

The primary mechanisms responsible for berberine's antioxidant and anti-inflammatory defense mechanisms are as follows:

1. Activation of the Nrf2 pathway, which influences signal pathways including P38, AMPK, and PI3K/Akt.
2. Inhibition of MAPK (mitogen-activated protein kinase), Rho GTPase, NF-κB, and AP-1 pathways.
3. Negative regulation of NADPH oxidase and positive regulation of UCP2 (uncoupling protein 2) and SOD.

Berberine directly inhibits MAPK, Rho GTPase, NF-κB, and AP-1 pathways. Each of these mechanisms contributes to the reduction of cytokine production that fuels inflammation and the subsequent inflammatory processes. Given berberine's control over Rho GTPase, it may also indirectly hinder NF-κB signaling (Jeong et al., 2009; Ma et al., 2018; Poudel et al., 2019). Diabetes mellitus (DM) is often associated with persistent subclinical inflammation, and numerous studies have demonstrated the significant role of inflammation in the development of type 2 diabetes mellitus (T2DM) and its associated vascular complications. This connection is widely recognized in modern medicine (Dregan et al., 2014). Proinflammatory cytokines and acute-phase proteins, such as tumor necrosis factor, interleukin-6, IL-1, inducible nitric oxide synthase, prostaglandins, matrix metalloproteinase-9, monocyte chemoattractant protein-1 (MCP-1), C-reactive protein (CRP), and COX-2, are known contributors to this process (Jeong et al., 2009). Berberine (BBR) mitigates inflammation through various pathways, including those regulated by AMPK, mitogen-activated protein kinase (MAPK), nuclear factor-kappa B (NF-κB), and the Rho GTPase signaling pathway (Li et al., 2014; Wang, 2014). The antinociceptive properties of berberine are evidenced by the reduction of heat hyperalgesia and an increase in the mechanical threshold. Berberine also diminishes the activity of astrocytes and microglia in the mouse spinal cord, along with suppressing the expression of proinflammatory cytokines like TNF-α, IL-6, and IL-1. Notably, in diabetic mice, this alkaloid was found to alleviate neuropathic pain (Liu et al., 2019).

Berberine's Effects on Intestinal Flora

Berberine holds potential for treating type 2 diabetes mellitus by modulating intestinal flora. This supplement alters the composition and metabolites of intestinal flora, creating an environment that may hinder certain substances such as LPS (Liu et al., 2018; Nie et al., 2019). By increasing the concentration of short-chain fatty acids in the colon, berberine's impact on intestinal flora could potentially mitigate the onset of obesity and insulin resistance. The alkaloids in berberine enable a broader range of bacterial strains to produce these beneficial short-chain fatty acids. These acids enhance the intestinal barrier function, curb inflammatory reactions, and provide protection against pathogen infections (Habtemariam, 2020a; Xu et al., 2015). Even brief exposure to berberine can lead to a reduction in the quantity of several Clostridium strains, along with a decrease in their bile salt hydrolase activity. This leads to an accumulation of taurocholic acid in the colon, subsequently activating the intestinal farnesoid X receptor (FXR). This receptor's activation is pivotal in governing the metabolic processes of bile acids, lipids, and glucose (Tian et al., 2019). Research indicates that when berberine is used alone, it generally does not cause severe side effects. However, when combined with other therapies, the dosage is often reduced to minimize any lingering symptoms (Yin et al., 2008).

Berberine's Effects on Lipid Metabolism

The development and progression of insulin resistance (IR) are significantly affected by the accumulation of fat. Multiple studies have demonstrated the vital role of BBR in regulating adipose tissues. BBR is crucial for enhancing the synthesis of bile acids and the metabolism of liver cholesterol, which are both essential to prevent the buildup of lipids and the subsequent release of free fatty acids. As a result of BBR's effects, there was a notable increase in levels of HDL cholesterol and NO, while blood total cholesterol, triglycerides, and LDL cholesterol exhibited significant decreases in the tested subjects. This indicates a substantial promotion of lipid catabolism (Kong et al., 2004; Li et al., 2017; Li et al., 2015; Tang et al., 2006; Wang et al., 2014). As the principal transcription factors responsible for these processes, PPARs govern differentiation and fat metabolism. Studies have revealed that post BBR treatment, there is a significant reduction in PPARc mRNA expression. This decrease results in lowered PPARc transcriptional activity, thereby reducing fat synthesis. To regulate lipid metabolism, notably higher levels of PPARα and ATP-binding cassette transporter A1 were observed, alongside a decrease in PPARc and PPARc co-activator-1 levels. Furthermore, there was also a decline in PPARc and PPARc levels (Liang & Wang, 2018; Zhang et al., 2010; Zhou et al., 2008). Notably, the activity of NR in feces may potentially function as a biomarker for berberine-based treatment of hyperlipidemia. Reportedly, gut bacteria NR plays a crucial role in facilitating berberine's intestinal absorption (Liang & Wang, 2018).

Toxicity and/or Side Effects

The Singaporean government has prohibited the use of BBR due to a deficiency of glucose 6-phosphate dehydrogenase, which can be worsened by the method and dosage of BBR administration, potentially leading to acute toxicity. Data indicates that the LD50 for intravenous (IV) and intraperitoneal (IP) injections were 9.0386 g/kg1 and 57.6103 g/kg1, respectively. Interestingly, intragastric injection showed no significant LD50. Notably, intragastric administration had no LD50, while LD50s for intravenous and intraperitoneal injections were 9.0386 g/kg1 and 57.6103 g/kg1, respectively. In the context of managing type 2 diabetes mellitus, the safety and effectiveness of berberine have been studied. Individuals treated with berberine alone or in combination with Western anti-diabetic medications did not experience hypoglycemic side effects, but did report moderate gastrointestinal issues. Comparatively, adverse reactions in the treated group did not significantly differ from those in the placebo and lifestyle intervention groups (He et al., 2021; Kheir et al., 2010; Pang et al., 2015).

Conclusion

Berberine exhibits hypoglycemic activity and is a natural compound known for its excellent safety profile. Extensive research has been conducted to understand how berberine works to treat diabetes, with a specific focus on five key factors: reducing blood sugar levels, countering oxidative and inflammatory stress, regulating lipid metabolism, and managing gut flora. The interplay between intestinal flora, oxidative stress, and inflammation in diabetic patients has garnered increased attention in research. However, berberine's potential as an antidiabetic agent is hindered by its limited bioavailability, attributed to its unfavorable pharmacokinetic profile. The molecular mechanisms underlying berberine's antidiabetic effects remain somewhat elusive, and some administration routes may only yield potential effects. As a result, future research efforts will require more comprehensive and in-depth exploration. The precise methodologies and substances employed in investigations into berberine's role in regulating gut dysbiosis and preventing diabetes are currently unclear. Further clarification in this area is needed to facilitate a deeper understanding of berberine's mechanisms and potential applications.

References

Alolga, R. N., Fan, Y., Chen, Z., Liu, L. W., Zhao, Y. J., Li, J., Chen, Y., Lai, M. D., Li, P., Qi, L. W. (2016). Significant pharmacokinetic differences of berberine are attributable to variations in gut microbiota between Africans and Chinese. *Scientific Reports*, 6(1), 27671.

Belwal, T., Bisht, A., Devkota, H. P., Ullah, H., Khan, H., Pandey, A., Bhatt, I. D., Echeverría, J. (2020). Phytopharmacology and clinical updates of Berberis species against diabetes and other metabolic diseases. Frontiers in Pharmacology, 11, 41.

Berger, J., Moller, D. E. (2002). The mechanisms of action of PPARs. *Annual Review of Medicine*, 53(1), 409-435.

Bhutada, P., Mundhada, Y., Bansod, K., Tawari, S., Patil, S., Dixit, P., Umathe, S., Mundhada, D. (2011). Protection of cholinergic and antioxidant system contributes to the effect of berberine ameliorating memory dysfunction in rat model of streptozotocin-induced diabetes. *Behavioural Brain Research*, 220(1), 30-41.

Cani, P. D., Delzenne, N. M. (2009). The role of the gut microbiota in energy metabolism and metabolic disease. *Current Pharmaceutical Design*, 15(13), 1546-1558.

Chen, C., Zhang, Y., Huang, C. (2010). Berberine inhibits PTP1B activity and mimics insulin action. *Biochemical and Biophysical Research Communications*, 397(3), 543-547.

Chen, Q. M., Xie, M. (1986). Studies on the hypoglycemic effect of Coptis chinensis and berberine. *Acta Pharmaceutica Sinica*, 21(6), 401-406.

Chueh, W. H., Lin, J. Y. (2011). Berberine, an isoquinoline alkaloid in herbal plants, protects pancreatic islets and serum lipids in nonobese diabetic mice. *Journal of Agricultural and Food Chemistry*, 59(14), 8021-8027.

Chueh, W. H., Lin, J. Y. (2012). Protective effect of berberine on serum glucose levels in non-obese diabetic mice. *International Immunopharmacology*, 12(3), 534-538.

Cole, L. K., Sparagna, G. C., Vandel, M., Xiang, B., Dolinsky, V. W., Hatch, G. M. (2021). Berberine elevates cardiolipin in heart of offspring from mouse dams with high fat diet-induced gestational diabetes mellitus. *Scientific Reports*, 11(1), 15770.

Derosa, G., Maffioli, P., Cicero, A. F. (2012). Berberine on metabolic and cardiovascular risk factors: an analysis from preclinical evidences to clinical trials. *Expert Opinion on Biological Therapy*, 12(8), 1113-1124.

Dregan, A., Charlton, J., Chowienczyk, P., Gulliford, M. C. (2014). Chronic inflammatory disorders and risk of type 2 diabetes mellitus, coronary heart disease, and stroke: a population-based cohort study. *Circulation*, 130(10), 837-844.

Feng, X., Wang, K., Cao, S., Ding, L., Qiu, F. (2021). Pharmacokinetics and excretion of berberine and its nine metabolites in rats. *Frontiers in Pharmacology*, 11, 594852.

García-Fontana, B., Morales-Santana, S., Díaz Navarro, C., Rozas-Moreno, P., Genilloud, O., Vicente Pérez, F., Pérez delPalacio, J., Muñoz-Torres, M. (2016). Metabolomic profile related to cardiovascular disease in patients with type 2 diabetes mellitus: a pilot study. *Talanta*, 148, 135-143.

Gu, Y., Zhang, Y., Shi, X., Li, X., Hong, J., Chen, J., Gu, W., Lu, X., Xu, G., Ning, G. (2010). Effect of traditional Chinese medicine berberine on type 2 diabetes based on comprehensive metabonomics. *Talanta*, 81(3), 766-772.

Guo, Y., Li, F., Ma, X., Cheng, X., Zhou, H., Klaassen, C. D. (2011). CYP2D plays a major role in berberine metabolism in liver of mice and humans. *Xenobiotica*, 41(11), 996-1005.

Habtemariam, S. (2020a). Berberine pharmacology and the gut microbiota: A hidden therapeutic link. *Pharmacological Research*, 155, 104722.

Habtemariam, S. (2020b). The quest to enhance the efficacy of berberine for type-2 diabetes and associated diseases: physicochemical modification approaches. *Biomedicines*, 8(4), 90.

Han, J., Lin, H., Huang, W. (2011). Modulating gut microbiota as an anti-diabetic mechanism of berberine. *Medical Science Monitor*, 17(7), RA164.

He, C., Jia, X., Zhang, L., Gao, F., Jiang, W., Wen, C., Chi, C., Li, X., Jiang, G., Mi, H., Liu, W., Zhang, D. (2021). Dietary berberine can ameliorate glucose metabolism disorder of Megalobramaamblycephala exposed to a high-carbohydrate diet. *Fish Physiology and Biochemistry*, 47, 499-513.

Hotamisligil, G. S. (2006). Inflammation and metabolic disorders. *Nature*, 444(7121), 860-867.

Hwang, J. T., Kwon, D. Y., Yoon, S. H. (2009). AMP-activated protein kinase: a potential target for the diseases prevention by natural occurring polyphenols. *New Biotechnology*, 26(1-2), 17-22.

Iwazaki, R. S., Endo, E. H., Ueda-Nakamura, T., Nakamura, C. V., Garcia, L. B., Filho, B. P. D. (2010). In vitro antifungal activity of the berberine and its synergism with fluconazole. *Antonie Van Leeuwenhoek*, 97, 201-205.

Jeong, H. W., Hsu, K. C., Lee, J. W., Ham, M., Huh, J. Y., Shin, H. J., Kim, W. S., Kim, J. B. (2009). Berberine suppresses proinflammatory responses through AMPK activation in macrophages. *American Journal of Physiology- Endocrinology and Metabolism*, 296(4), E955-E964.

Kahn, B. B., Alquier, T., Carling, D., Hardie, D. G. (2005). AMP-activated protein kinase: ancient energy gauge provides clues to modern understanding of metabolism. *Cell Metabolism*, 1(1), 15-25.

Khashayar, A., Bahari, Z., Elliyeh, M., Ghasemi, M. (2021). Therapeutic effects of berberine in metabolic diseases and diabetes mellitus. *Revista Brasileira de Farmacognosia*, 31(3), 272-281.

Kheir, M. M., Wang, Y., Hua, L., Hu, J., Li, L., Lei, F., Du, L. (2010). Acute toxicity of berberine and its correlation with the blood concentration in mice. *Food and Chemical Toxicology*, 48(4), 1105-1110.

Kim, S. H., Shin, E. J., Kim, E. D., Bayaraa, T., Frost, S. C., Hyun, C. K. (2007). Berberine activates GLUT1-mediated glucose uptake in 3T3-L1 adipocytes. *Biological and Pharmaceutical Bulletin*, 30(11), 2120-2125.

Ko, B. S., Choi, S. B., Park, S. K., Jang, J. S., Kim, Y. E., Park, S. (2005). Insulin sensitizing and insulinotropic action of berberine from Cortidisrhizoma. *Biological and Pharmaceutical Bulletin*, 28(8), 1431-1437.

Kong, W., Wei, J., Abidi, P., Lin, M., Inaba, S., Li, C., Wang, Y., Wang, Z., Si, S., Pan, H., Wang, S., Wu, J., Wang, Y., Li, Z., Liu, J., Jiang, J. D. (2004). Berberine is a novel cholesterol-lowering drug working through a unique mechanism distinct from statins. *Nature Medicine*, 10(12), 1344-1351.

Lao-ong, T., Chatuphonprasert, W., Nemoto, N., Jarukamjorn, K. (2012). Alteration of hepatic glutathione peroxidase and superoxide dismutase expression in streptozotocin-induced diabetic mice by berberine. *Pharmaceutical Biology*, 50(8), 1007-1012.

Lee, Y. S., Kim, W. S., Kim, K. H., Yoon, M. J., Cho, H. J., Shen, Y., Ye, J. M., Lee, C. H., Oh, W. K., Kim, C. T., Hohnen-Behrens, C., Gosby, A., Kraegen, E. W., James, D. E., Kim, J. B. (2006). Berberine, a natural plant product, activates AMP-activated protein kinase with beneficial metabolic effects in diabetic and insulin-resistant states. *Diabetes*, 55(8), 2256-2264.

Ley, R. E., Turnbaugh, P. J., Klein, S., Gordon, J. I. (2006). Human gut microbes associated with obesity. *Nature*, 444(7122), 1022-1023.

Li, D., Zheng, J., Hu, Y., Hou, H., Hao, S., Liu, N., Wang, Y. (2017). Amelioration of intestinal barrier dysfunction by berberine in the treatment of nonalcoholic fatty liver disease in rats. *Pharmacognosy Magazine*, 13(52), 677.

Li, X. Y., Zhao, Z. X., Huang, M., Feng, R., He, C. Y., Ma, C., Luo, S. H., Fu, J., Wen, B. Y., Ren, L., Shou, J. W., Guo, F., Chen, Y., Gao, X., Wang, Y., Jiang, J. D. (2015). Effect of Berberine on promoting the excretion of cholesterol in high-fat diet-induced hyperlipidemic hamsters. *Journal of Translational Medicine*, 13(1), 1-9.

Li, Y., Ren, G., Wang, Y. X., Kong, W. J., Yang, P., Wang, Y. M., Li, Y. H., Yi, H., Li, Z. R., Song, D. Q., Jiang, J. D. (2011). Bioactivities of berberine metabolites after transformation through CYP450 isoenzymes. *Journal of Translational Medicine*, 9(1), 1-10.

Li, Z., Geng, Y. N., Jiang, J. D., Kong, W. J. (2014). Antioxidant and anti-inflammatory activities of berberine in the treatment of diabetes mellitus. *Evidence-Based Complementary and Alternative Medicine*, 2014, 289264.

Liang, H., Wang, Y. (2018). Berberine alleviates hepatic lipid accumulation by increasing ABCA1 through the protein kinase C δ pathway. *Biochemical and Biophysical Research Communications*, 498(3), 473-480.

Liu, C. S., Zheng, Y. R., Zhang, Y. F., Long, X. Y. (2016). Research progress on berberine with a special focus on its oral bioavailability. *Fitoterapia,* 109, 274-282.

Liu, D., Zhang, Y., Liu, Y., Hou, L., Li, S., Tian, H., Zhao, T. (2018). Berberine modulates gut microbiota and reduces insulin resistance via the TLR4 signaling pathway. *Experimental and Clinical Endocrinology & Diabetes*, 126(08), 513-520.

Liu, L., Deng, Y., Yu, S., Lu, S., Xie, L., Liu, X. (2008). Berberine attenuates intestinal disaccharidases in streptozotocin-induced diabetic rats. *Die Pharmazie*, 63(5), 384-388.

Liu, L., Yu, Y. L., Yang, J. S., Li, Y., Liu, Y. W., Liang, Y., Liu, X. D., Xie, L., Wang, G. J. (2010). Berberine suppresses intestinal disaccharidases with beneficial metabolic effects in diabetic states, evidences from in vivo and in vitro study. *Naunyn-Schmiedeberg's Archives of Pharmacology*, 381, 371-381.

Liu, M., Gao, L., Zhang, N. (2019). Berberine reduces neuroglia activation and inflammation in streptozotocin-induced diabetic mice. *International Journal of Immunopathology and Pharmacology*, 33, 2058738419866379.

Liu, Y. T., Hao, H. P., Xie, H. G., Lai, L., Wang, Q., Liu, C. X., Wang, G. J. (2010). Extensive intestinal first-pass elimination and predominant hepatic distribution of berberine explain its low plasma levels in rats. *Drug Metabolism and Disposition*, 38(10), 1779-1784.

Liu, Y., Hao, H., Xie, H., Lv, H., Liu, C., Wang, G. (2009). Oxidative demethylenation and subsequent glucuronidation are the major metabolic pathways of berberine in rats. *Journal of Pharmaceutical Sciences*, 98(11), 4391-4401.

Lu, S. S., Yu, Y. L., Zhu, H. J., Liu, X. D., Liu, L., Liu, Y. W., Wang, P., Xie, L., Wang, G. J. (2009). Berberine promotes glucagon-like peptide-1 (7-36) amide secretion in streptozotocin-induced diabetic rats. *Journal of Endocrinology*, 200(2), 159.

Ma, J. Y., Feng, R., Tan, X. S., Ma, C., Shou, J. W., Fu, J., Huang, M., He, C. Y., Chen, S. N., Zhao, Z. X., He, W. Y., Wang, Y., Jiang, J. D. (2013). Excretion of berberine and its metabolites in oral administration in rats. *Journal of Pharmaceutical Sciences*, 102(11), 4181-4192.

Ma, X., Chen, Z., Wang, L., Wang, G., Wang, Z., Dong, X., Wen, B., Zhang, Z. (2018). The pathogenesis of diabetes mellitus by oxidative stress and inflammation: its inhibition by berberine. *Frontiers in Pharmacology*, 9, 782.

Nie, Q., Chen, H., Hu, J., Fan, S., Nie, S. (2019). Dietary compounds and traditional Chinese medicine ameliorate type 2 diabetes by modulating gut microbiota. *Critical Reviews in Food Science and Nutrition*, 59(6), 848-863.

Pang, B., Zhao, L. H., Zhou, Q., Zhao, T. Y., Wang, H., Gu, C. J., Tong, X. L. (2015). Application of berberine on treating type 2 diabetes mellitus. *International Journal of Endocrinology*, 2015, 905749.

Poudel, A., Zhou, J. Y., Mekala, N., Welchko, R., Rosca, M. G., Li, L. (2019). Berberine hydrochloride protects against cytokine-induced inflammation through multiple pathways in undifferentiated C2C12 myoblast cells. *Canadian Journal of Physiology and Pharmacology*, 97(8), 699-707.

Rodríguez-Gutiérrez, R., Salcido-Montenegro, A., González-González, J. G. (2018). Early clinical expressions of insulin resistance: the real enemy to look for. *Diabetes Therapy*, 9, 435-438.

Singh, I. P., Mahajan, S. (2013). Berberine and its derivatives: a patent review (2009–2012). *Expert Opinion on Therapeutic Patents*, 23(2), 215-231.

Singh, J., Kakkar, P. (2009). Antihyperglycemic and antioxidant effect of Berberis aristata root extract and its role in regulating carbohydrate metabolism in diabetic rats. *Journal of Ethnopharmacology*, 123(1), 22-26.

Tan, X. S., Ma, J. Y., Feng, R., Ma, C., Chen, W. J., Sun, Y. P., Fu, J., Huang, M., He, C. Y., Shou, J. W., He, W. Y., Wang, Y., Jiang, J. D. (2013). Tissue distribution of berberine and its metabolites after oral administration in rats. *PLoS One*, 8(10), e77969.

Tang, L. Q., Wei, W., Chen, L. M., Liu, S. (2006). Effects of berberine on diabetes induced by alloxan and a high-fat/high-cholesterol diet in rats. *Journal of Ethnopharmacology*, 108(1), 109-115.

Tian, Y., Cai, J., Gui, W., Nichols, R. G., Koo, I., Zhang, J., Anitha, M., Patterson, A. D. (2019). Berberine directly affects the gut microbiota to promote intestinal farnesoid X receptor activation. *Drug Metabolism and Disposition*, 47(2), 86-93.

Vuddanda, P. R., Chakraborty, S., Singh, S. (2010). Berberine: a potential phytochemical with multispectrum therapeutic activities. *Expert Opinion on Investigational Drugs*, 19(10), 1297-1307.

Wang, K., Chai, L., Feng, X., Liu, Z., Liu, H., Ding, L., Qiu, F. (2017). Metabolites identification of berberine in rats using ultra-high performance liquid chromatography/quadrupole time-of-flight mass spectrometry. *Journal of Pharmaceutical and Biomedical Analysis*, 139, 73-86.

Wang, Y. (2014). Attenuation of berberine on lipopolysaccharide-induced inflammatory and apoptosis responses in β-cells via TLR4-independent JNK/NF-κB pathway. *Pharmaceutical Biology*, 52(4), 532-538.

Wang, Y., Yi, X., Ghanam, K., Zhang, S., Zhao, T., Zhu, X. (2014). Berberine decreases cholesterol levels in rats through multiple mechanisms, including inhibition of cholesterol absorption. *Metabolism*, 63(9), 1167-1177.

Wang, Z. Q., Lu, F. E., Leng, S. H., Fang, X. S., Chen, G., Wang, Z. S., Dong, L. P., Yan, Z. Q. (2008). Facilitating effects of berberine on rat pancreatic islets through modulating hepatic nuclear factor 4 alpha expression and glucokinase activity. *World Journal of Gastroenterology*, 14(39), 6004.

Wang, Z., Wu, J., Zhou, Q., Wang, Y., Chen, T. (2015). Berberine nanosuspension enhances hypoglycemic efficacy on streptozotocin induced diabetic C57BL/6 mice. *Evidence-Based Complementary and Alternative Medicine*, 2015, 239749.

Xia, X., Yan, J., Shen, Y., Tang, K., Yin, J., Zhang, Y., Yang, D., Liang, H., Ye, J., Weng, J. (2011). Berberine improves glucose metabolism in diabetic rats by inhibition of hepatic gluconeogenesis. *PLoS One*, 6(2), e16556.

Xie, W., Du, L. (2011). Diabetes is an inflammatory disease: evidence from traditional Chinese medicines. *Diabetes, Obesity and Metabolism*, 13(4), 289-301.

Xu, J., Lian, F., Zhao, L., Zhao, Y., Chen, X., Zhang, X., Guo, Y., Zhang, C., Zhou, Q., Xue, Z., Pang, X., Zhao, L., Tong, X. (2015). Structural modulation of gut microbiota during alleviation of type 2 diabetes with a Chinese herbal formula. *ISME Journal*, 9(3), 552-562.

Yang, J., Yin, J., Gao, H., Xu, L., Wang, Y., Xu, L., Li, M. (2012). Berberine improves insulin sensitivity by inhibiting fat store and adjusting adipokines profile in human preadipocytes and metabolic syndrome patients. *Evidence-Based Complementary and Alternative Medicine*, 2012, 363845.

Yin, J., Xing, H., Ye, J. (2008). Efficacy of berberine in patients with type 2 diabetes mellitus. *Metabolism*, 57(5), 712-717.

Yin, J., Ye, J., Jia, W. (2012). Effects and mechanisms of berberine in diabetes treatment. *Acta Pharmaceutica Sinica B*, 2(4), 327-334.

Yin, J., Zhang, H., Ye, J. (2008). Traditional Chinese medicine in treatment of metabolic syndrome. *Endocrine, Metabolic & Immune Disorders-Drug Targets*, 8(2), 99-111.

Zhang, Q., Xiao, X., Feng, K., Wang, T., Li, W., Yuan, T., Sun, X., Sun, Q., Xiang, H., Wang, H. (2010). Berberine moderates glucose and lipid metabolism through multipathway mechanism. *Evidence-Based Complementary and Alternative Medicine*, 2011, 924851.

Zhang, W., XU, Y. C., Guo, F. J., Meng, Y., Li, M. L. (2008). Anti-diabetic effects of cinnamaldehyde and berberine and their impacts on retinol-binding protein 4 expression in rats with type 2 diabetes mellitus. *Chinese Medical Journal*, 121(21), 2124-2128.

Zhou, J. Y., Zhou, S. W. (2011). Protective effect of berberine on antioxidant enzymes and positive transcription elongation factor b expression in diabetic rat liver. *Fitoterapia*, 82(2), 184-189.

Zhou, J. Y., Zhou, S. W., Zhang, K. B., Tang, J. L., Guang, L. X., Ying, Y., Xu, Y., Zhang, L., Li, D. D. (2008). Chronic effects of berberine on blood, liver glucolipid metabolism and liver PPARs expression in diabetic hyperlipidemic rats. *Biological and Pharmaceutical Bulletin*, 31(6), 1169-1176.

Chapter 19

Charantin: A Promising Natural Compound for the Clinical Management of Diabetes - Exploring Mechanisms, Extraction Process and Clinical Aspects

Jabin T. Paul
Sameer Rastogi*
and K. M. Shabana
School of Pharmacy, Noida International University, Greater Noida, G. B. Nagar, Uttar Pradesh, India

Abstract

Charantin, a natural compound derived from bitter melon, has shown potential in managing diabetes. This review article examines the various mechanisms of action of charantin and its clinical aspects in diabetes treatment. It also includes previous docking studies, which offer insights into the molecular interactions between charantin and its target proteins. The physical and chemical properties of charantin are also discussed. Studies conducted on animals have demonstrated that charantin can improve insulin sensitivity and reduce blood glucose levels. It achieves this by promoting the expression of proteins involved in glucose uptake and reducing insulin resistance. However, more research is needed to determine the effectiveness and safety of charantin in treating type 2 diabetes in humans. Additionally, charantin has been found to possess antioxidant and anti-inflammatory properties, which may provide additional benefits in managing diabetes. Despite these

* Corresponding Author's Email: rastogisameer1982@gmail.com.

In: Naturally Occurring Chemicals …
Editors: A. Singh Grewal, G. Deswal, A. Kumar Dhingra et al.
ISBN: 979-8-89113-491-1

promising findings, there have been very few clinical trials and case studies evaluating the efficacy and safety of bitter gourd (M. charantia) in diabetes treatment. To establish the optimal dose and duration of treatment for charantin, more extensive clinical studies are required. Nonetheless, charantin represents a promising natural compound for the clinical management of diabetes, and further research in this area is warranted.

Keywords: charantin, saponins, alpha-amylase and alpha-glucosidase, DPP4 inhibitors, IRS-1, GLUT-4

Abbreviations

ADP	Adenosine diphosphate
ATP	Adenosine triphosphate
BGL	Blood glucose level
CEMC	Charantin extract of M. charantia
DM	Diabetes mellitus
DPP	Dipeptidyl peptidase
GLUT	Glucose transporter
IAAP	Islet amyloid polypeptides
IRS	Insulin receptor substrates
	Reactive oxygen species
STZ	Streptozotocin
T2DM	Type-2 diabetes mellitus.

Introduction

Diabetes mellitus (DM) is a chronic metabolic disease characterized by high blood sugar levels, which causes problems in various organs and systems of the body. There are two main types of diabetes: type 1 and type 2. Type 1 diabetes occurs when the insulin-producing beta cells in the body are destroyed, resulting in a complete deficiency of insulin. It is most commonly diagnosed in children and cannot be prevented. On the other hand, type 2 diabetes accounts for more than 90% of diabetes cases worldwide and can often be delayed or prevented. It is increasingly being diagnosed in older children and is associated with being overweight or obese. The symptoms of type 2 diabetes are usually less severe and may go unnoticed, leading to a significant number of undiagnosed cases. (Sharma et al., 2021). This can result in complications such as vision loss, slow-healing ulcers, heart disease, and stroke. Therefore, early detection and management of type 2 diabetes are crucial to prevent these complications. Insulin is essential for individuals with type 1 diabetes, while management of type 2 diabetes involves making lifestyle changes, taking medication, and sometimes using insulin therapy. To effectively manage and prevent complications of diabetes, it is important to raise awareness, undergo regular check-ups, and receive a timely diagnosis. Risk factors for type 2 diabetes include obesity, increasing age, ethnicity, and having a family history of the disease. The exact causes are not fully understood, but it is believed to involve both genetic and environmental factors. The prevalence of diabetes is on the rise, with an estimated 537 million people worldwide affected in 2021. This number has significantly increased since 2019 and is projected to reach 783 million by 2045. Diabetes is associated with various complications, including cardiovascular disease, neuropathy, retinopathy, renal disease, and cognitive impairment. Risk factors such as insulin resistance, obesity, chronic inflammation, and abnormal blood sugar levels contribute to the cognitive implications of diabetes. Healthcare providers must recognize and address the cognitive implications of diabetes to provide comprehensive care. Efforts to prevent, diagnose, and treat diabetes are crucial in improving health outcomes and reducing the burden of complications. In terms of treatment, there are various drugs available in the market for type 2 diabetes mellitus (T2DM). One interesting compound that has been studied is charantin, which is found in bitter gourd (Momordica charantia Linn). Further research is needed to better understand the potential use of charantin in the treatment of diabetes.

Charantin

With characteristics similar to those of insulin, the cucurbitane-type triterpenoid charantin exists as an equal mixture of stigmasterol glucoside and sitosterol glucoside (1:1) (Figures 1 and 2). It has blood sugar-lowering properties similar to insulin (Çiçek, 2022; Desai & Tatke, 2015; Mahwish et al., 2021; Singh et al., 2011).

Description: White crystalline, neutral, and tasteless compound.
Molecular formula: $C_{35}H_{60}O_6$ (Singh et al., 2011).
Molecular Weight: 576 amu/ 9.7 kDa (Singh et al., 2011).

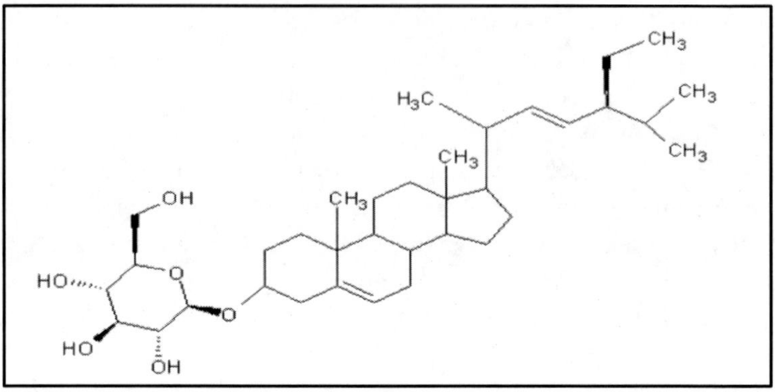

Figure 1. Stigmasterol glucoside structure.

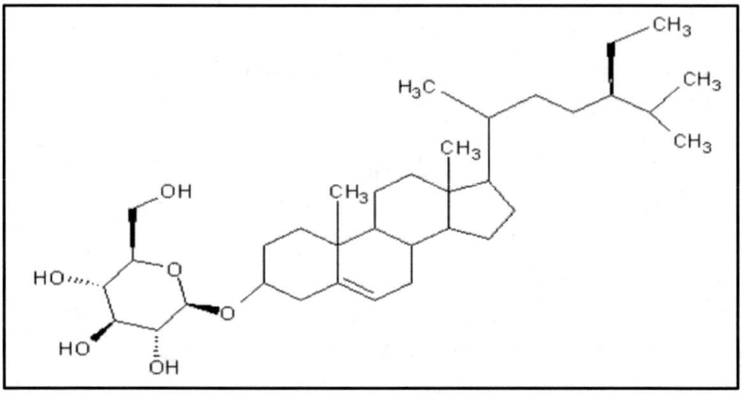

Figure 2. β-sitosterol glucoside structure.

Solubility: Challenging due to the presence of both aglycone and sugar moieties; slightly soluble in polar solvents like ethanol or methanol, but soluble in non-polar solvents like chloroform and dichloromethane; soluble for ether.

Melting range: 266-268°C.

Phytochemistry:

1. Gives violet color changing to blue, green, and yellow with Libermann-Burchard test.
2. Produces glucose and sterol on hydrolysis with acid
3. Gives violet-blue color with anisaldehyde sulphuric acid reagent
4. Gives pink color with vanillin sulphuric acid reagent (Desai & Tatke, 2015).

Indication

While a 2006 study did not find significant antihyperglycemic activity in charantin, subsequent in vitro and in vivo animal studies have shown its potential as an antidiabetic agent. These studies suggest that charantin may help regulate blood glucose levels by improving insulin sensitivity, increasing glucose uptake by cells, and reducing glucose production by the liver. However, further research is needed to confirm its efficacy and safety as a therapeutic option for diabetes (Çiçek, 2022; Desai & Tatke, 2015; Harinantenaina et al., 2006; Mahwish et al., 2021; Nagappan et al., 2018; Singh et al., 2011; Wang et al., 2014). Charantin has a chemical structure and properties similar to insulin and has been found to lower blood sugar levels equivalently to insulin (Desai & Tatke, 2015; Nagappan et al., 2018; Wang et al., 2014). It also exhibits anti-sialogogue activity, reducing saliva secretion. In anaesthetized cats, a dose of 800 mg/kg of charantin was found to lower blood pressure by 5-10% (Desai & Tatke, 2015). Bitter melon, which contains charantin, has been shown to be effective in managing post-prandial hyperglycemia (PPHG) in humans (Nagappan et al., 2018). Furthermore, charantin has been found to have antifertility effects in rabbits (Çiçek, 2022). Supplementation of bitter melon in normal rats has also shown improvement in managing the onset of diabetes (Mahwish et al., 2021). In addition, charantin has been reported to have antioxidant, hypoglycemic, anticancer, hypolipidemic, and antiviral properties (Richter et al., 2023).

Mechanism of Action

Two mechanisms have been identified to explain the anti-hyperglycemic activity of charantin: blocking metabolic enzymes in the small intestine, charantin slows down the absorption of carbohydrates (Çiçek, 2022), while CEMC has been found to increase the expression of GLUT4 and IRS-1 in the skeletal muscle and liver of KK/HIJ mice, respectively (Wang et al., 2014).

Charantin Action on Metabolic Enzymes (Alpha-Amylase and Alpha-Glucosidase)

Alpha-amylase is the primary enzyme found in saliva that helps break down starch in the mouth. Proper chewing and mastication are important for the enzyme to effectively penetrate the food and begin digestion. Alpha-amylase breaks down amylose, a complex carbohydrate, into smaller units like maltose and glucose. However, it cannot break down maltose itself. As amylose breaks down, intermediate dextrins are formed. Alpha-amylase can also break down amylopectin and glycogen, creating unbranched and branched oligosaccharides. Exoenzyme-glucosidase, similar to glucoamylase, works on disaccharides, oligosaccharides, and aryl glucosides (Hanefeld, 2018; Tomasik & Horton, 2012).

Mechanism of Charantin in Improving Insulin Resistance

Action of Charantin on GLUT4 in Skeletal Muscles

Glycogen synthase, hexokinase, and glucose transporter 4 (GLUT4) are the three main enzymes that regulate the intake of glucose and the production of glycogen. GLUT4 is responsible for transporting glucose from the bloodstream into cells, particularly muscle and fat cells. When insulin interacts with the insulin receptor (INSR) in muscle cells, GLUT4 is mobilized from intracellular compartments to the plasma membrane. This enables glucose absorption and lowers blood glucose levels. If there are low levels of INSR or GLUT4 expression, or deficiencies in the upstream or downstream signaling pathways, the muscles may not be able to effectively absorb glucose. This can result in elevated blood sugar levels. For insulin to affect glucose metabolism, the INSR tyrosine kinase activity must be activated. This is achieved by the phosphorylation of the -subunit of the INSR on several tyrosine residues after insulin binding. Mutations in the critical phosphorylation sites can affect insulin's ability to influence skeletal muscle and the activity of INSR tyrosine kinase. In insulin resistance, cells become less responsive to insulin, leading to reduced stimulation of GLUT4 transporters to move to the cell surface in response to insulin. This impairs the ability of cells to uptake glucose from the bloodstream, resulting in elevated blood glucose levels (Galicia-Garcia et al., 2020). Charantin having insulin-like properties increases GLUT4 expression in the skeletal muscle (Wang et al., 2014).

Table 1. Various studies of charantin covering their extraction and clinical parameters

First Author	Extraction source	Participants	Dose	Efficacy
Çiçek, 2022	Fruit of bitter gourd	Rabbits	180-315 g of fruit	Inhibitory effects on the enzyme α-amylase, with IC50 values of 28 μM.
Mahwish et al., 2021	Flesh part (0.16-0.02 mg/g)	Sprague Dawley rats	Potent dose = 300 mg/kg of whole fruit	Cured renal hypertrophy, polyuria, glycosuria, polydipsia, and improved glomerular filtration rate. Blood glucose levels decreased by 31.64%, and insulin levels rose by 27.35%.
Desai & Tatke, 2015	Present in the fruits and seeds of M. charantia	Cats	50 mg/kg oral dose	More potent than tolbutamide having similar effect on blood sugar level. Blood sugar levels decreased by 42% and 28%, respectively, at the fourth and fifth hours after an oral dosage of 50 mg/kg.
Ahamad et al., 2019	*M. charantia* Linn	Wistar albino mice (30-40 g)	20 mg/kg, b.w. oral dose	Strong alpha-glucosidase (IC_{50} 1.82±0.15 mg/mL) and mild apha-amylase (IC_{50} 2.71± 0.21 mg/mL) inhibitory activity. More potent than oral tolbutamide in alloxan-induced diabetic. Reduced starch and sucrose.
Wang et al., 2014	Fruit part of M. charantia	KK/HIJ mice (T_2D) were induced high-fat diet-ICR mice (T_1D) were induced STZ	CEMC (200 mg/kg/day) orally	Significant hypoglycemic effect and promoted insulin sensitivity in skeletal muscle in KK/HIJ mice, but no effect in ICR mice. In male ddY mice (400 mg/kg) with alloxan-induced diabetes, charantin did not have any hypoglycemic effects. Protected pancreatic cells against the cytotoxicity caused by high glucose, but the protective effect was no longer present after 72 hours. Significant reductions in insulin resistance, plasma glucose intolerance, and non-fasting blood glucose were observed in KK/HIJ mice.
Nagappan et al., 2018	Fruit part of *M. charantia*	Rabbits	50 mg/kg	The typical blood sugar drop over 5 hours was 28%. Despite being more powerful than tolbutamide, both substances produced a similar pattern of blood sugar change. A reduction of 42% in blood sugar levels was observed at the fourth hour when administered at a dose of 50 mg/kg.

Action of Charantin on Insulin Receptor Substrates (IRS) in the Liver

IRS (insulin receptor substrate) proteins are a group of cytoplasmic adaptor proteins that are found in various cells and tissues in the body, such as adipose tissue, liver, skeletal muscle, and the brain. They play a vital role in mediating the signaling of insulin, which is a hormone involved in regulating glucose metabolism. When the insulin receptor is activated, it phosphorylates IRS proteins. Once phosphorylated, IRS proteins act as docking sites for downstream signaling molecules. These downstream molecules bind to the IRS proteins and initiate signaling pathways that are important for regulating glucose metabolism, protein synthesis, and cell growth. The discovery of IRS proteins was made when researchers observed a 185 kD phosphoprotein in anti-phosphotyrosine immunoblots after insulin stimulation. This protein was later identified as IRS-1, which was the first member of the IRS protein family to be identified (Galicia-Garcia et al., 2020). In the liver, insulin controls lipid metabolism more extensively in addition to controlling the generation and utilization of glucose.

Clinical Aspects and Extraction Process of Charantin

Various studies of charantin covering extraction and clinical parameters are presented in Table 1.

Conclusion

Bitter gourd juice and extracts have been found to lower blood sugar levels in animals, but the effectiveness of dried fruit powder in human studies has been inconsistent, possibly because there is no standardized method of preparation. However, certain compounds found in bitter gourd, such as cucurbitane-type triterpenoids, have shown promising effects in tests related to glucose uptake, insulin sensitivity, and insulin secretion. Another compound called charantin has demonstrated its ability to inhibit carbohydrate enzymes and regulate blood sugar levels in mice and rabbits. This indicates that charantin may have potential as a treatment for diabetes. However, more clinical research is needed to determine its effectiveness and safety as an antidiabetic agent. Additionally, methods for cultivating, synthesizing, and isolating charantin should be improved, and new analytical techniques should be developed to accurately detect its components. It may also be beneficial to explore novel drug delivery systems, such as nanoparticles and microspheres, to enhance the efficacy of bitter gourd compounds in diabetes treatment.

References

Ahamad, J., Mir, S. R., Amin, S. (2019). Antihyperglycemic activity of charantin isolated from fruits of Momordica charantia Linn. *International Research Journal of Pharmacy*, 10(1), 61–64.

Desai, S., Tatke, P. (2015). Charantin: An important lead compound from Momordica charantia for the treatment of diabetes. *Journal of Pharmacognosy and Phytochemistry*, 3(6), 163–166.

Galicia-Garcia, U., Benito-Vicente, A., Jebari, S., Larrea-Sebal, A., Siddiqi, H., Uribe, K. B., Ostolaza, H., Martín, C. (2020). Pathophysiology of type 2 diabetes mellitus. *International Journal of Molecular Sciences*, 21(17), 1–34.

Hanefeld, M. (2018). Treatment: Alpha glucosidase inhibitors. *Encyclopedia of Endocrine Diseases*, 2018, 238–244.

Harinantenaina, L., Tanaka, M., Takaoka, S., Oda, M., Mogami, O., Uchida, M., Asakawa, Y. (2006). Momordica charantia constituents and antidiabetic screening of the isolated major compounds. *Chemical and Pharmaceutical Bulletin*, 54(7), 1017–1021.

IDF Diabetes Atlas 2021 | *IDF Diabetes Atlas*. (2021). Retrieved April 29, 2023, from https://diabetesatlas.org/atlas/tenth-edition/.

Mahwish, Saeed, F., Tauseef Sultan, M., Riaz, A., Ahmed, S., Bigiu, N., Amarowicz, R., Manea, R. (2021). Bitter Melon (Momordica charantia L.) Fruit Bioactives Charantin and Vicine Potential for Diabetes Prophylaxis and Treatment. *Plants*, 2021, 10(4), 730.

Malik, A., Ahmed, M., Mansoor, S., Ambreen, S., Usman, B., Shehryar, M. (2022). Cognitive Impairment in Type 2 Diabetes Mellitus. *Cureus*, 14(2), 59.

Nagappan, K., Anoop, K., Kowmudi, G. (2018). Charantin: A Neglected Antidiabetic Compound from Momordica charantia L. *International Journal of Pharmaceutical Sciences Review and Research*, 51(2), 35–40.

Richter, E., Geetha, T., Burnett, D., Broderick, T. L., Babu, J. R. (2023). The effects of Momordica charantia on type 2 diabetes mellitus and Alzheimer's disease. *International Journal of Molecular Sciences*, 24(5), 4643.

Sharma, P., Singh, S., Thakur, V., Sharma, N., Grewal, A. S. (2021). Novel and emerging therapeutic drug targets for management of type 2 diabetes mellitus. *Obesity Medicine*, 23, 100329.

Singh, J., Cumming, E., Manoharan, G., Kalasz, H., Adeghate, E. (2011). Medicinal chemistry of the anti-diabetic effects of Momordica charantia: active constituents and modes of actions. *Open Medicinal Chemistry Journal*, 5(Suppl 2), 70.

Tomasik, P., Horton, D. (2012). Enzymatic conversions of starch. *Advances in Carbohydrate Chemistry and Biochemistry*, 68, 59–436.

Wang, H. Y., Kan, W. C., Cheng, T. J., Yu, S. H., Chang, L. H., Chuu, J. J. (2014). Differential anti-diabetic effects and mechanism of action of charantin-rich extract of Taiwanese Momordica charantia between type 1 and type 2 diabetic mice. *Food and Chemical Toxicology*, 69, 347–356.

Chapter 20

Curcumin in the Management of Diabetes Mellitus

Aakriti Saini[1,*]
Diksha Gulati[1]
Deepshi Arora[1]
Janhavi Singh[2]
Sangya Dubey[2]
Chaitanay Vinayak Narayan[2]
Neelam Singh[2]
Gaurav Chaudhary[2]
Sweta Pundir[2]
Raj Kumari[2]
Meenakshi Sharma[2]
and Rohit Malik[3]
[1]Guru Gobind Singh College of Pharmacy, Yamuna Nagar, Haryana, India
[2]I. T. S. College of Pharmacy, Muradnagar, Ghaziabad, Uttar Pradesh, India
[3]Veer Kunwar College of Pharmacy, Bijnor, Uttar Pradesh, India

Abstract

A group of metabolic disorders, known as diabetes mellitus, has reached pandemic levels worldwide. Managing patients with this complex illness, who require continuous medication and lifestyle

---

* Corresponding Author's Email: sainiakki16041991@gmail.com.

In: Naturally Occurring Chemicals …
Editors: A. Singh Grewal, G. Deswal, A. Kumar Dhingra et al.
ISBN: 979-8-89113-491-1

adjustments, poses a significant challenge. It is widely known that diabetes mellitus can be prevented, and reducing the number of new cases could help lessen its burden on the world. Current research supports the effectiveness of herbal supplements in preventing and controlling diabetes mellitus. One increasingly studied medicinal plant is curcumin, found in the rhizome of the turmeric plant, Curcuma longa. Turmeric, a natural product with extensive medicinal properties, has been predominantly linked to the therapeutic effects of curcuminoids on various diseases, including cancer, diabetes, and neurodegenerative, hepatic, and renal damage. Curcumin has been shown to improve the metabolic profile and related issues of diabetes mellitus, functioning as a hypoglycemic drug or as an adjuvant. It is important to investigate any potential interactions between curcumin and conventional antidiabetic medications for the treatment of diabetes mellitus.

Keywords: diabetes mellitus, turmeric, neurodegenerative, curcuminoids, hypoglycaemic agents

Introduction

Diabetes, specifically type II diabetes, is a complex chronic metabolic condition that affects the production and utilization of insulin, thereby impacting the metabolism of proteins, carbohydrates, and fats, and leading to persistent hyperglycemia (Alberti & Zimmet, 1998; Roglic, 2016). In the United States, dealing with Type 2 diabetes cost $245 million in 2012 (Petersen, 2013). This condition can have adverse effects during pregnancy, such as fetal mortality, preeclampsia, and eclampsia. The key characteristics of diabetes include dysfunction of pancreatic β-cells and insulin resistance, although various studies have elucidated the intricate nature of diabetes mellitus (Wu et al., 2016). To cope with the disease, pancreatic β-cells may undergo changes in the function of their regulatory components and gene expression patterns (Kendall et al., 2009). One important process involved in cell preservation, regulation of apoptosis, and modulation of antioxidant agent concentrations is the activation of AMP-activated protein kinase (AMPK), which triggers the PI3K/protein kinase B (Akt)/mammalian targeting of rapamycin (mTOR) pathway. Another significant intracellular pathway is mediated by IKK, which activates the transcription of the pro-inflammatory cytokine-controlling nuclear factor-kB (NF-kb) (Lawlor et al., 2017). The forkhead box protein O 1 (FoxO1), involved in cell cycle progression, redox balance, and glucose and lipid metabolism, plays a role in regulating apoptosis as well (Liang et al., 2017). Additionally, GLP-1 is known to promote insulin synthesis and reduce the production of pro-inflammatory cytokines (Mackenzie et al., 2014). B-cell dysfunction manifests at the cellular level as progressive B-cell failure and structural abnormalities, resulting in a decrease in both the number and insulin-secreting ability of B-cells (Oguiza et al., 2015). Current medications for B-cell dysfunction not only impose a financial burden on society but also have various negative consequences such as obesity, congestive heart failure, hypoglycemia, and changes in digestive glands. To alleviate these adverse effects and leverage the nutritional and therapeutic benefits of specific plants and their constituent chemicals, natural products have gained significant attention globally (Peng et al., 2008). One such natural product is turmeric, scientifically known as Curcuma longa, a short, herbaceous plant belonging to the Zingiberaceae family. Turmeric is predominantly cultivated in tropical and subtropical climates and has been traditionally used in Chinese and Indian medicine for its curative properties (Lavin et al., 2016). Commercial curcumin, derived from turmeric, mainly consists of approximately 77% curcumin (curcumin I), 17% desmethoxycurcumin (curcumin II), 3% bisdemethoxycurcumin (curcumin III), and cyclocurcumin (curcumin IV) (Saraswati et al., 2018). Apart from curcuminoids, turmeric also contains 69.4% sugars, 6.3% amino acids, 5.1% fat, and 5.8% essential oils (Tsuchiya & Ogawa, 2017). Curcumin exhibits therapeutic potential in the treatment of diabetes mellitus, progressive liver failure, renal diseases, neurological disorders, and vascular conditions (Guo et al., 2016).

Antihyperglycemic Properties of Turmeric

Curcumin has gained considerable attention in the past decade for its potential anti-diabetic properties. Several studies, mostly conducted in animal models and in vitro, have explored the use of curcumin as an alternative to currently prescribed medications for diabetes mellitus (Ferrannini, 2010). In one study using rats, the administration of theracurmin (a formulation that increases the bioavailability of curcumin when taken orally) resulted in a reduction in glucose intolerance. This effect was reversed when the rats were treated with GW1000, an antagonist of the G protein-coupled receptor (GPR) 40/120, and neomycin, an anti-phospholipase C. The increased secretion of glucagon-like peptide-1 (GLP-1) was identified as the mechanism behind this effect, as GLP-1 stimulates the release of insulin, leading to a reduction in blood glucose (Cinti et al., 2016). Curcumin's efficacy in insulin resistance models has been evaluated both in vivo and in vitro. For example, curcumin has been shown to reduce insulin resistance in rats with polycystic ovarian syndrome or a metabolic disorder, as well as in human hepatic HepG2 cells (Vetere et al., 2014). Furthermore, studies have investigated the effects of curcumin on animal models of disease. By activating the IRS/PI3K/Akt system and increasing the expression of glucose transporters (GLUT) 1 and 3 genes, curcumin has been demonstrated to decrease insulin resistance (Weir, 2013). Another significant target of curcumin in diabetes management is the enzyme GSK-3b, which plays a role in glycogen formation through phosphorylation. A computer-simulated docking study revealed that curcumin can bind to the enzyme GSK-3b's binding region, inhibiting its activity and increasing glycogen production in fasting mice (Tangvarasittichai, 2015). Curcumin has also been shown to prevent high glucose-induced apoptosis in newborn rat cardiomyocytes in culture by increasing Akt and GSK-3β phosphorylation (Back, 2012). Additionally, curcumin has been found to decrease glucose levels and coronary artery disease, as well as improve other heart characteristics such as fibrosis, in a mouse model of type 2 diabetes, in vivo (Back, 2012). The relationship between diabetes mellitus and obesity is well-established, and adipokines released by adipose tissue have been linked to insulin resistance and glucose dysregulation (Masini et al., 2017). Leptin, a hormone that typically suppresses appetite and enhances insulin sensitivity (Mulder & Ling, 2009), may become resistant in cases of overweight, hyperleptinemia, and type 2 diabetes, leading to increased food intake, fat accumulation, and disruptions in glucose and lipid metabolism (Wu et al., 2017). Additionally, curcumin has been found to activate the Wnt/b-catenin pathway (Kim & Lee, 2014). In hamsters fed a high-fat diet, curcumin has been found to decrease the expression of fatty acid synthase and hepatic fatty acid b-oxidation, potentially preventing hyperlipidemia (Hogan & Hull, 2017). In rats with elevated cholesterol levels, metabolic disorders, and diabetes, curcumin has been shown to alter the lipid profile by reducing triglycerides in the blood and potentially increasing HDL cholesterol levels (Hogan & Hull, 2017). In a study conducted on rats with diabetic complications caused by streptozotocin, a comparison was made between a modified form of curcumin and native curcumin. The modified form showed better results in the sugar tolerance test, was more effective at lowering blood sugar levels, and delivered a higher amount of curcumin in vitro experiments (Westwell Roper, 2014).

However, in pancreatic tissue, both the modified form and native curcumin were found to lower triglyceride and cholesterol levels to comparable levels, without affecting the concentration of insulin (Portero McLellan et al., 2014). Curcumin has also been shown to counteract oxidative stress, which is a characteristic of diabetes, by enhancing the functioning of antioxidant enzymes like paraoxonase-1, super oxygen dismutase 1 (SOD1), catalase, and glutathione peroxidase (Hogan & Hull, 2017). There have been studies conducted to evaluate the relative biological activity of different curcuminoids present in Curcuma longa, the plant from which curcumin is derived (Sylvetsky et al., 2017). From the three main curcuminoids, curcumin has demonstrated the greatest anti-inflammatory power, followed by bisdemethoxycurcumin and desmethoxycurcumin. Although bisdemethoxycurcumin showed the strongest anti-inflammatory effect, both the DPPH and FRAP assays indicated a decrease in inflammation. Curcumin has been proven to combat oxidative stress and inflammation, both of which are characteristic of diabetes (Holstein, 2009). By inhibiting the breakdown of alpha b inhibitors (IkBa) and reducing oxidative load-sympathetic enzymes (ERK 1/2 and p38), curcumin effectively manages oxidative stress and inflammation in the muscles of rats fed fructose. This prevents the activation of nuclear hormone significant effects-light-chain-enhancer of B cells (NF-kb) when pro-inflammatory cytokines such as tumor necrosis factor-alpha (TNFa) and C-reactive protein are present, thereby reducing inflammation (Gul et al., 2016). Curcumin's suppression of the NF-kb signaling cascade during diabetes benefits not only the pancreatic tissue but also other organs such as lymphatic vessels, kidneys, liver function, and adipose tissue. This suppression contributes to reducing the complications typically associated with diabetes mellitus (Li et al., 2017). It is worth noting that GSK-3b also plays a role in controlling NF-kb activity, which is closely related to the pathogenesis of diabetes (Prasad et al., 2014). Another important pathway through which curcumin exerts its effects in diabetes is the nuclear factor E2-related factors 2 (Nrf2)/Keap1/ARE pathway. This pathway regulates the expression of over 100 genes associated with oxidative damage, cell survival, and disease (Ríos, 2015). Numerous in vivo and in vitro studies have demonstrated that curcumin can reverse the negative effects on Nrf2 signaling, with the kidney being particularly responsive (Varzakas et al., 2016). Curcumin has also been shown to enhance the activity of antioxidant enzymes, reduce the levels of inflammatory cytokines such as TNF-a and IL-1b, and improve both immune response and antioxidant profile. Additionally, curcumin may have potential benefits when used alongside bone marrow transplantation (Panwar, 2014).

Curcumin's Effects on Diabetic Nephropathy

In both the US and Europe, diabetes mellitus is a significant cause of morbidity and mortality, and it is now the leading global cause of chronic renal failure. Studies have shown that approximately 40% of diabetic patients develop diabetic nephropathy, a microvascular complication (Ding et al., 2016). Diabetic nephropathy is characterized by alterations in renal hemodynamic conditions and structural damage, primarily affecting the glomeruli and tubules. Although the exact mechanisms contributing to the development of diabetic nephropathy are unknown, several factors associated with high blood sugar levels have been proposed, such as increased protein glycosylation, heightened aldose reductase activity, activation of cytokines and growth factors, and the production of oxidative stress (Gunnink et al., 2016). The management of diabetic nephropathy has been a major focus for the development of effective methods utilizing therapeutic substances with nutritional and medicinal properties. Treatment with curcumin in diabetic rats has shown promising results, including reduced kidney structural abnormalities, improved creatinine clearance, and decreased levels of urinary protein excretion. Additionally, curcumin treatment suppressed the inflammatory response in rats by reducing renal macrophage infiltration and the release of macrophage-associated factors such as peptides-1, IL-1b, IL-6, and TNF-α (Kalaycio & Erim, 2017). The kidney-protective effect of curcumin therapy is attributed to its ability to decrease caveolin-1 phosphorylated at Tyr14 and inhibit the kinase activity of toll-like receptor 4. Additionally, it has been discovered that curcumin can regulate the interactions between caveolin-1, activation, and reactive oxygen species (ROS), which can in turn lessen the effects of high glucose on podocyte death in vitro and diabetic renal disease in rats (Kaur & Chintamaneni, 2016). Curcumin has also been found to inhibit several epithelial-mesenchymal transition-related events in NRK-52E, including an increase in the levels of α-smooth muscle actin associated with Nrf2 activation and subsequent heme oxygenase-1 induction, and a decrease in the production of the protein E-cadherin (Panahi et al., 2017). Additionally, curcumin blocks the effects of transforming growth factor-beta 1 (TGF-β1), fibronectin, and IV collagen in protecting against diabetic nephropathy. It also inhibits the activity of inflammasomes due to its potent antifibrotic effects. The inflammasome consists of the proteins caspase-1, NOD-like receptor 3, and the adaptor protein apoptotic cell death-associated speck-like protein with a CARD domain.

Curcumin's Effects on Diabetic Cardiomyopathy

Diabetes mellitus often leads to diabetic cardiomyopathy, which is dysfunction in the left ventricle of the heart during diastole or systole (Amalraj et al., 2017). Factors such as apoptosis, inflammation, hypertrophy, and oxidative damage contribute to negative effects on the heart in individuals with Type 2 diabetes. However, studies conducted on rats have demonstrated that curcumin can help mitigate these effects. In one study, rats were given a moderate dose of streptozotocin and treated with 300 milligrams/kg/day of curcumin for 16 weeks. The results showed reduced heart tissue fibrosis, particularly decreased deposition of both type I and type III collagen (Castro et al., 2014). Additional information gathered from the treatment of human heart fibroblasts with 30 mmol/l of glucose followed by curcumin provided further understanding of the potential mechanism of action. Curcumin was found to block TGF-b1 and its subsequent processes, both dependent and independent of the protein Smad. These processes stimulate myofibroblast activation, increase the formation of the extracellular matrix, and slow down its breakdown (Poole et al., 2015). Curcumin has been found to prevent myocyte hypertrophy, a symptom of diabetes, by reversing the lowered activity of PPARg and Akt in vitro. This protective effect helps shield the cells from the negative morphological and functional changes caused by excessive glucose levels. In a study conducted on rats, the harmful effects induced by streptozotocin in their hearts – including increased body weight and oxidative stress – were effectively reversed by curcumin administration at a dosage of 200 µg/ml/kg/day for six weeks. Furthermore, curcumin restored the levels of several antioxidant enzymes, such as catalase SOD1 and antioxidants-S-transferase, as well as glutathione. Moreover, curcumin alleviated the streptozotocin-induced elevation in enzyme activity, which is indicative of heart injury (Trujillo et al., 2016).

Clinical Trials Provide Evidence for the Antihyperglycemic Effects of Curcumin

The use of curcumin in laboratory and animal models has demonstrated a multitude of potential mechanisms, but clinical studies have had inconsistent results (Trujillo, 2013). Curcumin is a natural polyphenol found in turmeric that has been used in traditional medicine for centuries to treat various ailments, including diabetes. Recent research suggests that curcumin may have antihyperglycemic properties and can help decrease blood sugar levels in individuals with diabetes. Clinical studies have explored the antihyperglycemic effects of curcumin in humans, and one study found that supplementing with curcumin significantly improved beta-cell function and reduced the risk of developing type 2 diabetes in individuals with prediabetes (Sylvester et al., 2015). However, it is important to note that curcumin may interact with certain medications and may not be suitable for everyone, so consulting a healthcare professional before taking any supplements is advised (Guo, 2017).

Future Perspectives

Future studies may investigate the potential benefits of administering turmeric alongside other antidiabetic medications, such as metformin or insulin. This combined therapy could potentially offer even greater advantages than using either treatment alone. Furthermore, researchers could explore the development of new curcumin formulations, such as nanoparticles or liposomes, which could enhance its bioavailability and effectiveness. These advancements could make turmeric a more attractive option for managing diabetes.

Conclusion

Although curcumin has shown promising results in treating diabetes mellitus, further studies are needed to fully understand its mechanisms of action and determine the optimal dosages and formulations for therapeutic use. Curcumin, the main component of turmeric, has been found to be beneficial in managing diabetes mellitus. Studies have demonstrated its ability to reduce blood glucose levels, improve insulin sensitivity, and decrease the risk of diabetes-related complications. However, to fully grasp how curcumin functions and establish the most effective dosages and preparations for clinical practice, more research is required.

References

Alberti, K. G. M, Zimmet, P. Z. (1998). Definition, diagnosis, and classification of diabetes mellitus and its complications. Part 1: Diagnosis and classification of diabetes mellitus. *Diabetes Care*, 15, 539-553.

Amalraj A., Pius., Gopi, S. (2017). Biological activities of curcuminoids, other biomolecules from turmeric and their derivatives- a review. *Journal of Traditional and Complementary Medicine*, 7(2), 205-223.

Back, S. H., Kaufman, R. J. (2012). Endoplasmic reticulum stress and type 2 diabetes. *Annual Review of Biochemistry*, 81, 767-793.

Castro, C. N., Barcala Tabarrozzi, A. E., Winnewisser, J., Gimeno, M. L., Antunica Noguerol, M., Liberman, A. C., Paz, D. A., Dewey R. A., Perone, M. J. (2014). Curcumin ameliorates autoimmune diabetes: Evidence in accelerated murine models of type 1 diabetes. *Clinical and experimental Immunology*, 177, 149-160.

Cinti, F., Bouchi, R., Kim-Muller, J. Y., Ohmura Y., Sandoval, P. R., Masini, M., Marselli, L., Suleiman, M., Ratner, L. E., Marchetti, P., Accili D. (2016). Evidence of B-cell dedifferentiation in human type 2 diabetes. *Journal of Clinical Endocrinology & Metabolism*, 101, 1044-1054.

Ding, L., Li, J., Song, B., Xiao, X., Zhang, B., Qi, M., Huang, W., Yang, L., Wang, Z. (2016). Curcumin rescues high-fat diet-induced obesity and insulin sensitivity in mice by regulating SREBP pathway. *Toxicology and Applied Pharmacology*, 304, 99-109.

Sylvetsky, A. C., Edelstein, S. L., Walford, G., Boyko, E. J., Horton, E. S., Ibebuogu, U. N., Knowler, W. C., Montez, M. G., Temprosa, M., Hoskin, M., Rother, K. I., Delahanty, L. M., Diabetes Prevention Program Research Group. (2017). A high-carbohydrate, high-fiber, low-fat diet results in weight loss among adults at high risk of type 2 diabetes. *Journal of Nutrition*, 147(11), 2060-2066.

Ferrannini, E. (2010). The stunned b cell: a brief history. *Cell Metabolism*, 11, 349-352.

Guo, S., Liu, F., Yang, Y., Zhao, X., Fan, Y., Ma, W., Yang, D., Yang, A., Yu, Y. (2017). Curcumin-induced autophagy anticancer effects on human lung adenocarcinoma cell line A549. *Oncology Letters*, 14, 2775-2782.

Gunnink, L. K., Alabi, O. D., Kuiper, B. D., Gunnink, S. M., Schuiteman, S. J., Strohbehn, L. E., Hamilton, K. E., Wrobel, K. E., Louters, L. L. (2016). Curcumin directly inhibits the transport activity of GLUT1. *Biochimie*, 125, 179-185.

Gul, K., Singh, A. K., Jabeen, R. (2016). Nutraceuticals and functional foods: The foods for the future world. *Critical Reviews in Food Science and Nutrition*, 56(13), 2617-2627.

Guo, C., Huang, T., Chen, A., Chen, X., Wang, L., Shen, F., Gu, X. (2016). Glucagon-like peptide 1 improves insulin resistance in vitro through the anti-inflammation of macrophages. *Brazilian Journal of Medical and Biological Research*, 2016, 49.

Holstein, A., Beil, W. (2009). Oral antidiabetic drug metabolism: pharmacogenomics and drug interactions. *Expert Opinion on Drug Metabolism & Toxicology*, 5(2), 225-241.

Hogan, M. F., Hull, R. L. (2017). The islet endothelial cell: A novel contributor to beta cell secretory dysfunction in diabetes. *Diabetologia*, 60, 952-959.

Kim, K. S., Lee, H. J., Jeong, S. H., Chung, K. H., Kim, B. I. (2017). Antibacterial photodynamic therapy with curcumin and Curcuma xanthorrhiza extract against Streptococcus mutans. *Photodiagnosis and Photodynamic Therapy*, 19, 300-309.

Kaur, G., Invally, M., Chintamaneni, M. (2016). Influence of piperine and quercetin on antidiabetic potential of curcumin. *Journal of Complementary and Integrative Medicine*, 13, 247-255.

Kalaycio_glu, Z., Gazio_glu, I., Erim, F. B. (2017). Comparison of antioxidant, anticholinesterase, and antidiabetic activities of three curcuminoids isolated from Curcuma longa L. *Natural Product Research*, 2017, 1-4.

Kim, K. H., Lee, M. S. (2014). Autophagy - a key player in cellular and body metabolism. *Nature Reviews Endocrinology*, 10, 322-337.

Kendall, D. M., Cuddihy, R. M., Bergenstal, R. M. (2009). Clinical application of incretin-based therapy: therapeutic potential, patient selection and clinical use. *The American Journal of Medicine*, 122(6 Suppl), S37-S50.

Lawlor, N., Khetan, S., Ucar, D., Stitzel, M. L. (2017). Genomics of islet (Dys)function and type 2 diabetes. *Trends in Genetics*, 33, 244-255.

Liang, Y., Li, J., Lin, Q., Huang, P., Zhang, L., Wu, W., Ma, Y. (2017). Research progress on signaling pathway-associated oxidative stress in endothelial cells. *Oxidative Medicine and Cellular Longevity*, 2017, 7156941.

Lavin, D. P., White, M. F., Brazil, D. P. (2016). IRS proteins and diabetic complications. *Diabetologia*, 59, 2280-2291.

Li, W., Yuan, G., Pan, Y., Wang, C., Chen, H. (2017). Network pharmacology studies on the bioactive compounds and action mechanisms of natural products for the treatment of diabetes mellitus: A review. *Frontiers in Pharmacology*, 8, 74.

Lestari, Y., Velina, Y., Rahminiwati, M. (2015). Metabolites activity of endophytic Streptomyces sp. IPBCC. b.15.1539 from Tinospora crispa l. miers: a-glucosidase inhibitor and anti-hyperglycemic in mice. *International Journal of Pharmaceutics and Pharmaceutical Sciences*, 7, 235-239.

Masini, M., Martino, L., Marselli, L., Bugliani, M., Boggi, U., Filipponi, F., Marchetti, P., De Tata, V. (2017). Ultrastructural alterations of pancreatic beta cells in human diabetes mellitus. *Diabetes & Metabolism*, 33, E2894.

Mulder, H., Ling, C. (2009). Mitochondrial dysfunction in pancreatic beta-cells in Type 2 Diabetes. *Molecular and Cellular Endocrinology*, 297, 34-40.

Mackenzie, R. W., Elliott, B. T. (2014). Akt/PKB activation and insulin signaling: a novel insulin signaling pathway in the treatment of type 2 diabetes. *Diabetes, Metabolic Syndrome and Obesity: Targets and Therapy*, 7, 55-64.

Petersen, M. (2013). Economic costs of diabetes in the U.S. in 2012. *Diabetes Care*, 39, 1033-1046.

Peng, F., Wu, D., Gao, B., Ingram, A. J., Zhang, B., Chorneyko, K., McKenzie, R., Krepinsky, J. C. (2008). RhoA/Rho-kinase contribute to the pathogenesis of the diabetic renal disease. *Diabetes*, 57(6), 1683-1692.

Portero McLellan, K. C., Wyne, K., Villagomez, E. T., Hsueh, W. A. (2014). Therapeutic interventions to reduce the risk of progression from prediabetes to type 2 diabetes mellitus. *Therapeutics and Clinical Risk Management*, 10, 173-188.

Prasad, S., Gupta, S. C., Tyagi, A. K., Aggarwal, B. B. (2014). Curcumin, a component of golden spice: from bedside to bench and back. *Biotechnology Advances*, 32(6), 1053-1064.

Panwar, H., Calderwood, D., Grant, I. R., Grover, S., Green, B. D. (2014). Lactobacillus strains isolated from infant faeces possess potent inhibitory activity against intestinal alpha-and beta-glucosidases suggesting anti-diabetic potential. *European Journal of Nutrition*, 53(7), 1465-1474.

Poole, K. M., Nelson, C. E., Joshi, R. V., Martin, J. R., Gupta, M. K., Haws, S. C., Kavanaugh, T. E., Skala, M. C., Duvall, C. L. (2015). ROS-responsive microspheres for on demand antioxidant therapy in a model of diabetic peripheral arterial disease. *Biomaterials*, 41, 166-175.

Panahi, Y., Khalili, N., Sahebi, E., Namazi, S., Karimian, M. S., Majeed, M., Sahebkar, A. (2017). Antioxidant effects of curcuminoids in patients with type 2 diabetes mellitus: a randomized controlled trial. *Inflammopharmacology*, 25, 25-31.

Ríos, J. L., Francini, F., Schinella, G. R. (2015). Natural products for the treatment of type 2 diabetes mellitus. *Planta Medica*, 81(12-13), 975-994.

Roglic, G., World Health Organization (Eds.). (2016). *Global Report on Diabetes*. Geneva, Switzerland: World Health Organization.

Saraswati, A. P., Ali Hussaini, S. M., Krishna, N. H., Babu, B. N., Kamal, A. (2018). Glycogen synthase kinase-3 and its inhibitors: potential target for various therapeutic conditions. *European Journal of Medicinal Chemistry*, 144, 843-858.

Sylvester, W. S., Son, R., Lew, K. F., Rukayadi, Y. (2015). Antibacterial activity of java turmeric (Curcuma xanthorrhiza Roxb.) extract against Klebsiella pneumoniae isolated from several vegetables. *International Food Research Journal*, 22(5), 1770-1776.

Tsuchiya, K., Ogawa, Y. (2017). Forkhead box class O family member proteins: the biology and pathophysiological roles in diabetes. *Journal of Diabetes Investigation*, 8, 726-734.

Tangvarasittichai, S. (2015). Oxidative stress, insulin resistance, dyslipidemia and type 2 diabetes mellitus. *World Journal of Diabetes*, 6, 456.

Trujillo, J., Molina-Jijón, E., Medina-Campos, O. N., Rodríguez-Muñoz, R., Reyes, J. L., Loredo, M. L., Barrera-Oviedo, D., Pinzón, E., Rodríguez-Rangel, D. S., Pedraza-Chaverri, J. (2016). Curcumin prevents cisplatin-induced decrease in the tight and adherens junctions: Relation to oxidative stress. *Food & Function*, 7(1), 279-293.

Trujillo, J., Chirino, Y. I., Molina-Jijón, E., Andérica-Romero, A. C., Tapia, E., Pedraza-Chaverrí, J. (2013). Renoprotective effect of the antioxidant curcumin: Recent findings. *Redox Biology*, 1, 448-456.

Vetere, A., Choudhary, A., Burns, S. M., Wagner, B. K. (2014). Targeting the pancreatic β-cell to treat diabetes. *Nature Reviews Drug Discovery*, 13, 278-289.

Varzakas, T., Zakynthinos, G., Verpoort, F. (2016). Plant food residues as a source of nutraceuticals and functional foods. *Foods*, 5(4), 88.

Wu, E. T., Nien, F. J., Kuo, C. H., Chen, S. C., Chen, K. Y., Chuang, L. M., Li, H. Y., Lee, C. N. (2016). Diagnosis of more gestational diabetes lead to better pregnancy outcomes: comparing the international association of the diabetes and pregnancy study group criteria, and the carpenter and Coustan criteria. *Journal of Diabetes Investigation*, 7, 121-126.

Weir, G. C., Aguayo-Mazzucato, C., Bonner-Weir, S. (2013). β-cell dedifferentiation in diabetes is important, but what is it? *Islets*, 5, 233-237.

Wu, J., Luo, X., Thangthaeng, N., Sumien, N., Chen, Z., Rutledge, M. A., Jing, S., Forster, M. J., Yan, L. J. (2017). Pancreatic mitochondrial complex I exhibit aberrant hyperactivity in diabetes. *Biochemistry and Biophysics Reports*, 11, 119-129.

Westwell-Roper, C., Nackiewicz, D., Dan, M., Ehses, J. A. (2014). Toll-like receptors and NLRP3 as central regulators of pancreatic islet inflammation in type 2 diabetes. *Immunology and Cell Biology*, 92, 314-323.

Chapter 21

Gallic Acid in the Management of Diabetes Mellitus

Junaid Tantray[1,*]
Akhilesh Patel[1]
Sourabh Kosey[2]
Ankur Agrawal[3]
and Puneet Chauhan[1]
[1]NIMS Institute of Pharmacy, NIMS University, Jaipur, Rajasthan, India
[2]I. S. F. College of Pharmacy, Moga, Punjab, India
[3]Jai Institute of Pharmaceutical Sciences and Research, Gwalior, Madhya Pradesh, India

Abstract

Gallic acid, a natural compound found in many plant-based foods, has been studied for its potential in managing diabetes. This chapter explores the current research on gallic acid and its effects on blood sugar control, insulin sensitivity, and complications related to diabetes. Animal and cell studies have shown that gallic acid may lower blood sugar levels by inhibiting enzymes involved in carbohydrate metabolism. Furthermore, gallic acid has antioxidant and anti-inflammatory properties, which could be beneficial in managing complications such as neuropathy, retinopathy, and nephropathy. While more research is necessary to determine the safety and effectiveness of gallic acid in humans with diabetes, these findings indicate that gallic acid could be a promising natural treatment for diabetes. Potential aspects of gallic acid in diabetes include its ability to lower blood sugar

* Corresponding Author's Email: junaidtantray22@gmail.com.

In: Naturally Occurring Chemicals …
Editors: A. Singh Grewal, G. Deswal, A. Kumar Dhingra et al.
ISBN: 979-8-89113-491-1

levels, act as an antioxidant, reduce inflammation, and prevent glycation.

Keywords: diabetes mellitus, oxidative stress, inflammation, gallic acid

Abbreviations

AGEs	Advanced glycation end-products
COX	Cyclooxygenase
DM	Diabetes mellitus
FRG	Free radical generation
GA	Gallic acid
GA3P	glyceraldehyde-3-phosphate
IRS1	insulin receptor substrate 1
LOX	Lipoxygenase
MAPK	Mitogen-activated protein kinases
OS	Oxidative stress
PKC	Protein kinase C
PPAR	Peroxisome proliferator-activated receptors
ROS	Reactive oxygen species
T1DM	Type 1 diabetes mellitus
T2DM	Type 2 diabetes mellitus
TNFα	Tumour necrosis factor α
WHO	World Health Organisation.

Introduction

Insufficient insulin production, reduced insulin effectiveness, or both contribute to the high levels of blood sugar seen in diabetes mellitus, a group of metabolic diseases. Diabetes mellitus is a chronic condition that impairs the body's ability to metabolize glucose, which leads to significant health effects. The World Health Organization recognizes two main types of diabetes: Type 1 (DM1) and Type 2 (DM2). DM1 is characterized by a complete lack of insulin, usually resulting from the loss of pancreatic beta cells. DM2, on the other hand, is caused by insulin resistance or decreased insulin secretion. In DM1, the body either does not produce enough insulin or does not utilize it effectively. Without insulin, glucose cannot enter the cells and builds up in the blood, causing high blood sugar levels, known as hyperglycemia. This excess glucose is then excreted in the urine, a condition called glycosuria. There are various complications associated with diabetes. Microvascular complications include retinopathy (damage to the retina), nephropathy (kidney damage), and neuropathy (nerve damage). Macrovascular complications include ischemic heart disease (reduced blood flow to the heart), stroke, and peripheral vascular disease, all of which can have serious effects on multiple parts of the body. The global incidence of diabetes has been steadily increasing, largely due to the rising rates of obesity. Diabetes is a significant public health concern because it is associated with early morbidity, increased mortality, reduced life expectancy, and burdensome financial costs for patients, caregivers, and healthcare systems (Forouhi and Wareham, 2010).

Mechanisms of Oxidative Stress (OS) Development in Diabetes Mellitus

Diabetes is strongly linked to oxidative stress (OS), a condition where the body produces more reactive oxygen species (ROS) than it can counteract with antioxidants. ROS are highly reactive molecules that can harm DNA, proteins, and lipids, leading to tissue damage and cellular abnormalities. Various factors influence OS in diabetes: High blood sugar levels trigger ROS production through metabolic pathways like the polyol pathway, advanced glycation end product (AGE) production, and protein kinase C (PKC) activation. Mitochondrial dysfunction and chronic low-grade inflammation also contribute to ROS production. Furthermore, the reduced antioxidant defenses in people with diabetes aggravate OS. Effective treatment of OS is crucial for preventing and managing diabetes-related issues. Increased blood glucose levels and OS are linked to vascular problems, and different metabolic pathways, such as glycolysis, AGE formation, PKC activation, and impairment of the insulin signaling pathway, contribute to OS in hyperglycemic conditions. The accumulation of glyceraldehyde-3-phosphate (GA3P) speeds up the oxidation of glucose, resulting in the production of glyoxal, a precursor to AGEs, and an increase in OS within cells (Bigagli et al., 2010).

Role of OS in the Development and Complications of DM

ROS, or reactive oxygen species, are molecules that are highly reactive and are produced during cellular metabolism. They include both non-radical molecules like hydrogen peroxide and singlet oxygen, as well as free radicals like superoxide anions and hydroxyl radicals. While ROS plays important roles in physiological processes such as cell signaling, excessive production of ROS can result in oxidative stress (OS), which can damage important biomolecules like DNA, proteins, and lipids. It is crucial to maintain a balance between ROS production and the antioxidant defence system to promote overall health.

In conditions like diabetes mellitus (DM), hyperglycemia, or high blood sugar levels, triggers various metabolic pathways that contribute to the production of ROS and OS. These pathways include the polyol pathway, advanced glycation end products (AGEs), and protein kinase C (PKC). The resulting oxidative stress in diabetes can lead to complications in multiple tissues and organs, including neuropathy, retinopathy, nephropathy, and cardiovascular disease. Managing and controlling high blood sugar levels through lifestyle changes, medications, and antioxidant therapy can help prevent diabetes-related complications and reduce their incidence. Acute episodes of hyperglycemia can promote the generation of reactive oxygen species and further disturb the physiological balance, potentially leading to vascular dysfunction. Research suggests a connection between oxidative stress and hyperglycemia, with evidence of decreased antioxidant defences and increased markers of oxidative stress in response to acute episodes of high blood sugar. Dysfunction of vascular endothelial cells and the resulting glycoxidation stress contribute to the development of diabetes complications (Nkanu et al., 2007).

OS in Insulin Resistance with Its Consequences

The overproduction of reactive oxygen species (ROS) in liver cells of obese mice is associated with insulin resistance, which is an indicator of the risk of developing metabolic syndrome and diabetes. Researchers have discovered that removing hydrogen peroxide, a type of ROS, helps reduce insulin resistance. When mitochondria produce higher levels of ROS, oxidative stress (OS) in the body increases. Elevated levels of OS and glucose are specifically associated with type 1 and type 2 diabetes. ROS can disrupt cell signaling by activating various stress-sensitive pathways in cells. Stress kinases in different cell lines can be activated by micromolar concentrations of hydrogen peroxide. These stress kinases include c-Jun N-terminal kinase, p38, IB kinase, and extracellular receptor 1/2 kinase. Activation of stress kinases can impair physiological responses to insulin, reducing its ability to increase glucose uptake, glycogen formation, and protein production. The downregulation of oxidized cells is a complex process involving multiple mechanisms. Insulin receptor substrate 1 (IRS1) undergoes increased serine/threonine phosphorylation in response to insulin, while protein kinase B phosphorylation decreases and GLUT4 translocation to the plasma membrane is reduced (Bloch-Damti et al., 2005). Insulin resistance (IR) is a common characteristic of metabolic syndrome and diabetes. When cells face stress, they activate various cellular responses such as the ubiquitin-proteasome pathway, DNA damage response, unfolded protein response, apoptosis, inflammasome activation, and pyroptosis. Dysregulation of processes like autophagy induction, heat shock response, and signaling pathways involving erythroid nuclear factor 2 (ERF2) may occur. Insulin target cells also contribute to cellular stress by releasing certain chemicals that increase the accumulation and activation of myeloid cells, leading to chronic inflammation. Targeting specific triggers and pathways of the stress response through drugs has the potential to prevent or improve insulin resistance (Onyango, 2018).

Effects of Inflammation and Oxidative Stress

Inflammation plays a crucial role in the development of insulin resistance and type 2 diabetes (DM2). Higher levels of inflammatory markers during the initial stages of inflammation have been linked to insulin resistance and DM2. Moreover, the persistent inflammation throughout the body that accompanies insulin resistance worsens the metabolic problems associated with diabetes. When cells or tissues are damaged, immune cells can trigger an inflammatory response. Reactive oxygen species (ROS) are believed to contribute to oxidative stress, which is involved in sustaining inflammation. Excessive ROS can activate transcription factors and enhance the production of pro-inflammatory cytokines, thus perpetuating the cycle of inflammation and metabolic dysfunction (Oguntibeju et al., 2019).

Gallic Acid (GA) Is a Naturally Occurring Antioxidant

GA, also known as 3,4,5-trihydroxy benzoic acid, is a secondary metabolite that can be found in various plants and nuts. The compound has gained popularity due to its potent anti-inflammatory properties. While GA is plentiful in plants, its extraction rate is relatively low, which limits its use in research and development. However, there are alternative methods to acquire GA. One method is through biological synthesis, where certain organisms are engineered to produce GA as a byproduct of their metabolic processes. Another method is chemical synthesis, which involves artificially creating GA in a laboratory setting. Several plant species have been identified as sources of GA. For instance, species such as Achillea (from the Asteraceae family), Mentha (from the Lamiaceae family), and Abutilon (from the Malvaceae family) have been found to contain GA in multiple parts of the plant. Among these species, Phyllanthus a. was found to have the highest concentration of GA (Bai et al., 2021).

GA Is a Natural Bioactive Metabolite

It has been found to possess specific anti-inflammatory properties, which is one of the reasons for its recent popularity. Researchers have discovered that GA can inhibit the activity of enzymes such as cyclooxygenase (COX) and lipoxygenase (LOX), which play a role in the production of inflammatory mediators like TNF-alpha, interleukin-6, and interleukin-1 beta. GA has also been shown to suppress the activation of transcription factors including NF-kappaB and AP-1, which are vital in regulating the expression of inflammatory genes (Rosas et al., 2019). GA is extracted from natural sources using a combination of polar solvents. It has been demonstrated to have various biological effects, such as anti-inflammatory, antibacterial, antioxidant, cardioprotective, antiviral, and anticancer properties (Rosas et al., 2019). These effects might be attributed to its potent antioxidant activity, which surpasses that of certain vitamins in absorbing and neutralizing free radicals. However, in rare cases, GA can potentially induce oxidative stress in cells and exhibit prooxidant activity, which can lead to cytotoxicity. Some studies have shown that GA-induced reactive oxygen species (ROS) facilitate apoptosis in cancer cell cultures grown in vitro (Govea-Salas et al., 2018).

Medicinal Properties of GA and Its Derivatives

GA and its analogues, such as lauryl gallate, propyl gallate, and hexadecyl gallate, have the ability to prevent oxidation and rancidity in oils and fats. This is due to their antioxidant and free radical scavenging capabilities. As a result, they can be utilized as effective food additives to prevent spoilage and extend shelf life. However, the benefits of GA and its derivatives extend beyond their culinary applications. Extensive research has been conducted to explore their biological and pharmacological effects, revealing a range of therapeutic properties. These include anti-inflammatory, cardioprotective, antioxidant, and neuroprotective properties. By analyzing the current biological and pharmacological activities of GA, this study aims to provide a comprehensive understanding of its therapeutic potential. This research will shed light on the various ways in which GA and its analogs can positively impact human health (Kahkeshani et al., 2019).

Mechanism of GA's Antioxidant and Anti-Inflammatory Action

Gallic acid (GA) has an antioxidant effect due to its ability to neutralize and eliminate free radicals, such as reactive oxygen species (ROS). It achieves this by donating hydrogen atoms to free radicals, transforming them into more stable molecules. This antioxidant activity helps protect DNA, proteins, and lipids from oxidative stress. In addition to its antioxidant properties, GA also exhibits anti-inflammatory activity. It can modulate various inflammatory pathways in the body, including the suppression of pro-inflammatory cytokines such as tumor necrosis factor-alpha (TNF-α), interleukin 1 beta (IL-1β), and interleukin 6 (IL-6). GA can also inhibit the activity of nuclear factor kappa B (NF-kB), a key transcription factor that controls the expression of various pro-inflammatory genes. Furthermore, GA can block the formation of several pro-inflammatory mediators by inhibiting the enzymes cyclooxygenase (COX) and lipoxygenase (LOX). These enzymes are responsible for generating prostaglandins and leukotrienes, which are potent inflammatory molecules. By inhibiting COX and LOX, GA helps reduce inflammation. Another way in which GA exerts its anti-inflammatory effects is by regulating the gut flora. Evidence suggests that GA can promote the growth of beneficial bacteria such as Lactobacillus and

Bifidobacterium in the gut. This can lead to reduced intestinal inflammation and better overall health.

GA for Diabetic Therapy

A high content of gallic acid (GA) may explain the historical success of the medicinal herb Emblica officinalis in treating diabetes and cardiovascular problems. GA, along with E. officinalis fruit juice, has been found to improve glucose homeostasis, and insulin sensitivity, reduce obesity, lower hypertension and cholesterol levels, and promote adipogenesis in 3T3-L1 adipocytes (Variya et al., 2020). In 3T3-L1 adipocytes, GA treatment promotes Glut4 translocation and increases PPAR expression through the activation of C/EBPs. Additionally, E. officinalis fruit juice shows dual stimulation of Akt and AMPK, while GA therapy enhances insulin sensitivity through the Akt signaling mechanism (Variya et al., 2020). Thiazolidinedione, an agonist for the peroxisome proliferator-activated receptor, is currently used in pharmaceutical treatment for diabetes. However, it is associated with side effects such as obesity and therapy failure. E. officinalis, a well-known Ayurveda herbal medication, contains various phytoconstituents, including gallo and ellago-tannins, sesquiterpenoids, and nor sesquiterpenoids. Research has shown that E. officinalis exhibits anti-diabetic potential in preclinical and clinical studies, as well as anti-diabetic and anti-hyperlipidemic activity (Variya et al., 2020). In vitro tests have demonstrated that GA activates C/EBP and PPAR- to promote adipogenesis and fat accumulation in 3T3-L1 adipocytes. Enhanced Glut4 translocation in 3T3-L1 cells leads to improved glucose uptake. Furthermore, GA has been shown to prevent weight gain in vivo animals by enhancing cholesterol metabolism and reducing hepatic lipids. It also reverses the effects of fructose on hyperglycemia and cholesterol levels (Variya et al., 2020). While E. officinalis fruit juice promotes insulin sensitivity through Akt and AMPK stimulation due to its diverse phytochemical composition, GA specifically improves insulin sensitivity. Based on these findings, it can be concluded that E. officinalis has anti-diabetic potential and can be used as a dietary supplement to prevent diabetes and its associated complications (Variya et al., 2020).

Conclusion

GA, also known as gallic acid, is a naturally occurring molecule found in many plant-based diets. Recent research has shown that GA has the potential to treat diabetes. It works by improving insulin sensitivity, reducing glucose levels, and protecting pancreatic beta cells from oxidative stress. Additionally, GA has been found to lower inflammation and oxidative stress, which can help in preventing complications associated with diabetes such as neuropathy, nephropathy, and retinopathy. While GA shows promise as a treatment for diabetes, more studies are needed to confirm these preliminary findings. Although there have been some positive results from research so far, a deeper understanding of the benefits and risks of GA is still required before it can be recommended as a primary medication for diabetes.

References

Bai, J., Zhang, Y., Tang, C., Hou, Y., Ai, X., Chen, X., Zhang, Y., Wang, X., Meng, X. (2021). Gallic acid: Pharmacological activities and molecular mechanisms involved in inflammation-related diseases. *Biomedicine & Pharmacotherapy*, 133, 110985.

Bigagli, E., Lodovici, M. (2019). Circulating oxidative stress biomarkers in clinical studies on type 2 diabetes and its complications. *Oxidative Medicine and Cellular Longevity*, 2019, 5953685.

Bloch-Damti, A., Bashan, N. (2005). Proposed mechanisms for the induction of insulin resistance by oxidative stress. *Antioxidants & Redox Signaling*, 7(11-12), 1553-1567.

Cohen, G., Riahi, Y., Alpert, E., Gruzman, A., Sasson, S. (2007). The roles of hyperglycaemia and oxidative stress in the rise and collapse of the natural protective mechanism against vascular endothelial cell dysfunction in diabetes. *Archives of Physiology and Biochemistry*, 113(4-5), 259-267.

Darenskaya, M. A., Kolesnikova, L. I., Kolesnikov, S. I. (2021). Oxidative stress: pathogenetic role in diabetes mellitus and its complications and therapeutic approaches to correction. *Bulletin of Experimental Biology and Medicine*, 171(2), 179-189.

Forouhi, N. G., Wareham, N. J. (2010). Epidemiology of diabetes. *Medicine*, 38(11), 602-606.

Giacco, F., Brownlee, M. (2010). Oxidative stress and diabetic complications. *Circulation Research*, 107(9), 1058-1070.

Govea-Salas, M., Rivas-Estilla, A. M., Ascacio-Valdés, J., Zugasti-Cruz, A., Rodríguez-Herrera, R., Belmares-Cerda, R., Morlett-Chávez, J. (2018). Gallic Acid as a putative antioxidant in usage against liver disease. In *The Liver* (pp. 317-322). Academic Press.

Greenfield, J. R., Campbell, L. V. (2006). Relationship between inflammation, insulin resistance and type 2 diabetes: 'cause or effect'? *Current Diabetes Reviews*, 2(2), 195-211.

Ighodaro, O. M. (2018). Molecular pathways associated with oxidative stress in diabetes mellitus. *Biomedicine & Pharmacotherapy*, 108, 656-662.

Kahkeshani, N., Farzaei, F., Fotouhi, M., Alavi, S. S., Bahramsoltani, R., Naseri, R., Momtaz, S., Abbasabadi, Z., Rahimi, R., Farzaei, M. H., Bishayee, A. (2019). Pharmacological effects of gallic acid in health and diseases: A mechanistic review. *Iranian Journal of Basic Medical Sciences*, 22(3), 225237.

Nkanu, E. E., Ujong, G., Okon, V., Bassey, I. E. (2018). In vivo efficacy of Dialium guineense fruit pulp on hemeoxygenase-1 and angiotensin converting enzyme in experimental diabetes. *Journal of Medicinal Plants Research*, 12(28), 483-492.

Oguntibeju, O. O. (2019). Type 2 diabetes mellitus, oxidative stress and inflammation: examining the links. *International Journal of Physiology, Pathophysiology and Pharmacology*, 11(3), 45.

Onyango, A. N. (2018). Cellular stresses and stress responses in the pathogenesis of insulin resistance. *Oxidative Medicine and Cellular Longevity*, 2018, 4321714.

Rolo, A. P., Palmeira, C. M. (2006). Diabetes and mitochondrial function: role of hyperglycemia and oxidative stress. *Toxicology and Applied Pharmacology*, 212(2), 167-178.

Rosas, E. C., Correa, L. B., das Graças Henriques, M. (2019). Antiinflammatory properties of Schinus terebinthifolius and its use in arthritic conditions. In *Bioactive food as dietary interventions for arthritis and related inflammatory diseas*es (pp. 489-505). Academic Press.

Sies, H. (1997). Oxidative stress: oxidants and antioxidants. *Experimental Physiology: Translation and Integration*, 82(2), 291-295.

Variya, B. C., Bakrania, A. K., Patel, S. S. (2020). Antidiabetic potential of gallic acid from Emblica officinalis: Improved glucose transporters and insulin sensitivity through PPAR-γ and Akt signaling. *Phytomedicine*, 73, 152906.

Chapter 22

Hesperidin in the Management of Diabetes Mellitus

Neelam Singh[1,*]
Chaitanya Vinayak Narayan[1]
Puneet Gupta[2]
and Charu Bharti[3]
[1]I. T. S. College of Pharmacy, Muradnagar, Ghaziabad, Uttar Pradesh, India
[2]Amity Institute of Pharmacy, Amity University, Noida, Uttar Pradesh, India
[3]Department of Pharmaceutics, School of Pharmacy, Bharat Institute of Technology, Meerut, Uttar Pradesh, India

Abstract

The intake of phytophagous, which refers to consuming plant-based foods, is crucial for promoting good health, especially in the control and prevention of chronic diseases. One such disease is diabetes mellitus, a metabolic condition that affects a large number of people worldwide. According to the International Diabetes Federation (IDF), there were around 415 million diabetic individuals in the world in 2015, and this number is projected to increase to 642 million by 2040. Therefore, there is a significant need for safe and effective alternative medications to treat this condition. Flavonoids, a group of polyphenolic compounds found in plant fruits, flowers, and leaves, have been recognized for their potential health benefits. Hesperidin, a natural flavanone, is one of these compounds and has been shown to have antioxidant, anti-inflammatory, and anti-apoptotic effects in diabetic rats, among other beneficial effects. However, the mechanism of action of hesperidin is not well

* Corresponding Author's Email: singhneelam16@gmail.com.

In: Naturally Occurring Chemicals …
Editors: A. Singh Grewal, G. Deswal, A. Kumar Dhingra et al.
ISBN: 979-8-89113-491-1

understood. Nevertheless, growing evidence suggests that hesperidin can inhibit diabetes-related disorders. This chapter aims to explain the mechanisms by which hesperidin may be effective in treating diabetes mellitus. Hesperidin has been found to control AMPK and PPAR signaling pathways, which are involved in fat and glucose metabolism. It also regulates antioxidant levels and prevents cell death. Additionally, hesperidin can effectively regulate NF-κB activation, a signaling pathway that triggers inflammation, which is important in managing diabetes. Furthermore, supplementation with hesperidin-enriched products can significantly improve symptoms such as postprandial hyperglycemia (high blood sugar after meals) and hyperlipidemia (high levels of fats in the blood). There is a large body of in vivo and ex vivo research that supports the positive effects of hesperidin in treating and preventing diabetes. However, further clinical trials are needed to evaluate its effectiveness in reducing cholesterol levels and to assess its safety.

Keywords: hesperidin, citrus, flavonoids, inflammation, glucose metabolism, phenolic compounds

Abbreviations

BDNF	Brain derived neurotrophic factor
G6P	Glucose-6-Phosphate
Hst	Hespertin
IL-6	Interleukin-6
MDF	Malondialdehyde
PTP1B	Protein tyrosine phosphate 1B
STZ	Streptozotocin
TNF	Tumour necrosis factor.

Introduction

According to the most recent data from the International Diabetes Federation, approximately 463 million individuals aged between 20 to 79 years have diabetes worldwide, with the majority residing in economically developing countries. Diabetes is characterized by several major health issues, including retinopathy, nephropathy, and neuropathy, which can cause harm to internal organs such as the kidneys, tissues, heart, liver, and pancreas. This necessitates extensive medical attention and management. Additionally, diabetes has been identified as the primary contributor to various chronic metabolic illnesses (Gandhi et al., 2020). The development of diabetes occurs due to abnormal anabolism and catabolism of proteins, lipids, and carbohydrates caused by insulin resistance or hypoinsulinism. Glycemic dysregulation can further worsen vascular homeostasis and promote the occurrence of micro- and macrovascular disorders. Individuals with diabetes also face a higher risk of physical and cognitive impairment, cancer, tuberculosis, and distress (Al-Aubaidy et al., 2021). Although diabetes is a challenging condition, some research suggests that redox imbalance resulting from extremely high blood sugar levels plays a crucial role in the development of various virus-related disorders, such as sensitivity and arterial occlusive disease. Despite the creation of numerous synthetic drugs, none of the molecules developed so far have been able to offer a complete recovery (Gandhi et al., 2020). Because some synthetic substances have severe side effects when used continuously, there is still a need for accessible, non-toxic medications. Traditional remedies have always been highly regarded by humans as a viable medical option. These are used all throughout the world, proving that herbal remedies are becoming an integral part of modern medical practice. The World Health Organization (WHO) has registered an overall figure of 21,000 plant species as being used as medicines worldwide. More than 400 of these plants have been shown to be effective in treating diabetes. Despite this, only a small number of these plants have been put through scientific and medical review to ascertain their effectiveness in treating diabetes. Anti-diabetic methods include the suppression of α-1,4-glucosidase, α-salivary amylase, and PT1B activities. The active components derived from plants work to control blood sugar levels. Many scientists have been motivated to develop innovative compounds capable of treating diabetes due to the relatively low side-effect profiles of herbal treatments (Jugran et al., 2021).

Researchers are actively seeking new membrane-bound molecules extracted from botanical medicine for the management of diabetes. Citrus flavonoid hesperetin (Hst) has shown promise in treating diabetes and its complications. However, the studies conducted so far on Hst are scattered and disorganized. To evaluate the potential therapeutic benefits of Hst in managing diabetes and related complications, a literature review of research conducted over the past ten years was summarized (Yang et al., 2022). The primary active compounds found in citrus fruits are called flavonoids, which have numerous therapeutic advantages, particularly in managing diabetes.

These flavonoids affect various molecular markers such as blood sugar levels, lipid profiles, kidney function, liver enzymes, and antioxidant enzymes. They also influence signaling pathways that are associated with glucose absorption and insulin resistance, both of which play a role in the development of diabetes and its related complications (Zengin et al., 2019).

Hesperidin and Diabetes Mellitus

Hesperidin, derived from Citrus aurantium L. and other Rutaceae species, is a cost-effective flavone glycoside. It is one of the leading insignificant nutrients for humans and is a flavonoid and glycosidase identified within citrus fruits such as oranges, tangerines, lemons, and grapefruits (Gandhi et al., 2020). Its name is derived from the term 'hesperidium,' which refers to citrus fruits. In humans, hesperidin has been shown to affect systolic pressure and boost antioxidant status. This citrus flavanone is extensively used as a nutritional aid, either alone or in combination with other bioflavonoids, to reduce blood vessel permeability and treat or prevent circulatory system disorders. It is also useful as an anti-inflammatory, antioxidant, or cancer-fighting herb. The therapeutic benefits of hesperidin, such as reducing oxidative stress and inflammation, are largely attributed to its ability to control pro-inflammatory cytokines, including TNF-alpha, IL-1, and IL-6. Numerous animal models of inflammatory responses have demonstrated this (Ota & Ulrih, 2017). Diabetes is one of the most common chronic disorders that can be treated with this flavonoid, according to studies. Researchers have assessed the impact of hesperidin on molecular marker G6P and bone loss measures in marginal type 1 diabetic rats using an animal model of STZ-induced diabetes. Hesperidin reduced blood glucose and serum insulin levels while normalizing the enzymatic activity of glucose-6-phosphatase (G6Pase), glucokinase, and other hepatic enzymes involved in glucose management. Additionally, Mahmoud et al. showed that hesperidin treatment can reduce hyperglycemia-induced oxidative damage and suppress the production of pro-inflammatory cytokines like TNF-α and IL-6 in T2DM rats fed an HFD/STZ diet (Mahmoud et al., 2012). These findings support the oral treatment of hesperidin as a potential therapeutic option for diabetes, as it has been shown to lower blood sugar levels, reduce oxidative stress markers such as MDA, and decrease inflammatory markers like IL-6.

Table 1. Summary of previous *in vitro* studies on hesperidin (flavanone) for management of diabetes mellitus

Treatment Concentration and Duration	*In-Vitro* Models	Molecular Mechanisms and Their Effects	Reference
0, 25, 50, 100 μM; 48 hr	Human normal hepatocytes	By preventing DNMT1 from silencing miR-149, hesperidin reduced oxidative stress, mitochondrial dysfunction, and insulin resistance.	(Tian et al., 2021)
10 μM; 48 hr	L6 myotube cells	In L6 myotubes, hesperidine decreased PI3 kinase activity while increasing GLUT4, IRS, and AKT, suggesting a potential overlap with the insulin signalling pathway.	(Dhanya & Jayamurthy, 2020)
0.25, 0.5, 1, and 2 mg/mL; 1 and 24 h	Islets of the pancreas	The islet of pancrease produced and released more insulin when hesperidin and naringin were present.	(Mahmoud et al., 2015)
12.5, 25, and 50 μmol/L; 6 h	Retinal ganglion cell type 5 (RGC-5) cells	By inhibiting caspase-9, caspase-3, and Bax/Bcl-2, hesperidin protected cells against extensive damage caused by glucose-induced apoptosis. Moreover, in high glucose-fed RGC-5 cells, it dramatically suppressed c-Jun N-terminal kinases (JNK) phosphorylation and activated p38 MAPK.	(Liu et al., 2017)
40, 80, 120, 160, and 200 μM; 24 h	Rat hepatocytes	Hesperidin and Hst are flavonoids that have been shown to be beneficial in treating AST and ALT-mediated metabolic diseases, including diabetes mellitus. These flavonoids suppress the activity of two gluconeogenesis enzymes, alanine aminotransferase (ALT) and aspartate aminotransferase (AST).	(Zareei et al., 2017)

Table 2. Summary of previous *in vivo* studies on hesperidin (flavanone) for management of diabetes mellitus

Dose, Procedure, and Length of the Experiment	*In Vivo* Models	Molecular mechanisms and the effects	Reference
Animal food (10 g/kg diet) with hesperidin; 28 days	Wistar Rats	In STZ-immunized marginal diabetic weanling rats, hesperidin lesser high level of sugar and fat by lowering blood glucose and restoring normal gluconeogenesis enzyme activities, but it had no effect on bone tissue or bone metabolic parameters.	(Akiyama et al., 2010)
Oral administration (50 mg/kg); 28 and 30 days	Wistar Rats	Hesperidin and naringin standardised the altered blood glucose and antioxidant parameters in the liver, which in turn decreased the amount of pro-inflammatory cytokine production (tumour necrosis factor-alpha (TNF-) and interleukin (IL)-6) and increased antioxidant defences in a type 2 diabetic rat model.	(Mahmoud et al., 2012)
Oral dosage of 25, 50, or 100 mg/kg; 21 days	Wistar Rats	Hesperidin was successful in treating and controlling neurogenesis in diabetic rats by lowering hyperglycemia, lowering MDA and IL-6 levels, and increasing abrineurin and aminoalkane in the brain.	(El-Marasy et al., 2014)
Oral administration (25, 50, and 100 mg/kg); 28 days	Sprague-Dawley Rats	Hesperidin raised the nociceptive threshold, electromyograph velocity, electro-neurograph velocity, insulin levels, and sodium–potassium ATPase in the diabetic rats while decreasing the degree of STZ-induced hyperglycemia and pro-inflammatory cytokines.	(Visnagri et al., 2014)
Oral administration (50 mg/kg); 30 days	Wistar Rats	In diabetic rats, hesperidin and naringin dramatically increased adipose tissue glucose transporter type 4 (GLUT4) mRNA and protein expression, corrected the impaired characteristics of glucose metabolism, and hypoglycemia.	(Tian et al., 2021)
Oral administration (100 mg/kg); 15 days	Wistar Rats	The metabolism of insulin was positively impacted by hesperidin and quercetin. In experimental diabetic rats induced by STZ, they reduced the levels of triglycerides, MDA, TNF, and IL-6 and increased glutathione (GSH).	(Dokumacioglu et al., 2018)
Oral dosages of 25, 50, and 100 mg/kg; 21 days	Sprague-Dawley Rats	In STZ-induced diabetes, hesperidin reduced the elevated blood glucose, serum insulin, calorie, and fluid consumption. Additionally, it improved wound recovery in the prolonged diabetic foot ulcer condition in diabetic rats by stepping up ontogenesis and vasculogenesis via the upregulating of vascular permeability factor (VPF), Angiopoietin (Ang)-1/Tie-2, transforming growth factor (TGF-), and small mothers against decapentaplegic (Smad)-2/3 mRNA expression.	(Li et al., 2018)

Hesperidin also increased levels of the antioxidant GSH and brain-derived neurotrophic factor (BDNF) in the brains of diabetic rats, suggesting potential neuroprotective effects.

Furthermore, hesperidin was found to have beneficial effects on various biochemical parameters associated with diabetes, including reducing hyperglycemia, total cholesterol (TC), and serum triglycerides (TG), and increasing insulin levels (Table 1). These effects can have a positive impact on the management of diabetes and its associated cardiovascular and respiratory complications. Additionally, hesperidin demonstrated anti-inflammatory effects by reducing neutrophil and macrophage infiltration in the sciatic nerve and decreasing the expression of pro-inflammatory cytokines TNF-alpha and IL-1. This suggests that hesperidin may have a role in mitigating the development of diabetes-related inflammation (Hussain et al., 2020). Moreover, hesperidin improved the architecture of the sciatic nerve, which can be distorted in diabetic conditions. It attenuated necrosis, edema, and nerve fiber congestion induced by STZ; a chemical used to induce diabetes in animal models (Table 2). Hesperidin was also shown to have direct effects on glucose metabolism, including lowering fasting plasma glucose levels, improving insulin sensitivity, and increasing insulin release. It restored the activity of key metabolic enzymes involved in glucose metabolism, such as G6P, glycogen phosphorylase, and fructosephosphate, suggesting potential mechanisms by which hesperidin exerts its antidiabetic effects. Furthermore, hesperidin has been reported to enhance glucose absorption in isolated pancreatic cells and increase GLUT4 mRNA and protein expression in fatty tissue, further supporting its role in improving glucose homeostasis (Jugran et al., 2021). Oxidative stress is known to play a significant role in the development of diabetes, characterized by increased levels of reactive oxygen species (ROS) and lipid peroxidation marker MDA, along with decreased antioxidant enzyme activity. Hesperidin has been shown to reduce oxidative stress markers and restore antioxidant enzyme activity, suggesting its potential to counteract the oxidative stress associated with diabetes (Tian et al., 2021). Hesperidin has been shown to have a positive effect on various aspects of diabetes and associated complications. It reduces the levels of oxidative stress markers and protein damage in retinal cells exposed to high glucose levels. It also restores the activity of antioxidant enzymes, which are often dysregulated in metabolic syndrome, atherogenesis, and diabetes. Additionally, hesperidin has been found to inhibit certain liver enzymes associated with liver damage in rat liver cells. This suggests that it could be a promising treatment for hepatic damage associated with diabetes mellitus. Hesperidin has also been shown to be effective in treating diabetic foot ulcers, reducing weight loss and insulin concentrations, normalizing blood glucose levels, and improving antioxidant levels in diabetes-induced rats. Moreover, hesperidin has demonstrated beneficial effects in wound healing, reducing inflammation and promoting angiogenesis and vasculogenesis. Overall, these findings suggest that hesperidin may be a safe and effective treatment for diabetes and its associated complications, including hepatic damage and diabetic foot ulcers. (Carvalho et al., 2021). The effects described above can be attributed to hesperidin's ability to regulate important biomarkers such as VEGF-c and angiopoietin-1. Previously reported data on hesperidin were supported by the study, and new molecular findings suggested that hesperidin significantly reduced levels of serum total cholesterol, TG, LDL, VLDL, and MDA, while increasing GSH concentrations. However, HDL-C levels were not affected. The researchers also observed a decrease in pro-inflammatory cytokines in diabetic rats. The authors speculated that the targeted modulation of TNF-alpha and IL-6 levels in adipose tissue played a role in the weight loss management observed in diabetic rats treated with hesperidin (Dhanya & Jayamurthy, 2020). According to studies, higher production of TNF-alpha and IL-6 by subcutaneous adipose tissue corresponds with obesity and adiposity, and has also been linked to the onset of diabetic microvascular problems (Gandhi et al., 2020).

Hesperidin's Impact on the Metabolism of Glucose

Inhibiting hepatic gluconeogenesis and slowing the development of diabetes can be achieved by targeting impaired glucose metabolism-related genetic variations, which are influenced by obesity-modifiable factors. Glucose plays a vital role in providing the necessary carbon for the synthesis of essential components in daughter cells, including nucleotides, fatty acids, and amino acids (Xiong et al., 2019). The compound Hesperidin has been found to effectively lower glucose-6-phosphatase activity in HepG2 cells, thereby preventing the breakdown of amylose and amylopectin. Docking simulations have shown that Hesperidin blocks the entry of certain enzymes into the channel, leading to a decrease in the synthesis of oxaloacetate, pyruvate, and alpha-ketoglutarate. Studies conducted on diabetic rat and porcine models induced by streptozotocin have demonstrated that Hesperidin can reduce blood glucose levels. Furthermore, it has been observed that Hesperidin increases glycolysis and glycogenolysis in isolated perfused rat liver. By partially inhibiting the intestinal glucose transporter, Hesperidin may also alter the post-prandial glycemic response of orange juice, suggesting its potential use in preventing post-meal hyperglycemia. Hesperidin exerts its effects on glucose metabolism by regulating the activity of PPAR-c (Peroxisome proliferator-activated receptor) and reducing fat production. PPAR-c is a nuclear protein transcription factor that controls the metabolism of lipids and glucose. By directly or indirectly modulating the metabolism of glucose and insulin, Hesperidin helps improve the interaction between obesity and glucose metabolic diseases, making it a promising approach for combating obesity (Gandhi et al., 2020).

Hesperidin for Targeted Delivery

Although hesperidin (a bioflavonoid) has shown promising anti-diabetic effects, its poor bioavailability and solubility limit its absorption, requiring the use of delivery methods to achieve therapeutic results. To overcome this challenge, Sulaiman et al. used a chemical synthesis approach to create hesperidin-loaded gold nanoparticles (Hsp-AuNPs) (Sulaiman et al., 2020). The use of Hsp-AuNPs has demonstrated potential as an efficient technique in clinical cancer therapy and should be further investigated for drug delivery applications. In addition, the use of hesperidin nanoparticles has shown positive effects on blood glucose, insulin, HbA1c%, and lipid profile in diabetic rats. Moreover, these nanoparticles have also led to a significant reduction in TNF-alpha, IL-17, and MDA levels, while increasing catalase levels, indicating their potential as an anti-diabetic medication (Ali et al., 2019). To further enhance the efficacy of hesperidin, Jangde et al. developed hesperidin-loaded lipid-polymer hybrid nanoparticles. This formulation aims to disperse hesperidin to endogenous sites in the wound bed, enhancing its effectiveness (Jangde et al., 2022).

Conclusion and Future Prospects

Hesperidin has shown efficacy in preventing complications of diabetes, including high blood sugar levels, oxidative damage, and cell death caused by excessive glucose. Therefore, it may be considered as a potential medication for preventing diabetes. Supplementation of hesperidin has been found to enhance control over blood sugar levels and reduce insulin resistance. Citrus flavonoids, of which hesperidin is one, have demonstrated various protective effects against the development of diabetes. However, further research involving human trials is necessary to confirm the anti-diabetic benefits of hesperidin and other citrus flavonoids.

References

Akiyama, S., Katsumata, S. I., Suzuki, K., Ishimi, Y., Wu, J., Uehara, M. (2010). Dietary hesperidin exerts hypoglycemic and hypolipidemic effects in streptozotocin-induced marginal type 1 diabetic rats. *Journal of Clinical Biochemistry and Nutrition*, 46(1), 87–92.

Al-Aubaidy, H. A., Dayan, A., Deseo, M. A., Itsiopoulos, C., Jamil, D., Hadi, N. R., Thomas, C. J. (2021). Twelve-Week Mediterranean Diet Intervention Increases Citrus Bioflavonoid Levels and Reduces Inflammation in People with Type 2 Diabetes Mellitus. *Nutrients*, 13(4), 1133.

Ali, S. H., Sulaiman, G. M., Al-Halbosiy, M. M. F., Jabir, M. S., Hameed, A. H. (2019). Fabrication of hesperidin nanoparticles loaded by poly lactic co-Glycolic acid for improved therapeutic efficiency and cytotoxicity. *Artificial Cells, Nanomedicine, and Biotechnology*, 47(1), 378–394.

Carvalho, M. T. B., Araújo-Filho, H. G., Barreto, A. S., Quintans-Júnior, L. J., Quintans, J. S. S., Barreto, R. S. S. (2021). Wound healing properties of flavonoids: A systematic review highlighting the mechanisms of action. *Phytomedicine*, 90, 153636.

Dhanya, R., Jayamurthy, P. (2020). In vitro evaluation of antidiabetic potential of hesperidin and its aglycone hesperetin under oxidative stress in skeletal muscle cell line. *Cell Biochemistry and Function*, 38(4), 419–427.

Dokumacioglu, E., Iskender, H., Sen, T. M., Ince, I., Dokumacioglu, A., Kanbay, Y., Erbas, E., Saral, S. (2018). The Effects of Hesperidin and Quercetin on Serum Tumor Necrosis Factor-Alpha and Interleukin-6 Levels in Streptozotocin-induced Diabetes Model. *Pharmacognosy Magazine*, 14(54), 167–173.

El-Marasy, S. A., Abdallah, H. M. I., El-Shenawy, S. M., El-Khatib, A. S., El-Shabrawy, O. A., Kenawy, S. A. (2014). Anti-depressant effect of hesperidin in diabetic rats. *Canadian Journal of Physiology and Pharmacology*, 92(11), 945–952.

Gandhi, G. R., Vasconcelos, A. B. S., Wu, D. T., Li, H. B., Antony, P. J., Li, H., Geng, F., Gurgel, R. Q., Narain, N., Gan, R. -Y. (2020). Citrus Flavonoids as Promising Phytochemicals Targeting Diabetes and Related Complications: A Systematic Review of In Vitro and In Vivo Studies. *Nutrients*, 12(10), 2907.

Hussain, T., Tan, B., Murtaza, G., Liu, G., Rahu, N., Saleem Kalhoro, M., Hussain Kalhoro, D., Adebowale, T. O., Usman Mazhar, M., Rehman, Z. ur, Martínez, Y., Akber Khan, S., Yin, Y. (2020). Flavonoids and type 2 diabetes: Evidence of efficacy in clinical and animal studies and delivery strategies to enhance their therapeutic efficacy. *Pharmacological Research*, 152, 104629.

Jangde, R., Elhassan, G. O., Khute, S., Singh, D., Singh, M., Sahu, R. K., Khan, J. (2022). Hesperidin-Loaded Lipid Polymer Hybrid Nanoparticles for Topical Delivery of Bioactive Drugs. *Pharmaceuticals*, 15(2), 211.

Jugran, A. K., Rawat, S., Devkota, H. P., Bhatt, I. D., Rawal, R. S. (2021). Diabetes and plant-derived natural products: From ethnopharmacological approaches to their potential for modern drug discovery and development. *Phytotherapy Research*, 35(1), 223–245.

Li, W., Kandhare, A. D., Mukherjee, A. A., Bodhankar, S. L. (2018). Hesperidin, a plant flavonoid accelerated the cutaneous wound healing in streptozotocin-induced diabetic rats: Role of TGF-ß/Smads and Ang-1/Tie-2 signaling pathways. *EXCLI Journal*, 17, 399–419.

Liu, W. Y., Liou, S. S., Hong, T. Y., Liu, I. M. (2017). Protective Effects of Hesperidin (Citrus Flavonone) on High Glucose Induced Oxidative Stress and Apoptosis in a Cellular Model for Diabetic Retinopathy. *Nutrients*, 9(12), 1312.

Mahmoud, A. M., Ahmed, O. M., Ashour, M. B., Abdel-Moneim, A. (2015). In vivo and in vitro antidiabetic effects of citrus flavonoids; a study on the mechanism of action. *International Journal of Diabetes in Developing Countries*, 35(3), 250–263.

Mahmoud, A. M., Ashour, M. B., Abdel-Moneim, A., Ahmed, O. M. (2012). Hesperidin and naringin attenuate hyperglycemia-mediated oxidative stress and proinflammatory cytokine production in high fat fed/streptozotocin-induced type 2 diabetic rats. *Journal of Diabetes and Its Complications*, 26(6), 483–490.

Ota, A., Ulrih, N. P. (2017). An overview of herbal products and secondary metabolites used for management of type two diabetes. *Frontiers in Pharmacology*, 8, 436.

Sulaiman, G. M., Waheeb, H. M., Jabir, M. S., Khazaal, S. H., Dewir, Y. H., Naidoo, Y. (2020). Hesperidin loaded on gold nanoparticles as a drug delivery system for a successful biocompatible, anti-cancer, anti-inflammatory and phagocytosis inducer model. *Scientific Reports*, 10(1), Article 1.

Tian, M., Han, Y. B., Zhao, C. C., Liu, L., Zhang, F. L. (2021). Hesperidin alleviates insulin resistance by improving HG-induced oxidative stress and mitochondrial dysfunction by restoring miR-149. *Diabetology & Metabolic Syndrome*, 13(1), 50.

Visnagri, A., Kandhare, A. D., Chakravarty, S., Ghosh, P., Bodhankar, S. L. (2014). Hesperidin, a flavanoglycone attenuates experimental diabetic neuropathy via modulation of cellular and biochemical marker to improve nerve functions. *Pharmaceutical Biology*, 52(7), 814–828.

Xiong, H., Wang, J., Ran, Q., Lou, G., Peng, C., Gan, Q., Hu, J., Sun, J., Yao, R., Huang, Q. (2019). Hesperidin: a therapeutic agent for obesity. *Drug Design, Development and Therapy*, 13, 3855–3866.

Yang, H., Wang, Y., Xu, S., Ren, J., Tang, L., Gong, J., Lin, Y., Fang, H., Su, D. (2022). Hesperetin, a promising treatment option for diabetes and related complications: a literature review. *Journal of Agricultural and Food Chemistry*, 70(28), 8582–8592.

Zareei, S., Boojar, M. M. A., Amanlou, M. (2017). Inhibition of liver alanine aminotransferase and aspartate aminotransferase by hesperidin and its aglycone hesperetin: An in vitro and in silico study. *Life Sciences*, 178, 49–55.

Zengin, G., Stefanucci, A., Rodrigues, M. J., Mollica, A., Custodio, L., Aumeeruddy, M., Mahomoodally, M. F. (2019). Scrophularia lucida L. as a valuable source of bioactive compounds for pharmaceutical applications: In vitro antioxidant, anti-inflammatory, enzyme inhibitory properties, in silico studies, and HPLC profiles. *Journal of Pharmaceutical and Biomedical Analysis*, 162, 225–233.

Chapter 23

Kaempferol in the Management of Diabetes Mellitus

Swati Pahwa[1,*]
Geeta Deswal[1]
Neha Saini[1]
Shivanki Joshi[1]
Fatimah Jan[2]
Sonam Grewal[3]
and Vishakha Saini[4]
[1]Guru Gobind Singh College of Pharmacy, Yamuna Nagar, Haryana, India
[2]School of Pharmaceutical Sciences, CT University, Ludhiana, Punjab, India
[3]M. M. Institute of Pharmacy, M.M. (Deemed to be) University, Mullana, Haryana, India
[4]Ganpati Institute of Pharmacy, Bilaspur, Yamuna Nagar, Haryana, India

Abstract

Kaempferol, a natural flavonoid compound found in various fruits and vegetables, has garnered significant attention for its potential role in diabetes mellitus management. Kaempferol appears to possess anti-diabetic properties by enhancing insulin sensitivity and regulating blood glucose levels. It has demonstrated the capacity to increase glucose uptake in cells, facilitating glucose metabolism and thereby leading to improved glucose control. Additionally, kaempferol has been observed to inhibit α-glucosidase, the enzyme responsible for breaking down carbohydrates into glucose. This inhibition effectively reduces the post-

* Corresponding Author's Email: swatipahwa129@gmail.com.

In: Naturally Occurring Chemicals …
Editors: A. Singh Grewal, G. Deswal, A. Kumar Dhingra et al.
ISBN: 979-8-89113-491-1

meal surge in blood sugar levels. Moreover, kaempferol exhibits notable antioxidant and anti-inflammatory effects, both of which hold promise in diabetes management. Its ability to alleviate oxidative stress and inflammation can help shield against the detrimental effects of elevated blood sugar levels. Furthermore, researchers have explored kaempferol's potential in guarding against diabetic complications. Diabetes elevates the risk of cardiovascular ailments, kidney damage, and diabetic neuropathy. Studies suggest that kaempferol may mitigate these complications by reducing oxidative stress, enhancing endothelial function, and impeding the formation of advanced glycation end products, which play a role in diabetic vascular issues.

Keywords: Haemoglobin A1c (HbA1c), hyperglycemia, insulin resistance, diabetes mellitus, glucose metabolism, oxidative stress

Introduction

Diabetes mellitus (DM), a complex metabolic disorder characterized by persistently elevated blood glucose levels (hyperglycemia), affects the metabolism of carbohydrates, fats, and proteins. The root causes of hyperglycemia in DM involve abnormalities in insulin secretion and action (Banday et al., 2020). With the increasing prevalence of diabetes, there is a growing interest in developing innovative therapeutic approaches to address this condition. Recently, natural compounds like flavonoids have garnered considerable attention due to their potential health benefits, including their ability to influence insulin sensitivity and glucose regulation. Kaempferol, a flavonoid found in various plant-based foods such as tea, fruits, vegetables, and herbs, has gained recognition for its diverse pharmacological effects, including anti-inflammatory, anti-cancer, and cardioprotective properties (Calderon-Montano et al., 2011). Moreover, kaempferol has emerged as a promising candidate for the treatment of diabetes mellitus. Both experimental and clinical studies have suggested that kaempferol may enhance glucose homeostasis, improve insulin sensitivity, and positively impact various metabolic parameters in individuals with diabetes mellitus (Maurya et al., 2015; Meng et al., 2017). This chapter aims to provide a comprehensive overview of the current state of knowledge regarding kaempferol and its potential role in the management of diabetes mellitus.

Kaempferol

Kaempferol is classified as a flavonoid, specifically a flavonol, with the chemical name 3,5,7-trihydroxy-2-(4-hydroxyphenyl)-4H-1-benzopyran-4-one. Flavonoids represent a significant group of secondary plant metabolites known for their antioxidant properties. It's estimated that there are more than 104 distinct types of flavonoids (Periferakis et al., 2022). Kaempferol can be found in various natural sources, including Ginkgo biloba L., cruciferous vegetables, grapefruit, tea, and some edible berries. Notably, it has been extracted from Bauhinia forficata leaves and demonstrated impressive effects, comparable to insulin, in reducing elevated serum glucose levels and enhancing glucose uptake in rat soleus muscle. Kaempferol's beneficial effects are associated with several mechanisms, including improved cAMP signaling, anti-apoptotic effects on Akt and Bcl-2 protein expression, and enhanced insulin secretion and synthesis in pancreatic beta cells. It has also been shown to reduce the levels of pro-inflammatory cytokines such as IL-1 and TNF-α, decrease lipid peroxidation and nitrite production, enhance antioxidant defence, and promote body weight control. In studies involving oral administration, kaempferol has significantly lowered fasting blood sugar levels, reduced serum HbA1c levels (a marker of long-term glucose control), and improved insulin sensitivity. Its influence extends to the regulation of gene expression in the liver, specifically in the downregulation of PPAR-γ and SREBP-1c. These effects on obesity and diabetes are mediated through the activation of AMPK, a key metabolic regulator (Vinayagam et al., 2019).

Mechanism of Action of Antidiabetic Action of Kaempferol

Although the exact mechanism of action of kaempferol in DM is unknown, several theories have been put forth in light of experimental and clinical research. Several of the suggested mechanisms of action are listed below:

Antioxidant Activity

Kaempferol has shown robust antioxidant properties that could play a role in preventing oxidative stress, a factor in the development and advancement of diabetes mellitus (Ren et al., 2019). Oxidative stress can harm pancreatic beta cells, hindering insulin secretion and glucose regulation. Kaempferol has the potential to mitigate oxidative stress by scavenging free radicals in the body and enhancing the activity of antioxidant enzymes (Silva et al., 2016). This action may help protect pancreatic function and contribute to improved insulin sensitivity and glucose control.

Anti-Inflammatory Activity

Kaempferol possesses anti-inflammatory properties both in vitro and in vivo. Inflammation plays a significant role in the onset of diabetes mellitus. Kaempferol helps reduce inflammation by inhibiting the production of pro-inflammatory cytokines and chemokines and regulating the activity of inflammatory signaling pathways (Kim et al., 2010; Choi et al., 2011). This anti-inflammatory action of kaempferol can contribute to the management of diabetes by mitigating the inflammatory processes associated with the disease.

Modulation of Insulin Signalling

Kaempferol has been shown to enhance insulin sensitivity in animal models of diabetes. It achieves this by activating insulin receptor substrates (IRS) and increasing glucose uptake in peripheral tissues, thereby improving insulin signaling (Liu, X et al., 2015). This improvement in insulin sensitivity is a significant factor in the potential therapeutic benefits of kaempferol for managing diabetes mellitus.

Regulation Of Glucose Metabolism

Kaempferol may also play a role in regulating glucose metabolism by influencing the activity of enzymes involved in gluconeogenesis and glycogen synthesis. Specifically, kaempferol has been shown to inhibit the activity of glucose-6-phosphatase, an enzyme involved in gluconeogenesis, while simultaneously increasing the activity of glycogen synthase, an enzyme responsible for glycogen synthesis (Jo et al., 2015).

In summary, these studies collectively suggest that kaempferol holds promise as a potential therapeutic agent for managing diabetes mellitus. Its ability to reduce oxidative stress, combat inflammation, improve insulin sensitivity, and regulate glucose metabolism highlights its multifaceted potential in the treatment and management of this metabolic disorder.

Kaempferol Protects Pancreatic β Cells

In diabetes, β cells often face challenges such as loss of mass and apoptosis. This is typically induced by pro-inflammatory factors like IL-1β, interferon, and TNF-α. The primary mechanism behind β-cell apoptosis in response to inflammation is the intrinsic apoptotic pathway, mediated by caspases. TNF-α and IL-1β trigger the activation of NF-κB, which, in turn, leads to the upregulation of inducible nitric oxide synthase and the release of nitric oxide (NO). The presence of NO results in a depletion of calcium ions in the endoplasmic reticulum (ER), leading to ER stress, the induction of C/EBP homologous protein (CHOP), and ultimately, β-cell apoptosis. NF-κB activation in β cells promotes apoptosis when exposed to IL-1β or TNF-α. The IL-1β/NF-κB pathway is considered a common mechanism contributing to β-cell death in both type 1 and type 2 diabetes. Autophagy, a crucial process for maintaining cellular homeostasis, is disrupted in insulin resistance, obesity, and type 2 diabetes. High levels of fatty acids and glucose can impair autophagic flux in human islet β cells, leading to apoptotic cell death. Excessive activation of autophagy is associated with increased lipolysis, ectopic lipid accumulation, and lipotoxic damage in β cells. The mTOR/AMPK pathway and autophagy-related genes (ATGs) play crucial roles in regulating autophagy. Markers of autophagy include microtubule-associated protein light chain 3-II (LC3-II) and p62. Inhibiting mTOR, which is a negative regulator of autophagy, has been shown to improve insulin resistance and hepatic steatosis in type 2 diabetes models. Kaempferol has been found to enhance autophagy and facilitate intracellular lipid degradation, thereby reducing ER stress and protecting β cells from lipotoxic damage (Yang et al., 2022).

Role of Kaempferol in Geriatric and Paediatric Patients

Geriatric Patients

In a randomized, double-blind, placebo-controlled clinical trial, 40 senior adults with type 2 diabetes were administered either a 100 mg/day kaempferol supplement or a placebo. Kaempferol supplementation led to a significant improvement in glycemic control. This improvement was evident through reductions in fasting blood glucose levels and HbA1c levels when compared to the placebo group (Rahmani et al., 2019). Another study aimed to investigate the impact of kaempferol on oxidative stress and inflammation in elderly patients diagnosed with type 2 diabetes. This study involved the administration of kaempferol supplementation at a dosage of 100 mg/day for a duration of 8 weeks. The findings of this research revealed that kaempferol supplementation led to a significant reduction in markers of oxidative stress, such as malondialdehyde, as well as markers of inflammation, such as C-reactive protein (Pourmasoumi et al., 2020).

Pediatric Patients

Research conducted on diabetic rats revealed that kaempferol has the potential to enhance glucose tolerance and insulin sensitivity, while simultaneously reducing oxidative stress and inflammation in the liver. These findings indicate that kaempferol may hold promise for the management of diabetes in pediatric patients. However, it's important to note that further studies involving human subjects are necessary to validate these effects (Li et al., 2015). Another study delved into the impact of kaempferol on insulin resistance in obese children. This investigation found that a diet rich in kaempferol (providing 0.02% kaempferol) led to improved insulin sensitivity and a reduction in inflammation within adipose tissue when compared to a control diet. These results suggest that kaempferol could serve as a valuable dietary intervention for addressing insulin resistance and obesity in pediatric patients (Wang et al., 2020). Collectively, these studies propose that kaempferol might offer potential benefits in the management of diabetes mellitus, both in elderly and pediatric populations.

Benefits of Kaempferol in Various Diabetic Conditions

Type 1 Diabetes

In a study conducted by Kim et al., (2011), the impact of kaempferol on pancreatic β-cell function in type 1 diabetic rats was explored. The findings from this research revealed that kaempferol treatment led to several positive outcomes. It notably improved the function of pancreatic β-cells, reduced oxidative stress, and mitigated inflammation. These results collectively suggest that kaempferol may exert a protective influence on β-cells in the context of type 1 diabetes.

Type 2 Diabetes

In a meticulously conducted randomized, double-blind, and placebo-controlled study, 50 individuals who were overweight or obese and diagnosed with type 2 diabetes participated. They were assigned to receive either a kaempferol-rich extract or a control substance for a duration of 12 weeks. The study outcomes, which were subsequently published in the Journal of Functional Foods, demonstrated that the group receiving the kaempferol extract experienced significant reductions in fasting blood glucose levels, HbA1c levels, and insulin resistance when compared to the placebo group (Basu et al., 2015).

Diabetic Neuropathy

A study featured in the Journal of Ethnopharmacology delved into the impact of kaempferol on diabetic neuropathy using a rat model. The findings from this research indicated that administering kaempferol led to enhancements in nerve conduction velocity and reductions in oxidative stress and inflammation within the sciatic nerve. These outcomes suggest that kaempferol could potentially offer protective benefits against diabetic neuropathy (Singh et al., 2018).

Diabetic Retinopathy

Li et al., (2018) conducted a study on diabetic retinopathy utilizing a diabetic rat model. The study's findings demonstrated that treatment with kaempferol led to reductions in oxidative stress, inflammation, and apoptosis within the retina. These results suggest that kaempferol might offer protective effects against diabetic retinopathy.

Anti-Adipogenic Property

Kaempferol has demonstrated anti-adipogenic effects, which can be advantageous in the management of diabetes. Adipogenesis, the process of generating new fat cells, contributes to obesity and insulin resistance, worsening diabetes. Sterol regulatory element-binding proteins (SREBPs) are transcription factors involved in adipogenesis, with SREBP1c being the primary subtype expressed in most tissues. SREBP2 regulates cholesterol metabolism and is controlled through a negative feedback mechanism involving downstream products of the cholesterol biosynthesis pathway. In cases of insulin resistance, the liver protein kinase B (Akt)/mammalian target of rapamycin complex 1 (mTORC1)/SREBP1c pathway becomes overactivated, leading to excessive adipogenesis. This contributes to lipid metabolism disorders in diabetic individuals. However, it's important to note that the direct role of SREBP2 in kaempferol's regulation of lipid metabolism lacks experimental support and requires further investigation. It's also worth mentioning that ongoing research is delving into kaempferol's effects on SREBPs and the regulation of lipid metabolism. Overall, these trials indicate that kaempferol might be advantageous for people with both type 1 and type 2 diabetes, diabetic neuropathy, and diabetic retinopathy. However, further investigation is required to establish the ideal kaempferol dosage and course, as well as the drug's long-term safety and effectiveness (Yang et al., 2022).

Conclusion

Kaempferol, a flavonoid commonly found in various fruits, vegetables, and plants, has garnered significant attention for its therapeutic potential in managing various diseases, including diabetes. Diabetes, a chronic metabolic disorder characterized by elevated blood sugar levels (hyperglycemia), insulin resistance, and beta-cell dysfunction, has been on the rise globally and poses a significant public health challenge. Kaempferol has demonstrated anti-diabetic properties through multiple mechanisms, including its influence on glucose uptake, insulin secretion, insulin sensitivity, and the reduction of oxidative stress. These findings suggest that kaempferol holds promise as a potential therapeutic agent for managing diabetes. However, further preclinical and clinical research is essential to establish its safety and efficacy in the treatment of diabetes.

References

Banday, M. Z., Sameer, A. S., Nissar, S. (2020). Pathophysiology of diabetes: An overview. *Avicenna Journal of Medicine*, 10(4), 174-188.

Basu, A., Lucas, E. A., Sanchez, K., Wood, S. L. (2015). Kaempferol-enriched diet lowers blood glucose levels and enhances insulin sensitivity in diabetic rats. *Journal of Functional Foods*, 17, 782-791.

Calderon-Montano, J. M., Burgos-Moron, E., Perez-Guerrero, C., Lopez-Lazaro, M. (2011). The pharmacology of flavonoids. *British Journal of Pharmacology*, 162(8), 1414-1438.

Choi, H. Y., Lim, J. E., Hong, J. H., Park, J. K., Kim, J. R., Kim, S. J. (2011). Kaempferol suppresses lipid accumulation by inhibiting early adipogenesis in 3T3-L1 cells and zebrafish. *Food and Chemical Toxicology*, 49(7), 1673-1679.

Jin, Y., Liu, M., Zhang, S., Liu, Y., Liu, Y., Qin, Y., Wang, J. (2013). Kaempferol, a flavonoid compound from Gynura medica, rescues streptozotocin-induced diabetic nephropathy in rats. *Journal of Agricultural and Food Chemistry*, 61(33), 7976-7986.

Jo, S. H., Ha, K. S., Moon, K. S., Kim, Y. C. (2015). Kaempferol stimulates glucose uptake through AMPK activation in muscle cells. *Food & Function*, 6(7), 2506-2513.

Kim, J. A., Ahn, J. H., Kim, M., Hong, Y. S., Jung, S. H., Hwang, S. G. (2010). Kaempferol inhibits PMA-induced cyclooxygenase-2 expression in mouse skin by blocking NF-κB activation. *Journal of Nutritional Biochemistry*, 21(11), 1131-1135.

Kim, J. A., Choi, H. Y., Jeong, S. I. (2011). Kaempferol protects pancreatic β-cells from oxidative stress-induced apoptosis. *Journal of Agricultural and Food Chemistry*, 59(16), 8349-8356.

Li, Y., Yao, J., Han, C., Yang, J., Chaudhry, M. T., Wang, S., Yin, Y. (2015). Quercetin, inflammation and immunity. *Nutrients*, 7(10), 7116-7138.

Lin, C., Wu, F., Zheng, T., Wang, X., Chen, Y., Wu, X. (2019). Kaempferol attenuates retinal ganglion cell death by suppressing NLRP1/NLRP3 inflammasomes and caspase-8 via JNK and NF-κB pathways in acute glaucoma. *Eye*, 33(5), 777-784.

Luo, C., Yang, H., Tang, C., Yao, G., Kong, L., He, H., Zhou, Y. (2015). Kaempferol alleviates insulin resistance via hepatic IKK/NF-κB signal in type 2 diabetic rats. *International immunopharmacology*, 28(1), 744-750.

Maurya, A. K., Patel, R., Mishra, A., Jaiswal, D. (2015). Therapeutic potential of kaempferol: A review of preclinical and clinical evidence. *Phytotherapy Research*, 29(3), 185-199.

Meng, S., Cao, J., Feng, Q., Peng, J., Hu, Y. (2017). Kaempferol attenuates streptozotocin-induced diabetic nephropathy in rats through antioxidative stress, inflammation and anti-apoptosis. *Pharmaceutical Biology*, 55(1), 157-164.

Periferakis, A., Periferakis, K., Badarau, I. A., Petran, E. M., Popa, D. C., Caruntu, A., Costache, R. S., Scheau, C., Caruntu, C., Costache, D. O. (2022). Kaempferol: Antimicrobial Properties, Sources, Clinical, and Traditional Applications. *International Journal of Molecular Sciences*, 23(15), 15054.

Pourmasoumi, M., Hadi, A., Najafgholizadeh, A., Joukar, F. (2020). The effects of kaempferol supplementation on biomarkers of inflammation and oxidative stress: A systematic review and meta-analysis of randomized controlled trials. *European Journal of Pharmacology*, 882, 173270.

Rahmani, J., Kord-Varkaneh, H., Hekmatdoost, A., Sadeghi, M., Maleki, V., Panahi, Y. (2019). The effects of kaempferol supplementation on glycemic control, lipid profile, and inflammatory markers in patients with type 2 diabetes: A systematic review and meta-analysis of randomized controlled trials. *Phytotherapy Research*, 33(3), 491-500.

Ren, J., Lu, Y., Qian, Y., Chen, B., Wu, T., Ji, G. (2019). Recent progress regarding kaempferol for the treatment of various diseases (Review). *Experimental and Therapeutic Medicine*, 18, 2759-2776.

Singh, V. P., Patil, C. S., Kulkarni, S. K., Udayabanu, M. (2018). Protective effect of kaempferol against diabetic neuropathy in experimental rats. *Journal of Ethnopharmacology*, 227, 199-210.

Vinayagam, R., Xu, B. (2015). Antidiabetic properties of dietary flavonoids: a cellular mechanism review. *Nutrition & Metabolism*, 12, 60.

Wang, T., Wu, Q., Zhao, T. (2020). Preventive Effects of Kaempferol on High-Fat Diet-Induced Obesity Complications in C57BL/6 Mice. *BioMed Research International*, 2020, 4532482.

White, P. A., Oliveira, R. C., Oliveira, A. P., Serafini, M. R., Araújo, A. A., Gelain, D. P., Moreira, J. C., Almeida, J. R., Quintans, J. S., Quintans-Junior, L. J., Santos, M. R. (2014). Antioxidant activity and mechanisms of action of natural compounds isolated from lichens: a systematic review. *Molecules*, 19(9), 14496–14527.

Yang, Y., Chen, Z., Zhao, X., Xie, H., Du, L., Gao, H., Xie, C. (2022). Mechanisms of Kaempferol in the treatment of diabetes: A comprehensive and latest review. *Frontiers in Endocrinology*, 13, 990299.

Chapter 24

Quercetin in the Management of Diabetes Mellitus

Meenakshi Sharma[1,*]
Raj Kumari[1]
Rinu Rana[2]
Dev Raj Sharma[2]
Sanjay Kumar[2]
Mahendra Singh Ashawat[2]
Kalpana Garg[3]
Gagandeep Kaur[4]
and Sakshi Bajaj[3]
[1]I. T. S. College of Pharmacy, Muradnagar, Ghaziabad, Uttar Pradesh, India
[2]Laureate Institute of Pharmacy, Kathog, Jawalaji, Himachal Pradesh, India
[3]Ch. Devi Lal College of Pharmacy, Jagadhri, Haryana, India
[4]Chitkara University School of Pharmacy, Chitkara University, Himachal Pradesh, India

Abstract

Diabetes mellitus (DM) is a hormonal disorder characterized by chronically elevated blood sugar levels. It arises from either insufficient insulin secretion or resistance to insulin, resulting in impaired lipid and protein metabolism. Without appropriate and timely treatment, DM can lead to significant complications affecting the eyes, kidneys, blood vessels, brain, and cardiovascular system. The prevalence of diabetes

* Corresponding Author's Email: meenakshisharma3128@gmail.com.

In: Naturally Occurring Chemicals …
Editors: A. Singh Grewal, G. Deswal, A. Kumar Dhingra et al.
ISBN: 979-8-89113-491-1

has seen a significant and concerning increase worldwide in recent decades. Type 2 diabetes mellitus is currently managed with a variety of anti-diabetic medications, including metformin, sulfonylureas, thiazolidinedione, GLP-1 mimetics, SGLT2 inhibitors, and DPP-IV inhibitors. However, some of these medications are expensive and have noticeable side effects. Therefore, bioflavonoids have emerged as potential treatments for diabetes. Bioflavonoids have garnered significant interest in therapeutic research, particularly in relation to diabetes. Among the numerous beneficial flavonoids, quercetin stands out due to its remarkable ability to lower blood sugar levels. It achieves this by promoting stable and sustained insulin secretion and aiding in the regeneration of pancreatic islets in humans. Importantly, quercetin offers these hypoglycemic benefits without posing significant health risks. Quercetin affects various targets of diabetes and regulates important signaling pathways, allowing it to mitigate both the consequences and symptoms of type 2 diabetes.

Keywords: diabetes mellitus (DM), hypoglycemia, insulin, quercetin, bioflavonoids

Introduction

Diabetes mellitus (DM) is a leading cause of illness and mortality worldwide, and it is a chronic disease. It is diagnosed when there is an increase in blood glucose levels (hyperglycemia) due to insufficient insulin secretion, improper insulin action, or both. Anomalies in protein and lipid metabolism have also been linked to improper insulin regulation. If DM is not promptly and effectively treated, it can lead to severe damage to various parts of the body and the cardiovascular system, and it can even result in life-threatening conditions like nonketotic hyperosmolar syndrome and ketoacidosis (Kharroubi et al., 2015; American Diabetes Association, 2013). Metabolic disturbances occur due to reduced insulin levels or insulin resistance in skeletal muscles, adipose tissue, and other target tissues. There is a significant association between the development, pathophysiology, and complications of DM and higher levels of oxidative stress, free radicals, and other metabolic stressors (Lamb et al., 2009; Ansari et al., 2022). Reports from 2021 estimated that 465 million individuals worldwide have DM, and this number is projected to reach 700 million by 2045. Most people with DM come from middle- and low-income nations (Robertson et al., 2003; Akhtar et al., 2020). Diabetes is managed through various methods, including the consumption of nutritious foods and dietary management, the use of insulin injections, and conventional hypoglycemic medications. These approaches aim to support the survival of pancreatic islets and promote cell regeneration, often facilitated by islet neogenesis-related proteins (Krentz, 2006; Rafaeloff et al., 1997). Although current treatments for the disease can be effective, they may also have adverse side effects. It is common to believe that traditional herbal remedies can effectively prevent and treat diabetes with minimal to negligible side effects (Yin et al., 2008). Therefore, an increasing number of medicinal plants are favored as a natural source of medications for curing DM (Dhasarathan et al., 2011) because they are considered more readily available, less harmful, and safer than manufactured medications (Ramesh et al., 2006). In this context, quercetin, an essential polyphenolic flavonoid found in fruits and vegetables, has been researched for its role in improving health (David et al., 2016; Dabeek et al., 2019). Consuming quercetin has been shown to impact mitochondrial defects, enhance electron transport chain performance, reduce reactive oxygen generation, and increase energy production (Wei and Liu, 2009; Ray et al., 2009). Additionally, in recent years, researchers have dedicated themselves to investigating the potential disease-related mechanisms of onset and progression to develop efficient therapeutic approaches and address these pathological characteristics. There is mounting evidence that oxidative stress (Miranda-Diaz et al., 2018), inflammation cytokines (Ray et al., 2009), chemokines, apoptosis (Schattenberg and Schuchmann, 2009), autophagy (He et al., 2017), and ferroptosis (Cao et al., 2016; Dixon et al., 2014) play significant roles in the development of diabetes complications. Preventive measures are preferred over alternative therapeutic procedures for treating diabetic complications because they are often difficult to treat or even irreversible. Despite the fact that these widespread diseases affect millions of patients, our understanding of their pathogenesis is still limited. As a result, researchers still need to fully examine the pathophysiology of these disorders. In the realm of conventional medicine, identifying and developing effective and safe treatments to delay or prevent the complications of diabetes are currently a significant focus in clinical research. Throughout history, natural herbal plants have been a rich source of polyphenolic compounds, which are widely used for diabetes prevention and care because of their therapeutic advantages, versatility, and minimal risk of toxicity (Boots et al., 2008).

Quercetin's Chemistry

The name "quercetin" originates from the Latin word "Quercetum," which means "oak forest." Quercetin is primarily found in fruits, vegetables, and several medicinal plants. Its chemical formula is $C_{15}H_{10}O_7$, and it was initially identified as a flavonoid glycoside. Quercetin is yellow in color, soluble in alcohol and lipids, insoluble in cold water, and slightly soluble in hot water. It belongs to the flavonol subclass of flavonoids (Figure 1).

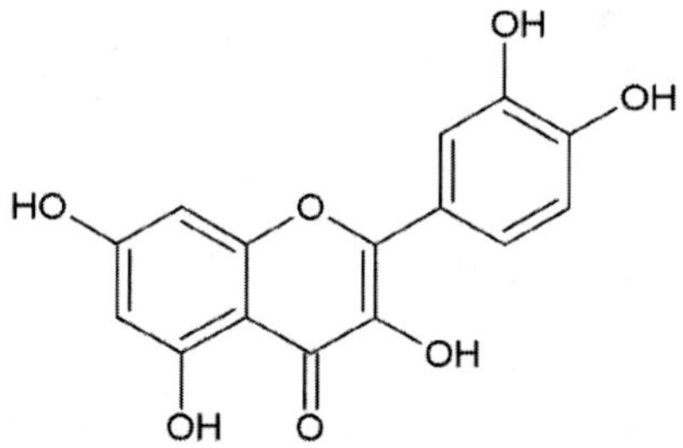

Figure 1. The chemical composition of quercetin.

Role in Diabetes

Quercetin, a naturally occurring flavonoid abundant in a variety of fruits, vegetables, and grains, has been the subject of several studies investigating its potential as an antidiabetic agent. In one study examining the impact of quercetin on rats with hyperglycemia, researchers explored its effects on oxidative stress and inflammation. The findings revealed that quercetin administration led to a reduction in blood sugar levels, an improvement in antioxidant status, and a suppression of inflammation. These effects were attributed to the inhibition of the NF-κB signaling pathway (Zhang et al., 2020). The results of a meta-analysis further supported the potential of quercetin. This analysis showed that quercetin supplementation had a significant impact on reducing fasting blood glucose levels and hemoglobin A1c (HbA1c) levels. These findings suggest that quercetin may hold promise as an adjunctive therapy for managing glycemic control in individuals with type 2 diabetes (Ostadmohammadi et al., 2019). In a controlled trial involving overweight participants with insulin resistance, the participants were divided into two groups, one receiving quercetin supplementation and the other receiving a placebo. The results of this trial demonstrated that the group receiving quercetin exhibited significant improvements in insulin resistance, reduced fasting blood glucose levels, and enhanced endothelial function compared to the placebo group. This suggests that quercetin supplementation has the potential to improve various aspects of metabolic health in individuals with insulin resistance. Another study investigated the impact of quercetin on metabolic syndrome and insulin resistance in rats. The findings indicated that quercetin improved glucose tolerance, enhanced insulin sensitivity, and upregulated the PI3K/AKT signaling pathway, which plays a crucial role in insulin signaling. These results suggest that quercetin may have beneficial effects on metabolic health and insulin resistance by modulating important signaling pathways (Hosseini et al., 2021). In a study involving type 2 diabetic mice, researchers investigated the effects of quercetin supplementation on insulin resistance and hepatic lipid accumulation. The study revealed that quercetin supplementation resulted in improvements in insulin resistance and a reduction in hepatic lipid accumulation. Furthermore, the researchers observed that quercetin increased IRS-1/PI3K/Akt-mediated insulin signaling. These findings indicate that quercetin may offer advantages in managing insulin resistance associated with type 2 diabetes by positively modulating key signaling pathways involved in insulin action (Salehi et al., 2020). In a study focusing on diabetic neuropathy, researchers examined the potential protective effects of quercetin. The study demonstrated that quercetin treatment resulted in a reduction in oxidative stress and an improvement in antioxidant enzyme activity within Schwann cells, leading to the alleviation of symptoms associated with diabetic neuropathy. These studies suggest that quercetin may hold promise as a therapeutic intervention for the prevention or treatment of diabetic neuropathy (Liu et al., 2020; Zhang et al., 2021). Another study investigated the effects of quercetin on insulin resistance induced by a high-fat diet in mice. The study revealed that supplementation with quercetin resulted in a reduction in adipose tissue inflammation and an improvement in insulin sensitivity. These effects were attributed to the modulation of the insulin signaling pathway. The results imply that quercetin may have advantages in reducing insulin resistance caused by a high-fat diet (Perdicaro et al., 2020). In a study exploring the potential protective effects of quercetin on pancreatic beta-cell function and mass in streptozotocin-induced diabetes (mice), the findings demonstrated that quercetin treatment effectively preserved pancreatic beta-cell function, reduced oxidative stress levels, and inhibited apoptosis. Consequently, these effects acted as a safeguard against the development of DM. Overall, the study suggests that quercetin holds promise as a potential therapeutic agent for protecting pancreatic beta-cells and preventing the onset of DM (Youl et al., 2010). Collectively, these studies highlight the potential of quercetin in addressing various aspects of DM, including insulin resistance, glycemic control, diabetic neuropathy, and pancreatic beta-cell function. Nevertheless, it is crucial to acknowledge that additional research is necessary to determine the ideal dosage, duration, and potential adverse effects of quercetin supplementation in the management of DM.

Hypoglycaemic Mechanism of Action of Quercetin

In-depth investigations into the anti-hyperglycemic properties of natural flavonoids have revealed a promising avenue for advancing diabetes research (Figure 2). Among the many flavonoids known for their anti-diabetic effects, quercetin has garnered the most attention. Quercetin's broad-reaching effects target various organs in the body, including muscles, the pancreas, the liver, and the small intestine. Notably, insulin-sensitive skeletal muscles play a pivotal role, responsible for absorbing over 80% of glucose in the human body. With the increasing interest in quercetin and its various derivatives for biomedical applications, this study primarily focuses on elucidating quercetin's anti-diabetic properties. Essentially, quercetin's action involves its effects on the liver, muscles, pancreas, and small intestine, collectively contributing to regulating blood glucose levels. It enhances the activity of glucose transporter 4 (GLUT 4) and insulin receptors in muscles, leading to increased glucose uptake and the maintenance of normal blood glucose levels. Additionally, quercetin augments glucokinase activity in the liver, resulting in improved glucose storage and regulated glycemia. It also increases beta cell regeneration in the pancreas through the MTOR pathway and decreases glucose absorption in the small intestine by acting on glucose transporters like Glut 2 and maltase (Eid & Haddad, 2017).

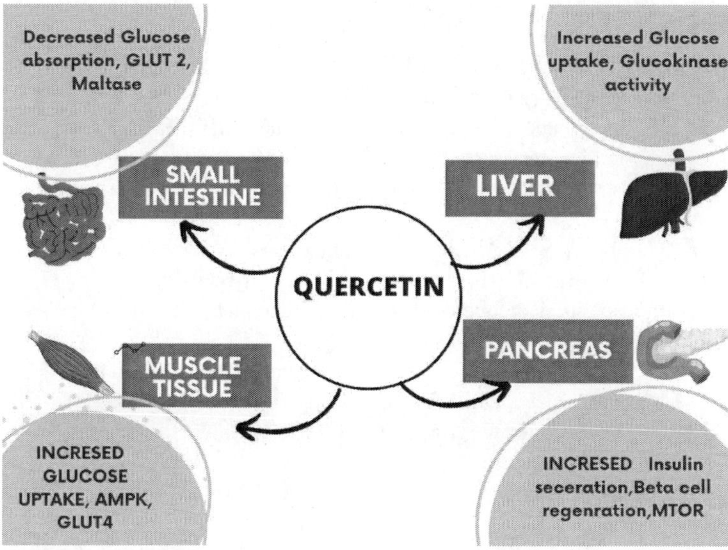

Figure 2. Mechanism of antidiabetic action of quercetin.

Conclusion

Quercetin, an important flavonoid with notable anti-inflammatory and antioxidant properties, has shown promise in the treatment of DM. Several studies have suggested that quercetin supplementation can lead to improvements in blood glucose levels, and lipid profiles, increased insulin sensitivity, and a reduced risk of diabetes-related complications. However, it's essential to note that the optimal dosage, duration, and safety of quercetin supplementation for individuals with diabetes still require further investigation. It's crucial to emphasize that quercetin should not be viewed as a replacement for standard diabetes treatments, including medications, dietary modifications, and exercise. Instead, it holds potential as a complementary therapy to enhance diabetes management. In summary, while quercetin exhibits promise as a potential adjunctive treatment for DM, additional research is necessary to comprehensively understand its potential benefits and limitations in the context of diabetes management.

References

Akhtar, S., Nasir, J. A., Sarwar, A., Nasr, N., Javed, A., Majeed, R., Salam, M. A., Billah, B. (2020). Prevalence of diabetes and pre-diabetes in Bangladesh: a systematic review and meta-analysis. *BMJ Open*, 10, e036086.

American Diabetes Association. (2013). Diagnosis and classification of diabetes mellitus. *Diabetes Care*, 37, S81-S90.

Ansari, P., Choudhury, S. T., Seidel, V., Rahman, A. B., Aziz, M. A., Richi, A. E., Rahman, A., Jafrin, U. H., Hannan, J. M. A., Abdel-Wahab, Y. H. A. (2022). Therapeutic potential of quercetin in the management of type-2 diabetes mellitus. *Life*, 12, 1146.

Bhatt, K., Flora, S. J. (2009). Protective effect of dietary quercetin on cadmium-induced toxicity in rats. *Environmental Toxicology and Pharmacology*, 28, 140.

Boots, A. W., Haenen, G. R., Bast, A. (2008). Health effects of quercetin: from antioxidant to nutraceutical. *European Journal of Pharmacology*, 585(2-3), 325-337.

Brahmachari, G. (2008). Bioactive natural products (Part III): furoquinoline alkaloids. *Natural Product Communications*, 3, 1337.

Bronner, C., Landry, Y. (1985). Kinetic analysis of human erythrocyte membrane-bound adenylate cyclase. *Agents and Actions*, 16, 147.

Cao, J. Y., Dixon, S. J. (2016). Mechanisms of ferroptosis. *Cell and Molecular Life Sciences*, 73, 2195-2209.

Dabeek, W. M., Marra, M. V. (2019). Dietary quercetin and kaempferol: Bioavailability and potential cardiovascular-related bioactivity in humans. *Nutrients*, 11, 2288.

David, A. V., Arulmoli, R., Parasuraman, S. (2016). Overviews of biological importance of quercetin: a bioactive flavonoid. *Pharmacognosy Reviews*, 10, 84-89.

Dhasarathan, P., Theriappan, P. (2011). Evaluation of anti-diabetic activity of Strychnos potatorum in alloxan induced diabetic rats. *Journal of Medical Sciences*, 2, 670-674.

Dixon, S. J., Patel, D. N., Welsch, M., Skouta, R., Lee, E. D., Hayano, M., Thomas, A. G., Gleason, C. E., Tatonetti, N. P., Slusher, B. S. (2014). Pharmacological inhibition of cystine–glutamate exchange induces endoplasmic reticulum stress and ferroptosis. *eLife*, 3, e02523.

Eid, H. M., Haddad, P. S. (2017). The antidiabetic potential of quercetin: underlying mechanisms. *Current Medicinal Chemistry*, 24(4), 355-364.

Gupta, A., Birhman, K., Raheja, I., Sharma, S. K., Kar, H. K. (2016). Quercetin: a wonder bioflavonoid with therapeutic potential in disease management. *Asian Pacific Journal of Tropical Disease*, 6, 248-252.

He, Y., Li, X., Xie, M., Xu, Y., Liu, X. (2017). Quercetin induces autophagy via FOXO1-dependent pathways and autophagy suppression enhances quercetin-induced apoptosis of PASMCs in hypoxia. *Free Radical Biology and Medicine*, 103, 165.

Hosseini, A., Razavi, B. M., Banach, M., Hosseinzadeh, H. (2021). Quercetin and metabolic syndrome: A review. *Phytotherapy Research*, 35(10), 5352-5364.

Krentz, A. J. (2006). Comparative safety of newer oral antidiabetic drugs. *Expert Opinion on Drug Safety*, 5, 827-834.

Lamb, M. M., Yin, X., Zerbe, G. O., Klingensmith, G. J., Dabelea, D., Fingerlin, T. E., Rewers, M., Norris, J. M. (2009). Height growth velocity, islet autoimmunity, and type 1 diabetes development: the diabetes autoimmunity study in the young. *Diabetologia*, 52, 2064-2071.

Li, X., Wang, R., Zhou, N., Wang, X., Liu, Q., Bai, Y., Bai, Y., Liu, Z., Yang, H., Zou, J., Wang, H., Shi, T. (2013). Quercetin improves insulin resistance and hepatic lipid accumulation in vitro in a NAFLD cell model. *Biomedical Reports*, 1(1), 71-76.

Liu, Y., Shao, S., Guo, H. (2020). Schwann cells apoptosis is induced by high glucose in diabetic peripheral neuropathy. *Life Sciences*, 2020, 248.

Miranda-Díaz, A. G., Padilla-Tejeda, D. E., Carrillo-Ibarra, S., Sifuentes-Franco, S. (2018). Oxidative stress, apoptosis, and mitochondrial function in diabetic nephropathy. *International Journal of Endocrinology*, 2018, 1-13.

Ostadmohammadi, V., Milajerdi, A., Ayati, E., Kolahdooz, F., Asemi, Z. (2019). Effects of quercetin supplementation on glycemic control among patients with metabolic syndrome and related disorders: A systematic review and meta-analysis of randomized controlled trials. *Phytotherapy Research*, 33(5), 1330-1340.

Perdicaro, D. J., Rodriguez Lanzi, C., Gambarte Tudela, J., Miatello, R. M., Oteiza, P. I., Vazquez Prieto, M. A. (2020). Quercetin attenuates adipose hypertrophy, in part through activation of adipogenesis in rats fed a high-fat diet. *Journal of Nutritional Biochemistry*, 79, 108352.

Rafaeloff, R., Pittenger, G. L., Barlow, S. W., Qin, X. F., Yan, B., Rosenberg, L., Duguid, W. P., Vinik, A. I. (1997). Cloning and sequencing of the pancreatic islet neogenesis associated protein (INGAP) gene and its expression in islet neogenesis in hamsters. *Journal of Clinical Investigation*, 99, 2100-2109.

Ramesh, B., Pugalendi, K. V. (2006). Anti-hyperglycemic effect of Umbelliferone in Streptozotocin diabetic rats. *Journal of Medicinal Plants*, 9, 562–566.

Ray, A., Huisman, M. V., Tamsma, J. T., Writing-Group, A., Van, A. G., Bingen, B. O., Broeders, E. A., Hoogeveen, E. S., Van H. F., Kwee, V. A. (2009). The role of inflammation on atherosclerosis, intermediate and clinical cardiovascular endpoints in type 2 diabetes mellitus. *European Journal of Internal Medicine*, 20, 253-260.

Robertson, R. P., Harmon, J., Tran, P. O., Tanaka, Y., Takahashi, H. (2003). Glucose toxicity in β-Cells: type 2 diabetes, good radicals gone bad, and the glutathione connection. *Diabetes*, 52, 581-587.

Salehi, B., Machin, L., Monzote, L., Sharifi-Rad, J., Ezzat, S. M., Salem, M. A., Merghany, R. M., El Mahdy, N. M., Kılıç, C. S., Sytar, O., Sharifi-Rad, M., Sharopov, F., Martins, N., Martorell, M., Cho, W. C. (2020). Therapeutic potential of quercetin: new insights and perspectives for human health. *ACS Omega*, 5, 11849-11872.

Scalbert, A., Williamson, G. (2000). Dietary intake and bioavailability of polyphenols. *Journal of Nutrition*, 130, 2073.

Schattenberg, J. M., Schuchmann, M. (2009). Diabetes and apoptosis: liver. *Apoptosis*, 14, 1459-1471.

Wei, W., Liu, Q. J., Tan, Y., Liu, L. C., Li, X. K., Cai, L. (2009). Oxidative stress, diabetes, and diabetic complications. *Hemoglobin*, 33, 370-377.

Yin, J., Zhang, H., Ye, J. (2008). Traditional Chinese medicine in the treatment of metabolic syndrome. *Endocrine, Metabolic & Immune Disorders Drug Targets*, 8, 99-111.

Youl, E., Bardy, G., Magous, R., Cros, G., Sejalon, F., Virsolvy, A., Richard, S., Quignard, J. F., Gross, R., Petit, P., Bataille, D., Oiry, C. (2010). Quercetin potentiates insulin secretion and protects INS-1 pancreatic β-cells against oxidative damage via the ERK1/2 pathway. *British Journal of Pharmacology*, 161(4), 799-814.

Zhang, F., Feng, J., Zhang, J., Kang, X., Qian, D. (2020). Quercetin modulates AMPK/SIRT1/NF-κB signaling to inhibit inflammatory/oxidative stress responses in diabetic high fat diet-induced atherosclerosis in the rat carotid artery. *Experimental and Therapeutic Medicine*, 20(6), 280.

Zhang, Q., Song, W., Zhao, B., Xie, J., Sun, Q., Shi, X., Yan, B., Tian, G., Liang, X. (2021). Quercetin attenuates diabetic peripheral neuropathy by correcting mitochondrial abnormality via activation of the AMPK/PGC-1α pathway in vivo and in vitro. *Frontiers in Neuroscience*, 15, 636172.

Chapter 25

Resveratrol in the Management of Diabetes Mellitus

Swati Joshi[1,*]
Mahendra Rana[1]
Satpal Singh Bisht[2]
Bhuwan Chandra Joshi[1]
Deepankar Bahuguna[3]
Amita Joshi Rana[1]
Meena Devi[4]
Jyoti[4]
Nisham Rani[4]
and Ritu Kataria[4]

[1]Department of Pharmaceutical Sciences, Faculty of Technology, Sir J. C. Bose Technical Campus, Kumaun University, Nainital, Uttarakhand, India
[2]Department of Zoology, D. S. B. Campus, Kumaun University, Nainital, Uttarakhand, India
[3]Department of Pharmaceutics, National Institute of Pharmaceutical Education and Research, Hyderabad, Telangana, India
[4]G. V. M. College of Pharmacy, Sonepat, Haryana, India

* Corresponding Author's Email: swatijoshi241@gmail.com.

In: Naturally Occurring Chemicals …
Editors: A. Singh Grewal, G. Deswal, A. Kumar Dhingra et al.
ISBN: 979-8-89113-491-1

Abstract

Resveratrol, a naturally occurring molecule found in grapes, peanuts, and mulberries, has gained significant popularity in recent times due to its diverse therapeutic effects. Scientific research has unveiled that its potential in treating and preventing various chronic diseases primarily stems from its antioxidant capabilities, making it a promising adjunct in chemotherapy. In recent years, extensive focus has been on resveratrol's role in diabetes management. It has been demonstrated to synergistically enhance the effects of anti-hyperglycemic medications. Numerous studies have unveiled its multifaceted mechanisms in controlling and managing diabetes, especially in animal models. Notably, resveratrol has exhibited the ability to ameliorate insulin resistance, facilitate glucose uptake, and safeguard the insulin-producing β cells within the Islets of Langerhans. Moreover, investigations have revealed that in the livers of diabetic rats, resveratrol induces cellular modifications that elevate the levels of GLUT4 and GLUT2 proteins – pivotal regulators of glucose transport. Clinical studies have also suggested that resveratrol supplementation might offer benefits to individuals with hyperglycemia and insulin resistance. This chapter delves into the factors driving the surging interest in resveratrol's role in diabetes management, examining its underlying mechanisms and potential benefits.

Keywords: resveratrol, antidiabetic, adjuvant, synergistic, anti-hyperglycemic, insulin resistance

Introduction

The rising prevalence of Diabetes Mellitus (DM) has become a significant global healthcare issue, prompting numerous epidemiological studies (Khan et al., 2020). It represents a worldwide burden of disease, contributing to an increase in diverse acute and chronic complications within the physiological system (Garg & Duggal, 2022). Several countries have conducted observational studies using their national database systems to assess hospitalization and mortality rates. The majority of these studies have documented a rise in both hospitalization and mortality rates among individuals with diabetes (Florencio et al., 2021). Impaired glucose homeostasis resulting in hyperglycemia is a hallmark of DM (Nandy et al., 2023). It is one of the characteristics of the life-threatening disorder metabolic syndrome (Fenwick et al., 2018). The primary forms of DM include Type 1 and Type 2. In Type 1 DM, an autoimmune reaction leads to the destruction of pancreatic β cells. Type 2 diabetes, on the other hand, is marked by irregularities in the gluco-receptors of β cells and reduced insulin sensitivity in peripheral tissues. Gestational Diabetes Mellitus (GDM), initially identified during pregnancy, represents a hyperglycemic condition primarily detected in the second trimester (Mcintyre et al., 2019). This condition arises from issues with both insulin production and peripheral resistance, and it frequently advances into Type 2 DM (Champion et al., 2022). The potential of natural supplements to address diabetes has garnered considerable attention in recent times. Resveratrol (RV) is among the compounds exhibiting ameliorative effects on DM.

Resveratrol

RV, a natural polyphenolic compound with the chemical formula 3,4′,5-trihydroxy-trans-stilbene, has been associated with beneficial effects not only in obesity, neurodegeneration, cancer, atherosclerosis, aging, inflammation, and oxidative stress but also in diabetes mellitus (Mahjabeen et al., 2022; Zhang et al., 2021). Research has unveiled that RV serves as a potent antioxidant, mitigating oxidative damage resulting from hyperglycemia (Santos et al., 2020).

Source and Structure

Significant quantities of RV can be found in the skin of red grapes, peanuts, and red wine (Wahab et al., 2017). RV has been first isolated from the roots of *Veratrum grandiflorum* (Grau et al., 2023). A traditional Chinese and Japanese remedy called *Polygonum cuspidatum* has also had RV extracted from its roots (He & Yan, 2013). Currently, red grapes stand as the primary source for extracting RV, mainly due to their abundant and high content of the compound (Tian & Liu, 2019). RV is present in various parts of different plant species, including roots, stems, leaves, flowers, fruits, and seeds. Achieving a high level of RV purity has led to its synthesis from glucose and ethanol, employing genetically engineered yeast *Saccharomyces cerevisiae* (Li et al., 2015). RV exist in cis or trans configurations (Figure 1) (Burns et al., 2002). Trans-RV-3-O-D-glucoside, commonly referred to as piceid or polydatin, represents a significant form of RV found in various plants (Jensen et al., 2010). Trans-RV has been documented as an effective therapeutic compound owing to its heightened biological activity against a range of ailments.

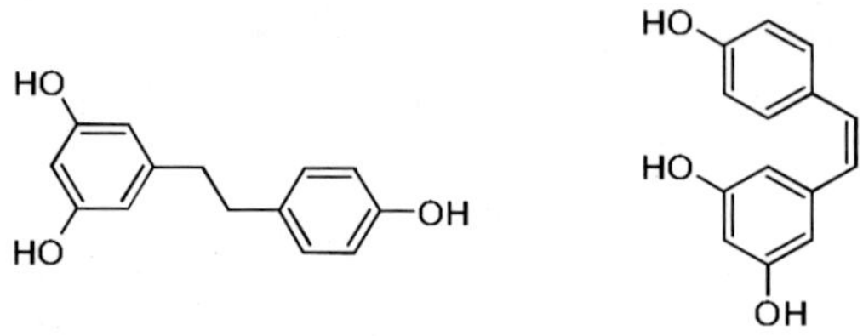

Figure 1. Trans (left) and cis (right) configurations of RV.

Metabolism, Bioavailability and Route of Administration

RV undergoes extensive metabolism in the liver and intestine. Due to its significant first-pass metabolism, when administered orally, its bioavailability is less than 1% (Shu et al., 2015). In a multiple-dose study, it was observed that trans-RV exhibited higher bioavailability when administered in the morning (Almeida et al., 2009, Vesely et al., 2021). In the liver, RV is known to interact with CYP P450 enzymes and Phase II enzymes (Surendran et al., 2019). The predominant metabolic pathways for RV involve Phase II processes such as glucuronidation and sulfation. This leads to the formation of metabolites including RV-3-O-D glucuronide, RV-4-O-D glucuronide, RV-3-sulfate, and RV-4-sulfate (Han et al., 2022). According to research, RV functions as a potent antioxidant, mitigating oxidative damage caused by hyperglycemia. According to the Biopharmaceutics Classification System (BCS) for drugs, RV falls under the category of BCS class II drugs (Chimento et al., 2019). Class II drugs are characterized by low solubility and high permeability. RV is commonly administered orally, and the documented range for dosages spans from 0.073 mg to 5 g (Huang et al., 2019). In the recent years, various novel methodologies have been employed to modify the kinetics of RV in order to enhance its bioavailability. An approach focused on the development of nanotechnology-based formulations, such as liposomes, emulsions, micelles, metallic nanoparticles, and solid lipid nanoparticles, has been adopted to improve its oral bioavailability (Robertson et al., 2022; Annaji et al., 2021).

Side Effects and Safety

Clinical trials that have explored different dosage concentrations of RV with small cohort sizes have reported side effects including nausea, diarrhea, skin rashes, headaches, dizziness, and abdominal discomfort (Singh et al., 2019; Almeida et al., 2009). Preclinical evidence of acute oral and dermal toxicity for trans-RV indicates that its LD50 is observed at dose levels of 2 g/day (Ratz-łyko & Arct, 2018). Numerous studies have consistently shown that both higher and lower doses of RV are well tolerated in preclinical investigations. Based on safety and tolerability evidence in mice, the recommended maximum daily dose for long-term usage should be 1g (Cai et al., 2021). According to a clinical investigation by Brown et al., (2010), consumption of 29 daily dosages of 0.5-5g is safe. Human clinical studies have demonstrated the safety of consuming RV, with single doses of up to 5 g being considered safe (Khattar et al., 2022; Boocock et al., 2007).

Marketed Dose

RV is available in the market in various dosage forms, including tablets, capsules, and powder (Annaji et al., 2021). It is also accessible for topical applications in the form of cream (Pentek et al., 2017). The RV supplements that are available come in doses ranging from 50 to 500 mg (Khattar et al., 2022). From the National Library of Medicine database, several RV-marketed products are listed, such as the VINE VERA Resveratrol Cabernet Replenishing Moisture Cream, ASCUOLI capsule, ASCUOLI lozenge, ALPHA9 powder, CO-BALAMIN capsule, and NMN.5S tablet.

Anti-Diabetic Effect of RV on Rodents

In-vivo investigations have demonstrated that RV holds promise for treating both the complications of DM and many of its symptoms by targeting various insulin signaling pathways and facilitating glucose uptake (as summarized in Table 1) (Szkudelska et al., 2019). Streptozotocin (STZ) is the most prevalent model employed to induce both type 1 and type 2 diabetes in rodents (Furman, 2021). According to in vivo investigations, STZ induces hyperglycemia-mediated oxidative stress. Due to their associated side effects, oral hypoglycemic medications are typically avoided during pregnancy. In a study on pregnant female rats, Zhang et al., (2021) discovered that RV increases insulin secretion in a dose-dependent manner, reduces glucose levels and body weight, regulates blood lipid levels, and affects plasma adipokines. Additionally, a study suggests that RV could potentially stimulate the growth of microorganisms utilizing glycolysis, with the aim of restoring glucose homeostasis in diabetic mice (Cai et al., 2020). Pregnant women with gestational diabetes mellitus (GDM) are at a higher risk of developing type 2 diabetes. In pregnant mice, RV has been shown to alleviate the symptoms of GDM. Intake of RV results in improvements such as hypoglycemia, enhanced insulin sensitivity, increased fetal survival rates, and reduced body weight in comparison to GDM pregnant females who do not receive RV treatment (Yao et al., 2015). To address GDM, an innovative approach was employed to enhance the bioavailability of RV. This was achieved by forming a resveratrol-metal combination and then encapsulating it within chitosan nanoparticles (Du et al., 2020). The study revealed that the chitosan-zinc oxide-resveratrol (CS-ZnO-RS) compound significantly lowered blood sugar levels. It also reduced inflammatory markers such as MCP-1 and IL-6, along with endoplasmic reticulum stress factors like GRP78, p-eIF2α, p-IRE1α, and p-PERK. Additionally, substantial inhibition of α-glucosidase (77.32%) and α-amylase (78.4%) was observed. Administering maternal RV can also help prevent symptoms of GDM in rat offspring (Brawerman et al., 2019). In the GDM group during the 3rd trimester, plasma insulin levels were decreased by up to 50% due to islet cell dysfunction. This impairment was partially ameliorated in GDM offspring treated with RV, leading to the restoration of glucose tolerance. Maternal supplementation with RV at a dose of 147 mg/kg per day was administered. Certain reports suggest that RV might offer benefits for complicated pregnancies (Darby et al., 2019).

RV is purported to enhance insulin sensitivity, protect cells, and reduce blood glucose levels in the STZ group through various signaling pathways (Szkudelski & Szkudelska, 2011). The majority of research studies have documented a positive impact of RV on diabetes mellitus (DM) based on their analyses. However, some investigations do not agree with the notion of RV having an anti-diabetic effect. Sadi et al., (2015) reported no change in blood glucose level of diabetic rats receiving RV.

Table 1. RV supplementation effects on diabetic rodents

Animal Strain	Inducing Model	RV Dose & Route	Treatment Duration	Outcomes of RV	Reference
Male wistar rats	STZ	20mg/kg, orally (Daily)	1 week	Improved glycemic control by lowering blood sugar to 25.46%; increased HDL by 13.23%; decreased LDL by 21.02%	Raskovic et al., 2019
Male albino wistar rats	STZ-nicotinamide	5mg/kg, orally (Daily)	30 days	No change in body weight; decreased blood glucose; reduced glycosylate; decreased haemoglobin, urea, uric acid and creatinine	Palsamy & Subramanian, 2008
Male and female mice	STZ	50 mg/L orally in drinking water (Daily)	2 weeks	Increased insulin sensitivity in absence of Sirt1	Rodriuez et al., 2015
Sprague Dawley male rats	STZ	10mg/kg intra-venous (Daily)	8 weeks	Decreased glucose, triglyceride along with inflammatory factors as TNF-α, IL-6, VCAM-1, MCP-1 and ICAM-1	Huo et al., 2019
Female wistar rats	STZ	5 mg/kg intra-venous (Daily)	4 weeks	Increased GLUT4, SIRT1, and PGC-1α gene expression	Akgun-unal et al., 2023
Male wistar rats	STZ-Nicotinamide	5mg/kg, orally (Daily)	4 weeks	Decreased glucose level ($p < 0.001$) and insulin resistance; increased GLP1 and antioxidant capacity	Pegah et al., 2021
Albino rats of same sex	Alloxan	30mg/kg, orally (Daily)	30 days	Highly significant hypoglycemic effect as decrease blood glucose & insulin resistance; increase GSH, CAT and SOD	Rehman et al., 2018
Male BALB/c albino mice	STZ	50 mg/kg, i.p. (Daily)	12 days	Mortality dropped from 40% to 20%; lowered blood glucose, total cholesterol, triglycerides, serum insulin; reduced CXCL16/NF-κB p65, CD45 expression	Darwish et al., 2021

Table 1. (Continued)

Animal Strain	Inducing Model	RV Dose & Route	Treatment Duration	Outcomes of RV	Reference
C57BL/6J male mice	High fat diet	15 mg/kg i.p. (Daily)	10 weeks	Enhanced hepatic and muscle glycogen synthesis; accelerated adipocyte lipolysis; decreased glucose, TG, body weight	Gong et al., 2020
Male wistar rats	STZ	30 mg/kg Orally (Daily)	16 weeks	Increased activation of SIRT1/ FOXO3; prevented increase in SOD and MDA level; increased, markedly elevated CAT levels	Wang et al., 2016
Female sprague dawley rats	STZ	60, 120, and 240 mg/kg	2 weeks	Increased insulin secretion; decreased blood glucose and body weight; Leptin, resistin, IL-6 and TNF-α, plasma levels in gestational diabetic rats markedly decreased	Zhang et al., 2021

Table 2. Clinicaltrials.gov reported completed RV supplement clinical studies for diabetes

Study Title	Daily Consumption	Study Duration	Outcome Measures	Identifier No.
Effects of Resveratrol in Patients with Type 2 Diabetes	3g for 12 weeks	Jan 2013-July 2016	Skeletal muscle sirtuin 1 (SIRT1) expression, Insulin sensitivity, Glycated hemoglobin (HbA1c), Skeletal muscle 5'-AMP-activated protein kinase (AMPK) expression	NCT01677611
Effects of high dose Resveratrol in Non-diabetic obese males	1g three times a day for 2 weeks	July 2009-October 2012	Change from baseline in insulin resistance via Homeostasis Model Assessment (HOMA) 2 calculator at 2 weeks, Beta cell function, B (%), Insulin sensitivity, S (%), Insulin resistance	NCT02247596
Pilot Study of the Effects of Resveratrol on Endothelial Function in Subjects with Type 2 Diabetes Mellitus	90mg & 270mg for 2 weeks	Jan 2010-Dec 2010	Brachial artery flow-mediated dilation, Blood markers of inflammation, oxidative stress, insulin resistance	NCT01038089
Effect of Resveratrol Administration on Metabolic Syndrome, Insulin Sensitivity and Insulin Secretion	500 mg thrice per day for 90 days	April 2012-September 2013	Fasting Glucose Levels, Total Insulin Secretion, Total Insulin Sensitivity, Body Mass Index, Total Cholesterol at Week 12	NCT02114892
Resveratrol and Metabolic Syndrome	1000 mg BID for 30 days	October 2012- July 2018	Reduction in Insulin resistance, Reduction in serum cytokines/chemokines, Changes in HOMA-IR, Changes in gene expression in adipose tissue	NCT01714102
Effect of Resveratrol in Age-related Insulin Resistance and Inflammation in Humans	1,000mg twice for 4 weeks	Mar 2008-Sep 2017	Peripheral Insulin Sensitivity, Endogenous Glucose Production with Resveratrol or Placebo at Baseline and at 4 Weeks	NCT01354977
Effect of Resveratrol and Pharmacist Intervention on Diabetes Mellitus and Its Neuropathic Complication	500 mg for 12 weeks	Dec 2021-Dec 2022	Visual analog scale, Electroneurography mean change in fasting blood glucose, HbA1c	NCT05172947
Effects of Resveratrol on Inflammation in Type 2 Diabetes Patients	4omg & 500mg for 6 months	Oct 2013-Feb 2016	C-reactive protein (CRP), Metabolic and oxidative markers (Interleukin-6, Pentraxin-3, total antioxidant status, fasting glucose, insulin, glycated hemoglobin, total and HDL-cholesterol, triglycerides, adiponectin)	NCT02244879

Table 2. (Continued)

Study Title	Daily Consumption	Study Duration	Outcome Measures	Identifier No.
Resveratrol and First-degree Relatives of Type 2 Diabetic Patients	150mg for 30 days	April 2014- July 2017	Insulin sensitivity: overall, muscle- and liver specific, muscle mitochondrial oxidative capacity (in vivo and ex vivo)	NCT02129595
Resveratrol's Effects in Diabetic Nephropathy (ReDNeph)	500mg for 12 weeks	Mar 2016- Feb 2017	Urine albumin level, Serum creatinine, Fasting blood sugar, Glycosylated hemoglobin, Serum insulin level	NCT02704494
Resveratrol for the Treatment of Non-Alcoholic Fatty Liver Disease and Insulin Resistance in Overweight Adolescents	Daily dose of 150 mg for 30 days	August 2015 - March 2017	Primary side effect profile determined by participant interview and serum biochemistry. Side effect profile determined by serum biochemistry: AST, ALT, total and conjugated bilirubin, creatinine, sodium, potassium, calcium, magnesium, chloride and TC02, haemoglobin, haematocrit, white blood cell and platelet counts, erythrocytes, and fasting lipid levels. Fasting glucose and insulin levels. PT/INR and PTT levels.	NCT02216552

Hypoglycaemic Effect of RV in Isolated Cells

Starch and disaccharides are converted into glucose through the action of α-glucosidase (Tang et al., 2022). L6 rat myocytes treated with RV oligomers (E-resveratrol and α-viniferin), extracted from the stem bark of *Hopea ponga*, exhibited remarkable α-glucosidase inhibitory activity, as indicated by their IC50 values. Moreover, these RV oligomers significantly increased glucose uptake within cells by substantially elevating AMPK levels (Sasikumar et al., 2019). In response to RV therapy, glycogen levels in diabetic HepG2 cells increased. This was attributed to the enhancement of insulin sensitivity and glucose uptake (Poonprasartporn & Chan, 2022). When palmitic acid-induced insulin-resistant HepG2 cells were treated with RV for a duration of 24 hours, the treatment resulted in a reduction of liver endoplasmic reticulum stress and an improvement in insulin sensitivity (Zhao et al., 2022). The utilization of RV-loaded nanoliposomes for treating diabetic pancreatic β-cells demonstrated effectiveness in examining the interplay between insulin and glucose levels (Yucel et al., 2018). The results of this study revealed that these cells exhibited the ability to elevate insulin levels, reduce elevated glucose levels, and exert antioxidant effects by enhancing the expression of enzymes that deactivate reactive oxygen species (ROS). When exposed to the culture medium for 24 to 72 hours, diabetic human pancreatic β-cells treated with RV demonstrated a notable enhancement in insulin production in response to glucose stimulation. The observed effect was entirely attributed to the overexpression of SIRT1 in these cells, as demonstrated by the fact that inhibiting SIRT1 hindered this effect (Vetterli et al., 2011). RV has been observed to exert a protective effect on isolated islet β-cells of diabetic mice, contributing to the reduction of pancreatic hypertrophy. The primary mechanism underlying this protective role was the promotion of increased β-cell apoptosis (Zhang et al., 2012).

Evidenced Clinical Trials for Hypoglycemic Effect of RV

A meta-analysis of data from eleven studies revealed that the consumption of RV led to reductions in fasting insulin, blood sugar levels, and insulin resistance (IR). Consequently, it was concluded that RV significantly enhances insulin sensitivity and glucose control in individuals with diabetes, while those without diabetes did not experience the same effects (Liu et al., 2014). In a cohort study involving overweight adults, administering 150mg of RV supplements per day for a duration of up to 6 months did not demonstrate any impact on insulin sensitivity (Ligt et al., 2020). In a double-blind trial conducted by Brasyno et al., in 2011, the effectiveness of RV was investigated in individuals with type 2 diabetes. The study involved a dosage of 5mg RV administered twice daily for up to 4 weeks. By utilizing the HOMA-IR method, the trial found that RV reduced insulin resistance (IR) and improved the ratio of phosphorylated protein kinase B (pAkt) to protein kinase B (Akt) in the platelets of these individuals (Marko et al., 2011). Several clinical trial reports are enumerated in Table 2.

Studies Targeting Key Molecular Mechanisms of RV Effect

RV serves as a dual modulator, exerting inhibitory or stimulatory effects within the insulin signaling cascade through diverse pathways, contributing to its beneficial impacts in diabetes mellitus (DM). This modulation involves transcription factors, kinases, cytokines, and enzymes, which are some of the molecular targets of RV discussed here.

Anti-Inflammatory Effect of RV in Diabetes

Chronic inflammation, by suppressing the insulin signaling pathway, contributes to the onset and progression of diabetes mellitus (DM) (Sajid et al., 2013). Defective immune responses lead to the production of cytokines such as interleukins (IL) and tumor necrosis factor (TNF). These inflammatory mediators, in conjunction with activated T cells, contribute to the dysfunction of pancreatic β-cells (Tsalamandris et al., 2019). Immunohistochemistry studies linked to the diverse anti-diabetic effects of RV have shown that it significantly reduces plasma levels of lipopolysaccharides (LPS) and proinflammatory mediators such as interferon-γ (IFN-γ), tumor necrosis factor-alpha (TNF-α), and interleukin-6 (IL-6) (Cai et al., 2020). RV's anti-inflammatory effect diminishes macrophage infiltration and impedes the NF-κB p65 signaling pathway within islet cells. This action targets inflammation and immune responses in type 1 DM (Darwish et al., 2021). NF-κB signaling pathway through transcription regulates the release of cytokines (TNF-α, IL-1β, and IL-6), chemokines and reactive oxygen species (ROS) (Coutinho et al., 2018). RV affects the AMPK pathway by inhibiting it, which leads to a reduction in the release of proinflammatory cytokines (Hassan et al., 2019). Activation of AMPK can also facilitate the nuclear translocation of Nrf2, ultimately leading to the inhibition of the release of proinflammatory cytokines (Huang et al., 2020). MAPK, a cellular signaling pathway, is another target of RV's action. Inhibition of this pathway by RV contributes to its anti-inflammatory response (Meng et al., 2021). The majority of insulin receptors are located in hepatic cells, where they promote the storage of glucose as glycogen (Qaid et al., 2016). In diabetic rodents subjected to a high-fructose diet, there is an elevated expression of the NLRP3 inflammasome, which contributes to hepatic inflammation in the context of type 2 DM (Rai et al., 2020). Compared to the diabetic group, RV therapy led to a decrease in the transcript level of NLRP3. Hyperglycemia activates the NLRP3 signaling cascade through the activation of caspase proteins, resulting in the production of pro-inflammatory cytokines in hepatic and pancreatic cells (Yang et al., 2012).

Effect of RV on Insulin Resistance

The transport of glucose from the bloodstream to the liver, muscles, and adipose tissues is regulated by the hormone insulin (Maechler et al., 2013). In individuals with type 2 diabetes mellitus (DM), insulin resistance (IR) is typically marked by reduced insulin-mediated glucose uptake in the liver, adipose tissue, and skeletal muscles. The three main signaling pathways involved in the expression of glucose transporter 4 (GLUT4) are the AMP-activated protein kinase (AMPK), PI3K/Akt, and PKC pathways (Tang et al., 2022). The presence of the significant glucose transporter protein GLUT4 in adipose tissue and skeletal muscle is crucial for reducing blood sugar levels and enhancing insulin resistance (IR). In type 2 diabetes mellitus, disruptions in insulin receptor signaling pathways such as PI3K-AKT and Extracellular Signal Regulated kinase (ERK) lead to insulin resistance (Agnese et al., 2022). Insulin resistance (IR) triggers modifications in regular intracellular processes. The primary abnormalities in type 2 DM involve hepatic insulin resistance coupled with significantly elevated plasma insulin levels (Cherrington et al., 2005). The accumulation of fat in tissues responsible for glucose and lipid metabolism leads to insulin resistance (IR). Retrospective research has unveiled a connection between the accumulation of fat in the pancreas and the malfunctioning of β-cells in diabetic patients (Wen et al., 2022). The reports were analyzed by assessing biochemical parameters and MRI images. Dysfunctional adipocytes trigger lipolysis, which elevates the levels of free fatty acids (FFAs) in the bloodstream (Yu et al., 2002). Chronic lipolysis, through the production of FFAs, is believed to contribute to insulin resistance (IR) in the liver and skeletal muscles. Metabolites of FFAs, including ceramides, acyl-CoA, and diacylglycerol (DAG), induce the phosphorylation of insulin receptor substrate (IRS) through the actions of protein kinase C (PKC), nuclear factor kappa B (NFκB), and inhibitory kappa B kinase beta (IKKβ) (Delarue et al., 2007). This process eventually leads to the inhibition of insulin signaling through protein kinase B/Akt. A study conducted by Zhao et al., in 2016 investigated RV's impact on insulin resistance in adipose 3T3-L1 and muscle C2C12 cell lines. The findings indicated that RV mitigated muscle insulin resistance by attenuating lipolysis and reducing inflammation in hypoxic adipose tissue. Subsequently, the DAG pathway activates insulin-PI3K signaling, contributing to insulin resistance. Activation of Protein Kinase C (PKC) within the DAG pathway decreases the stimulation of IRS-1-associated PI3-kinase activity, resulting in reduced glucose transport (Jimenez et al., 2018, Yu et al., 2002). Hence, RV's capacity to diminish insulin resistance (IR) also involves the activation of the AKT signaling pathway. The activation of AMPK signaling in diabetes mellitus therapy can be perceived as a protective mechanism (Wang et al., 2020). The AMPK cascade enhances the translocation of GLUT4 to cell membranes in specific tissues, subsequently leading to a decrease in serum glucose levels (Entezari et al., 2022). Insulin's ability to enhance cellular glycogen production and reduce gluconeogenesis is compromised by insulin resistance (IR) in the liver. Moreover, in insulin-resistant HepG2 cell lines, RV and its metabolites (RSV-3-O-glucuronide and RSV-4-O-glucuronide) significantly altered insulin signaling and increased insulin sensitivity by modifying the IRS-1/AMPK signaling pathway (Teng et al., 2018). Consequently, RV and its derivatives directed the insulin-resistant HepG2 cells to enhance intracellular glycogen production by influencing this pathway. Additionally, the study's outcomes demonstrated that as the concentration of RV increased, the respective treated groups also exhibited a higher percentage of glucose uptake. Another potential target for insulin resistance therapy is sirtuins (SIRTs) (Jiang et al., 2008). RV is recognized for its ability to activate its homolog SIRT1 in various tissues such as skeletal muscle, adipose tissue, pancreas, and brain (Borra et al., 2005). One of the most significant causes of IR is dysfunctional mitochondria (Huang et al., 2020). SIRT1 and SIRT3 activation leads to improvement of glucose uptake (Breen et al., 2008, Huang et al., 2020). Through Sirt1, RV enhances glucose absorption in insulin-resistant adipocytes (Chen et al., 2018). The literature highlights that RV activates SIRT1, which subsequently triggers the activation of AMPK, leading to AKT phosphorylation. This phosphorylation cascade results in the translocation of FOXO1 from the nucleus to the cytoplasm, leading to a reduction in the expression of resistin and an enhancement of insulin sensitivity. In diabetic rats treated with STZ, RV supplementation has been observed to mediate the activation of SIRT1, leading to the inhibition of the forkhead box protein (FOXO3) pathway (Akgun-unal et al., 2023).

Effect of RV on Oxidative Stress

Hyperglycemia leads to an increase in reactive oxygen species (ROS), which in turn triggers apoptosis in functioning cells (Luc et al., 2019). RV possesses the capability to suppress ROS, consequently promoting the gene expression of antioxidant enzymes, such as superoxide dismutase (SOD) and glutathione peroxidase (GPx) (Shoura et al., 2022). RV acts as an effective scavenger for reactive oxygen species (ROS), particularly superoxide anions and singlet oxygen (Chen et al., 2019). The major pathways that RV targets for its antioxidant mechanism are the SIRT1 and Nrf2 signaling pathways (Truong et al., 2017). These pathways are responsible for the transcription of a range of genes involved in cellular responses, encompassing inflammation, apoptosis, and oxidative stress. RV is recognized for activating SIRT1, which subsequently deactivates multiple proteins such as p53, FOXO, NF-kB, and proliferator-activated receptor gamma coactivator 1 alpha (PGC-1α). As a consequence, the inhibition of apoptosis and ROS generation occurs (Martinez et al., 2021). RV activates the Nrf2 signaling pathway, leading to the upregulation of antioxidant enzyme expression. This action aids in the scavenging of free radicals (Farkhondeh et al., 2020). Upon activation, the Nrf2 pathway targets the transcription of genes within the nucleus that are responsible for producing antioxidant effects. This includes genes such as NAD(P)H quinone oxidoreductase 1 (NQO1), catalase (CAT), and heme oxygenase 1 (HO-1) (Zhou et al., 2020). In the presence of RV, isolated human pancreatic islet cells exhibited a significant reduction in ROS levels, which were measured at intervals of 24 and 72 hours (Keshtkar et al., 2020).

The findings from Real-Time Quantitative PCR (qRT-PCR) analysis demonstrated that diabetic rats treated with RV exhibited increased mRNA gene expression levels of CAT, GPx, SIRT1, Nrf2, and NFkB (Sadi et al., 2014). NADPH oxidase facilitates the generation of ROS, whereas RV diminishes ROS production by inhibiting NADPH oxidase activity (Ungvari et al., 2011). Upon stimulation by RV, PI3K/Akt and AMPK pathways initiate Nrf2 nuclear translocation, subsequently leading to an increase in the expression of antioxidant enzymes (Brasnyo et al., 2011).

Effect of RV on Insulin Secretion

Insulin secretion is regulated by the membrane potential of β-cells. Depolarization of the pancreatic β-cell membrane triggers L-type Ca2+ channels, leading to elevated cytosolic Ca2+ levels and subsequent insulin secretion, resulting in the reduction of blood glucose levels. Chen et al., (2007) discovered that in diabetic mice insulinoma MIN6 cells, RV treatment increased insulin secretion by activating Ca2+-activated K+ channels and inhibiting ATP-sensitive and voltage-gated K+ channels. Membrane potential was monitored using the fluorescence of the voltage-sensitive dye bis-(1,3-dibutylbarbituric acid) pentamethine oxonol (DiBAC4(5)), which increases as the membrane potential becomes depolarized. The findings of another study demonstrate that treating diabetic human islets and insulinoma INS-1E cells with RV at 25μM for 24 and 72 hours increases insulin production through the SIRT1 mechanism. (Vetterli et al., 2011). Furthermore, it has been observed that RV enhances insulin production by inhibiting the activity of the protein kinase C enzyme (Woo et al., 2004). However, the results of studies investigating the effect of RV on insulin-producing cells are still inconclusive regarding whether it increases or decreases insulin production. There is evidence suggesting that RV impairs the ability of pancreatic cells to secrete insulin, and that it reduces insulin secretion in a dose-dependent manner. Additional research has documented this negative feedback mechanism of RV (Szkudelski et al., 2006).

Effect of Rv in Major Complications of Diabetes Related Deficits

Diabetic Nephropathy

Individuals with diabetes are at an elevated risk of developing nephropathy, a condition characterized by kidney damage. Various mechanisms lead to renal lesions that bring about structural and functional changes in the kidneys, resulting in nephropathy. RV has been shown to be effective in treating diabetic nephropathy by mitigating inflammation, oxidative stress, and the formation of advanced glycation end products (AGEs) (Gowd et al., 2020). Furthermore, RV stimulates autophagy and activates AMPK and SIRTs (sirtuins) (Li et al., 2021). A randomized controlled trial study assessed the therapeutic benefits of RV on this significant consequence of chronic diabetes (Sattarinezhad et al., 2018). Microalbuminuria serves as a marker for nephropathy, and in this study, the administration of 500mg/kg RV for a duration of 90 days was observed to reduce microalbuminuria levels in urine. In comparison to the placebo group, RV notably decreased levels of creatinine, insulin, and HbA1c. Renal dysfunction in diabetic rodents has been explored through various animal studies. RV significantly reduces serum creatinine, blood urea nitrogen, and 24-hour microalbuminuria levels in urine, thereby delaying the onset of diabetic nephropathy in diabetic rats. Elevated glucose levels lead to apoptosis of nephrotic cells through endoplasmic reticulum stress (Tian et al., 2020). RV prevented hyperglycemia-induced apoptosis in rat renal proximal tubular epithelial cells (NRK-52E) (Zhang et al., 2020).

Diabetic Neuropathy (DN)

It is characterized by the loss of sensations due to nerve damage and peripheral blood flow obstructions, leading to excruciating pain (Zaino et al., 2023). Hyperglycemia triggers the activation of multiple biochemical pathways, resulting in oxidative stress, inflammation, and apoptosis. All of these factors contribute to the deterioration of neurons (Paul et al., 2022). RV has been reported as an effective polyphenol in diabetic nephropathy (DN), exerting antioxidant effects and upregulating Nrf2 and SIRT1, while also suppressing NF-kB activity (Kumar et al., 2007). RV has been utilized to treat inflammation-induced diabetic nephropathy (DN) in rats by inhibiting the NF-kB inflammatory signaling cascade. In this context, RV reduced the levels of IL-6, TNF-α, COX-2, and NF-kB in the sciatic nerve of diabetic rats (Kumar et al., 2010).

Diabetic Retinopathy (DR)

Hyperglycemia leads to the destruction of blood vessels in the retina, resulting in vision loss (Shukla et al., 2023). Diabetes triggers an elevation of growth factors like vascular endothelial growth factor (VEGF) alongside inflammatory markers, exacerbating retinopathy. Researchers have identified the therapeutic potential of RV supplementation in diabetic retinopathy (DR) by reducing the expression of VEGF, chemokines, cytokines, and reactive oxygen species (ROS). In a study conducted by Soufi et al., in 2012, the quantification of NF-kB activity, apoptosis rate, and oxidative stress in the eyes of diabetic rats treated with RV was investigated. The results of this investigation demonstrated that oral administration of RV at a dose of 5 mg/kg daily for up to 4 months led to a reduction in retinal NF-kB activation, oxidative stress, and vascular cell death. In the treatment of diabetic retinopathy, Dong et al., (2019) employed RV-coated gold nanoparticles at a dose of 300 mg/kg daily for three continuous months. The findings of this study revealed that this approach lowered vascular permeability, growth factor (VEGF-1), chemokines (MCP-1, ICAM-1), and cytokines (TNFα, IL-6, IL-1β) in the retinal cells.

Conclusion

RV acts through targeting different molecular proteins responsible for translocating glucose transporters up to the cell membrane through insulin signaling pathway. In case of hyperglycemia expression of these proteins involved in insulin signaling pathways are suppressed. To lower blood sugar levels and IR, RV mimics the actions of insulin. Insulin resistance and decreased insulin secretion are caused by oxidative damage and chronic inflammation. RV has been reported to modulate its therapeutic effects mainly through SIRT1, NF-κB, Nrf2 and AMPK signaling cascade. RV has an immense antioxidant potential to scavenge ROS generated through hyperglycemia. Phosphorylation of transcription factors and antioxidant enzymes by RV increased their gene expression in diabetic models. It also protects dysfunction of pancreatic β-cells from inflammatory mediators. Despite of the poor bioavailability of RV alternative approaches are developed as novel drug delivery systems. To make it more effective and bioavailable by utilizing nanotechnology, which has proven useful in the relevant studies.

References

Agnese, A. D., Platt, J. M., Zheng, M. M., Friesen, M., Agnese, G. D., Blaise, A. M., Spinelli, J. B., Henninger, J. E., Tevonian, E. N., Hannett, N. M., Lazaris, C., Drescher, H. K., Bartsch, L. M., Kilgore, H. R., Jaenisch, R., Grif, L. G., Cisse, I. I., Jeppesen, J. F., Lee, T. I., Young, R. A. (2022). The dynamic clustering of insulin receptor underlies its signaling and is disrupted in insulin resistance. *Nature Communications*, 13, 7522.

Akgun-unal, N., Ozyildirim, S., Unal, O., Gulbahce-mutlu, E. (2023). The effects of resveratrol and melatonin on biochemical and molecular parameters in diabetic old female rat hearts. *Experimental Gerontology*, 172, 112043.

Almeida, L., Vaz-da-silva, M., Falco, A., Soares, E., Costa, R., Loureiro, A. I., Fernandes-lopes, C., Rocha, J., Nunes, T., Wright, L., Soares-da-silva, P. (2009). Pharmacokinetic and safety profile of trans - resveratrol in a rising multiple-dose study in healthy volunteers. *Molecular Nutrition & Food Research*, 53 Suppl 1, S7-S15.

Annaji, M., Poudel, I., Boddu, S. H. S., Tiwari, A. K., Babu, R. J., Arnold, R. D. (2021). Resveratrol-loaded nanomedicines for cancer applications. *Cancer Reports*, 4(3), e1353.

Boocock, D. J., Faust, G. E. S., Patel, K. R., Schinas, A. M., Brown, V. A., Ducharme, M. P., Booth, T. D., Crowell, J. A., Perloff, M., Gescher, A. J., Steward, W., Brenner, D. (2007). Phase I dose escalation pharmacokinetic study in healthy volunteers of resveratrol, a potential cancer chemopreventive agent. *Cancer Epidemiology, Biomarkers & Prevention*, 16(6), 1246-1252.

Borra, M. T., Smith, B. C., Denu, J. M. (2005). Mechanism of Human SIRT1 Activation by Resveratrol. *Journal of Biological Chemistry*, 280(17), 17187-17195.

Brasnyo, P., Molnar, G. A., Mohas, M., Marko, L., Laczy, B., Cseh, J., Mikolas, E., Szijarto, I. A., Merei A., Halmai R., Meszaros L. G., Sumegi, B., Wittmann, I. (2011). Resveratrol improves insulin sensitivity, reduces oxidative stress and activates the Akt pathway in type 2 diabetic patients. *British Journal of Nutrition*, 106, 383-389.

Brawerman, G. M., Kereliuk, S. M., Brar, N., Cole, L. K., Seshadri, N., Pereira, T. J., Xiang, B., Hunt, K. L., Fonseca, M. A., Hatch, G. M., Doucette, C. A., Dolinsky, V. W., Bennet, L., Morrison, J. (2019). Maternal resveratrol administration protects against gestational diabetes-induced glucose intolerance and islet dysfunction in the rat offspring. *Journal of Physiology*, 16, 4175-4192.

Breen, D. M., Sanli, T., Giacca, A., Tsiani, E. (2008). Stimulation of muscle cell glucose uptake by resveratrol through sirtuins and AMPK. *Biochemical and Biophysical Research Communications*, 374, 117-122.

Brown, V. A., Patel, K. R., Viskaduraki, M., Crowell, J. A., Perloff, M., Booth, T. D., Vasilinin, G., Sen, A., Schinas, A. M., Piccirilli, G., Brown, K., Steward, W. P., Gescher, A. J., Brenner, D. E. (2010). Repeat Dose Study of the Cancer Chemopreventive Agent Resveratrol in Healthy Volunteers: Safety, Pharmacokinetics, and Effect on the Insulin-like Growth Factor Axis. *Cancer Research*, 70(22), 9003-9011.

Burns, J., Yokota, T., Ashihara, H., Lean, M. J., Crozier, A. (2002). Plant Foods and Herbal Sources of Resveratrol. *Journal of Agricultural and Food Chemistry*, 50, 3337-3340.

Cai, H., Scott, E. N., Britton, R. G., Parrott, E., Ognibene, T. J., Malfatti, M., Khan, M., Steward, W. P., Brown, K. (2021). Distribution and metabolism of resveratrol in human prostate tissue after oral administration of a "dietary-achievable" or "pharmacological" dose: what are the implications for anticancer activity. *The American Journal of Clinical Nutrition*, 113(5), 1115-1125.

Cai, T. T., Ye, X. L., Li, R. R., Chen, H., Wang, Y. Y., Yong, H. J., Pan, M. L., Lu, W., Tang, Y., Miao, H., Snijders, A. M., Mao, J. H., Liu, X. Y., Lu, Y. B., Ding, D. F. (2020). Resveratrol Modulates the Gut Microbiota and Inflammation to Protect Against Diabetic Nephropathy in Mice. *Frontiers in Pharmacology*, 11, 1249.

Champion, M. L., Battarbee, A. N., Biggio, J. R., Casey, B. M., Harper, L. M. (2022). Postpartum glucose intolerance following early gestational diabetes mellitus. *American Journal of Obstetrics & Gynecology*, 4(3), 100609.

Chen, S., Zhao, Z., Ke, L., Li, Z., Li, W., Zhang, Z., Zhou, Y., Feng, X., Zhu, W. (2018). Resveratrol improves glucose uptake in insulin-resistant adipocytes via Sirt1. *Journal of Nutritional Biochemistry*, 55, 209-218.

Chen, W., Chi, T., Chuang, L., Su, M. (2007). Resveratrol enhances insulin secretion by blocking KATP and KV channels of beta cells. *European Journal of Pharmacology*, 568, 269-277.

Chen, Y., Meng, J., Li, H., Wei, H., Bi, F., Liu, S., Tang, K., Guo, H., Liu, W. (2019). Resveratrol exhibits an effect on attenuating retina inflammatory condition and damage of diabetic retinopathy via PON1. *Experimental Eye Research*, 181, 356-366.

Cherrington, A. D. (2005). The role of hepatic insulin receptors in the regulation of glucose production. *Journal of Clinical Investigation*, 115(5), 1136-1139.

Chimento, A., De Amicis, F., Sirianni, R., Sinicropi, M. S., Puoci, F., Casaburi, I., Saturnino, C., Pezzi, V. (2019). Progress to improve oral bioavailability and beneficial effects of resveratrol. *International Journal of Molecular Sciences*, 20(6), 1381.

Coutinho, D. D. S., Pacheco, M. T., Frozza, R. L. (2018). Anti-Inflammatory Effects of Resveratrol: Mechanistic Insights. *International Journal of Molecular Sciences*, 19(6), 1812.

Darby, J. R. T., Mohd, M. H. B., Regnault, T. R. H., Williams, M. T., Morrison, J. L. (2019). Systematic review: Impact of resveratrol exposure during pregnancy on maternal and fetal outcomes in animal models of human pregnancy complications — Are we ready for the clinic ? *Pharmacological Research*, 144, 264-278.

Darwish, M. A., Abo-Youssef, A. M., Messiha, B. A. S., Abo-Saif, A. A., Abdel-Bakky, M. S. (2021). Resveratrol inhibits macrophage infiltration of pancreatic islets in streptozotocin-induced type 1 diabetic mice via attenuation of the CXCL16/NF-κB p65 signaling pathway. *Life Sciences*, 272, 119250.

Delarue, J., Magnan, C. (2007). Free fatty acids and insulin resistance. *Current Opinion in Clinical Nutrition and Metabolic Care*, 10, 142-148.

Dong, Y., Wan, G., Yan, P., Qian, C., Li, F., Peng, G. (2019). Biology Fabrication of resveratrol coated gold nanoparticles and investigation of their effect on diabetic retinopathy in streptozotocin induced diabetic rats. *Journal of Photochemistry & Photobiology, B: Biology*, 195(1), 51-57.

Du, S., Lv, Y., Li, N., Huang, X., Liu, X., Li, H., Wang, C. (2020). Biological investigations on therapeutic effect of chitosan encapsulated nano resveratrol against gestational diabetes mellitus rats induced by streptozotocin. *Drug Delivery*, 27(1), 953-963.

Entezari, M., Hashemi, D., Taheriazam, A., Zabolian, A., Samarghandian, S. (2022). Biomedicine & Pharmacotherapy AMPK signaling in diabetes mellitus, insulin resistance and diabetic complications: A pre-clinical and clinical investigation. *Biomedicine & Pharmacotherapy*, 146, 112563.

Farkhondeh, T., Llorens, S., Pourbagher-shahri, A. M., Ashra, M., Samarghandian, S. (2020). The therapeutic effect of resveratrol: Focusing on the Nrf2 signaling pathway. *Biomedicine & Pharmacotherapy*, 127, 110234.

Fenwick, P. H., Jeejeebhoy, K., Dhaliwal, R., Royall, D., Brauer, P., Tremblay, A., Klein, D., Mutch, D. M. (2019). Lifestyle genomics and the metabolic syndrome: A review of genetic variants that influence response to diet and exercise interventions. *Critical Reviews in Food Science and Nutrition*, 59(13), 2028-2039.

Florencio, R. B., De, Araujo, Fonseca, L. G., Da, Silva, V. F. D., Lima, Í. N. D. F., Gualdi, L. P. (2021). Diabetes mellitus hospitalization and mortality rate according to a national database in Brazil: a longitudinal study. *BMC Public Health*, 21(1), 1-7.

Furman, B. L. (2021). Streptozotocin-induced diabetic models in mice and rats. *Current Protocols in Pharmacology*, 70, 1-20.

Garg, P., Duggal, N. (2022). Type 2 diabetes mellitus, its impact on quality of life and how the disease can be managed-a review. *Obesity Medicine*, 35, 100459.

Gong, L., Guo, S., Zou, Z. (2020). Resveratrol Ameliorates Metabolic Disorders and Insulin Resistance in High- Fat Diet-Fed Mice. *Life Sciences*, 242, 117212.

Gowd, V., Kang, Q., Wang, Q., Wang, Q., Chen, F., Cheng, K. W. (2020). Resveratrol: evidence for its nephroprotective effect in diabetic nephropathy. *Advances in Nutrition*, 11(6), 1555-1568.

Grau, L., Soucek, R., Pujol S. M. D. (2023). Resveratrol derivatives: Synthesis and their biological activities. *European Journal of Medicinal Chemistry*, 246, 114962.

Han, D., Seo, S., Choi, E., Kim, M., Yoo, J., Jung, Y., Yoon, I. (2022). Biomedicine & Pharmacotherapy Impact of route-dependent phase-II gut metabolism and enterohepatic circulation on the bioavailability and systemic disposition of resveratrol in rats and humans: A comprehensive whole body physiologically-based pharmacokinetic modeling. *Biomedicine & Pharmacotherapy*, 151, 113141.

Hassan, A. H. E., Yoo, S. Y., Lee, K. W., Yoon, Y. M., Ryu, H. W., Jeong, Y., Shin J., Kang, S. Y., Kim, S. Y., Lee, H. H., Park B. Y., Lee, K. T., Lee, Y. S. (2019). Repurposing mosloflavone/5,6,7-trimethoxyflavone-resveratrol hybrids: Discovery of novel p38-α MAPK inhibitors as potent interceptors of macrophage-dependent production of proinflammatory mediators. *European Journal of Medicinal Chemistry*, 180, 253-267.

He, S., Yan, X. (2013). From Resveratrol to Its Derivatives: New Sources of Natural Antioxidant. *Current Medicinal Chemistry*, 2013, 20, 1005-1017.

Huang, D. D., Shi, G., Jiang, Y., Yao, C., Zhu, C. (2020). A review on the potential of Resveratrol in prevention and therapy of diabetes and diabetic complications. *Biomedicine & Pharmacotherapy,* 125, 109767.

Huang, X. T., Li, X., Xie, M. L., Huang, Z., Huang, Y. X., Wu, G. X., Peng, Z. R., Sun, Y. N., Ming, Q. L., Liu, Y. X., Chen, J. P., Xu, S. N. (2019). Resveratrol: Review on its discovery, anti-leukemia effects and pharmacokinetics. *Chemico-Biological Interactions*, 306, 29-38.

Huo, X., Zhang, T., Meng, Q., Li, C., You, B. (2019). Resveratrol Effects on a Diabetic Rat Model with Coronary Heart Disease. *Medicine Science Monitor*, 25, 540-546.

Jensen, J. S., Wertz, C. F., Upsher-Smith, V. A. O. (2010). Preformulation Stability of trans-Resveratrol and trans-Resveratrol Glucoside (Piceid). *Journal of Agricultural Food Chemistry*, 58, 1685-1690.

Jiang, W. J. (2008). Sirtuins: Novel targets for metabolic disease in drug development. *Biochemical and Biophysical Research Communications*, 373(3), 341-344.

Jimenez, J. G. V., Guiberna, A. R., Mena, R. J., Reyes, J. A. O. (2018). Role of free fatty acids on insulin resistance. *Gaceta Medica de Mexico*, 153:773-783.

Keshtkar, S., Kaviani, M., Jabbarpour, Z., Abdullah, I. H. A. (2020). Nutrition, Metabolism & Cardiovascular Diseases Significant reduction of apoptosis induced via hypoxia and oxidative stress in isolated human islet by resveratrol. *Nutrition, Metabolism and Cardiovascular Diseases*, 30(7), 1216-1226.

Khan, M. A. B., Hashim, M. J., King, J. K., Govender, R. D., Mustafa, H., Al Kaabi, J. (2020). Epidemiology of Type 2 Diabetes - Global Burden of Disease and Forecasted Trends. *Journal of Epidemiology and Global Health*, 10(1), 107-111.

Khattar, S., Khan, S. A., Amir, S., Zaidi, A., Darvishikolour, M., Farooq, U. (2022). Resveratrol from Dietary Supplement to a Drug Candidate: An Assessment of Potential. *Pharmaceuticals*, 15(8), 957.

Kumar, A., Sharma, S. S. (2010). NF-κB inhibitory action of resveratrol: A probable mechanism of neuroprotection in experimental diabetic neuropathy. *Biochemical and Biophysical Research Communications*, 394(2), 360-365.

Kumar, A., Kaundal, R. K., Iyer, S., Sharma, S. S. (2007). Effects of resveratrol on nerve functions, oxidative stress and DNA fragmentation in experimental diabetic neuropathy. *Life Sciences*, 80, 1236-1244.

Li, K. X., Ji, M. J., Sun, H. J. (2021). An updated pharmacological insight of resveratrol in the treatment of diabetic nephropathy. *Gene*, 780, 145532.

Li, M., Kildegaard, K. R., Chen, Y., Rodriguez, A., Borodina, I., Nielsen, J. (2015). De novo production of resveratrol from glucose or ethanol by engineered Saccharomyces cerevisiae. *Metabolic Engineering*, 32, 1-11.

Ligt, M. De, Bergman, M., Fuentes, R. M., Essers, H., Moonen-kornips, E., Havekes, B. (2020). No effect of resveratrol supplementation after 6 months on insulin sensitivity in overweight adults: a randomized trial. *The American Journal of Clinical Nutrition*, 112(4), 1029-1038.

Liu, K., Zhou, R., Wang, B., Mi, M. (2014). Effect of resveratrol on glucose control and insulin sensitivity: a meta-analysis of 11 randomized controlled trials. *The American Journal of Clinical Nutrition*, 99(6), 1510-1519.

Luc, K., Schramm-Luc, A., Guzik, T. J., Mikolajczyk, T. P., (2019). Oxidative stress and inflammatory markers in prediabetes and diabetes. *Journal of Physiology and Pharmacology*, 70(6), 809-824.

Maechler, P. (2013). Molecular and Cellular Endocrinology Mitochondrial function and insulin secretion. *Molecular and Cellular Endocrinology*, 379(1-2), 12-18.

Mahjabeen, W., Khan, D. A., Mirza, S. A. (2022). Role of resveratrol supplementation in regulation of glucose hemostasis, inflammation and oxidative stress in patients with diabetes mellitus type 2: A randomized, placebo-controlled trial. *Complementary Therapies in Medicine*, 66, 102819.

Marko, L., Cseh, J., Molna, A., Me, A. (2011). Resveratrol improves insulin sensitivity, reduces oxidative stress and activates the Akt pathway in type 2 diabetic patients. *The British Journal of Nutrition*, 106(3), 383-389.

Martinez, B. I. G., Ramos, M, R., Chaverri, J. P., Osorio E. S., Nunez, V. M. M. (2021). Hypoglycemic Effect of Resveratrol: A Systematic Review and Meta-Analysis. *Antioxidants*, 10(1), 69.

Mcintyre, H. D., Catalano, P., Zhang, C., Desoye, G. (2019). Gestational diabetes mellitus. *Nature Reviews Disease Primers*, 5(1), 47.

Meng, T., Xiao, D., Muhammed, A., Deng, J., Chen, L., He, J. (2021). Anti-Inflammatory Action and Mechanisms of Resveratrol. *Molecules*, 26(1), 229.

Nandy, A. N., Virge, R., Hegde, H. V., Chattopadhyay, D. (2023). A review of patent literature on the regulation of glucose metabolism by six phytocompounds in the management of diabetes mellitus and its complications. *Journal of Integrative Medicine*, 21(3), 226-235.

Palsamy, P., Subramanian, S. (2008). Resveratrol, a natural phytoalexin, normalizes hyperglycemia in streptozotocin-nicotinamide induced experimental diabetic rats. *Biomedicine & Pharmacotherapy*, 62(9), 598-605.

Paul, A., Kumar, M., Das, P., Guha, N., Rudrapal, M., Zaman, K. (2022). Biomedicine & Pharmacotherapy Drug repurposing – A search for novel therapy for the treatment of diabetic neuropathy. *Biomedicine & Pharmacotherapy*, 156, 113846.

Pegah, A., Abbasi-oshaghi, E., Khodadadi, I., Mirzaei, F. (2021). Probiotic and resveratrol normalize GLP-1 levels and oxidative stress in the intestine of diabetic rats. *Metabolism Open*, 10, 100093.

Pentek, T., Newenhouse, E., O'Brien, B., Chauhan, A. S. (2017). Development of a Topical Resveratrol Formulation for Commercial Applications Using Dendrimer Nanotechnology. *Molecules*, 22(1), 137.

Poonprasartporn, A., Chan, K. L. A. (2022). Biosensors and Bioelectronics Label-free study of intracellular glycogen level in metformin and resveratrol-treated insulin-resistant HepG2 by live-cell FTIR spectroscopy. *Biosensors and Bioelectronics*, 212, 114416.

Qaid, M. M., Abdelrahman, M. M. (2016). Role of insulin and other related hormones in energy metabolism: A review. *Cogent Food & Agriculture*, 2(1), 1267691.

Rai, R. C., Bagulb, P. K., Banerjee, S. K. (2020). NLRP3 inflammasome drives inflammation in high fructose fed diabetic rat liver: Effect of resveratrol and metformin. *Life Sciences*, 253, 117727.

Raskovic, A., Ćucuz, V., Torovic, L., Tomas, A., Gojkovic-Bukarica, L., Ćebovic, T., Milijasevic, B., Stilinovic, N., Hogervorst, J. C. (2019). Resveratrol supplementation improves metabolic control in rats with induced hyperlipidemia and type 2 diabetes. *Saudi Pharmaceutical Journal*, 27(7):1036-1043.

Ratz-łyko, A., Arct, J. (2018). Resveratrol as an active ingredient for cosmetic and dermatological applications: a review. *Journal of Cosmetic and Laser Therapy*, 21(2), 84-90.

Rehman, K., Saeed, K., Mehak, S., Sajid, M., Akash, H. (2018). Resveratrol regulates hyperglycemia-induced modulations in experimental diabetic animal model. *Biomedicine & Pharmacotherapy*, 102, 140-146.

Robertson, I., Hau, T. W., Sami, F., Ali, M. S., Badgujar, V., Murtuja, S., Hasnain, M. S., Khan, A., Majeed, S., Ansari. M. T. (2022). The science of resveratrol, formulation, pharmacokinetic barriers and its chemotherapeutic potential. *International Journal of Pharmaceutics*, 618, 121605.

Rodriuez, A. G., Santamarıa, B., Gutierrez, J. A. M., Rada, P., Millan, E. F., Pardo, V., Alvarez, C., Cuadrado, A., Ros, M., Serrano, M., Valverde, A. M. (2015). Resveratrol treatment restores peripheral insulin sensitivity in diabetic mice in a sirt1-independent. *Molecular Nutrition & Food Research*, 59(8), 1431-1442.

Sadi, G., Bozan, D., Bekir, H. (2014). Redox regulation of antioxidant enzymes: post-translational modulation of catalase and glutathione peroxidase activity by resveratrol in diabetic rat liver. *Molecular and Cellular Biochemistry*, 393(1-2), 111-122.

Sadi, G., Pektas, M. B., Koca, H. B., Tosun, M., Koca, T. (2015). Resveratrol improves hepatic insulin signaling and reduces the inflammatory response in streptozotocin-induced diabetes. *Gene*, 570(2), 213-220.

Sajid, M., Akash, H., Rehman, K., Chen, S. (2013). Role of inflammatory mechanisms in pathogenesis of type 2 diabetes mellitus. *Journal of Cellular Biochemistry*, 114(3), 525-531.

Santos, M. A., Franco, F. N., Caldeira, C. A., De, Araujo, G. R., Vieira A., Chaves M. M., (2020). Antioxidant effect of Resveratrol: Change in MAPK cell signaling pathway during the aging process. *Archives of Gerontology and Geriatrics*, 92, 104266.

Sasikumar, P., Lekshmy, K., Sini, S., Prabha, B., Kumar, N. A., Sivan, V. V, Jithin, M. M., Jayamurthy, P., Shibi, I. G., Radhakrishnan, K. V. (2019). Isolation and characterization of resveratrol oligomers from the stem bark of Hopea ponga (Dennst.) Mabb. and their antidiabetic effect by modulation of digestive enzymes, protein glycation and glucose uptake in L6 myocytes. *Journal of Ethnopharmacology*, 236, 196-204.

Sattarinezhad, A., Roozbeh, J., Yeganeh, B. S., Omrani, G. R., Shams, M. (2018). Resveratrol reduces albuminuria in diabetic nephropathy: A randomized double-blind placebo-controlled clinical trial. *Diabetes and Metabolism*, 45(1), 53-59.

Shoura, S. M. S., Naghsh, N., Moslemi, E., Kavyani, Z., Moridpour, A. H., Musazadeh, V., Dehghan, P. (2022). Can resveratrol supplementation affect biomarkers of inflammation and oxidative stress? An umbrella meta-analysis. *Journal of Functional Foods*, 2022, 99.

Shu, X. H., Wang, L. L., Li, H., Song, X., Shi, S., Gu, J. Y., Wu, M. L., Chen X. Y., Kong, Q. Y., Liu, J. (2015). Diffusion efficiency and bioavailability of resveratrol administered to rat brain by different routes: therapeutic implications. *Neurotherapeutics*, 12(2), 491-501.

Shukla, U. V., Tripathy, K. (2023). *Diabetic Retinopathy*. StatPearls,

Singh, A. P., Verma, S. S., Rai, V., Kaschula, C. (2019). Health benefits of resveratrol: Evidence from clinical studies. *Medicinal Research Reviews*, 39(5), 1851-1891.

Soufi F. G., Mohammad-nejad D., Ahmadieh H. (2012). Resveratrol improves diabetic retinopathy possibly through oxidative stress nuclear factor κB – apoptosis pathway. *Pharmacological Reports*, 64(6), 1505-1514.

Surendran, S., Sapkal, R., Paul, D., Nanjappan, S. (2019). Effect of resveratrol on dipeptidyl peptidase-4 inhibitors pharmacokinetics: An in vitro and in vivo approach. *Chemico-Biological Interactions*, 315, 108909.

Szkudelska, K., Deniziak, M., Hertig, I., Wojciechowicz, T., Tyczewska, M., Jaroszewska, M., Szkudelski, T. (2019). Effects of Resveratrol in Goto-Kakizaki Rat, a model of type 2 diabetes. *Nutrients*, 11(10), 2488.

Szkudelski, T. (2006). Resveratrol inhibits insulin secretion from rat pancreatic islets. *European Journal of Pharmacology*, 552, 176-181.

Szkudelski, T., Szkudelska, K. (2011). Anti-diabetic effects of resveratrol. *Annals of the New York Academy of Sciences*, 1215, 34-39.

Tang, P., Yang, X., Chen, H., Zhang, T., Tang, H., Pang, K. (2022). Anti-diabetic activity of extract from Morus nigra L. twigs through activation of AMPK / PKC pathway in mice. *Journal of Functional Foods*, 99, 105358.

Teng, W., Yin, W., Zhao, L., Ma, C., Huang, J., Ren, F. (2018) Resveratrol metabolites ameliorate insulin resistance in HepG2 hepatocytes by modulating IRS-1/AMPK. *Royal Society of Chemistry*, 8(63), 36034-36042.

Tian, J., Mo, J., Xu, L., Zhang, R., Qiao, Y., Liu, B., Jiang, L., Ma, S., Shi, G. (2020). Scoulerine promotes cell viability reduction and apoptosis by activating ROS-dependent endoplasmic reticulum stress in colorectal cancer cells. *Chemico-Biological Interactions*, 327, 109184.

Tiana, B., Liu, J. (2020). Resveratrol: a review of plant sources, synthesis, stability, modification and food application. *Journal of Science & Food Agricultural*, 100(4), 1392-1404.

Truong, V., Jeong, W. (2017). Role of resveratrol in regulation of cellular defense systems against oxidative stress. *BioFactors*, 44(1), 36-49.

Tsalamandris, S., Antonopoulos, A. S., Oikonomou, E., Papamikroulis, G. A., Papaioannou, G. V. S., Deftereos, S., Tousoulis, D. (2019). Risk factors and cardiovascular disease prevention the role of inflammation in diabetes: current concepts and future perspectives. *European Cardiology Review*, 14(1), 50-59.

Ungvari, Z., Sonntag, W. E., de Cabo, R., Baur, J. A., Csiszar, A. (2011) Mitochondrial protection by resveratrol. *Exercise and Sport Sciences Reviews*, 39(3), 128-132.

Vesely, O., Baldovska, S., Kolesarova, A. (2021). Enhancing bioavailability of nutraceutically used resveratrol and other stilbenoids. *Nutrients*, 13(9), 3095.

Vetterli, L., Brun, T., Giovannoni, L., Bosco, D., Maechler, P. (2011). Resveratrol Potentiates Glucose-stimulated Insulin Secretion in INS-1E β-Cells and Human Islets through a SIRT1-dependent Mechanism. *Journal of Biological Chemistry*, 286(8), 6049-6060.

Vetterli, L., Brun, T., Giovannoni, L., Bosco, D., Maechler, P. (2011). Resveratrol Potentiates Glucose-stimulated Insulin Secretion in INS-1E β-Cells and Human Islets through a SIRT1-dependent Mechanism. *Journal of Biological Chemistry*, 286(8), 6049-6060.

Wahab, A., Gao, K., Jia, C., Zhang, F., Tian, G., Ghulam, M., Chen, J. (2017). Significance of Resveratrol in Clinical Management of Chronic Diseases. *Molecules*, 22(8), 1329.

Wang, X., Meng, L., Zhao, L., Wang, Z., Liu, H., Liu, G., Guan, G. (2016). Resveratrol ameliorates hyperglycemia-induced renal tubular oxidative stress damage via modulating the SIRT1/FOXO3a pathway. *Diabetes Research and Clinical Practice*, 126, 172-181.

Wang, Y., Rijal, B., Xu, M., Li, Z., An, Y., Zhang, F., Lu, C. (2020). Renal denervation improves vascular endothelial dysfunction by inducing autophagy via AMPK / mTOR signaling activation in a rat model of type 2 diabetes mellitus with insulin resistance. *Acta Diabetologica*, 57(10), 1227-1243.

Wen, Y., Chen, C., Kong, X., Xia, Z., Kong, W., Si, K., Han, P., Vivian, W., Li, X. (2022). Pancreatic fat infiltration, β-cell function and insulin resistance: A study of the young patients with obesity. *Diabetes Research and Clinical Practice*, 187, 109860.

Woo, J. H., Lim, J. H., Kim, Y. H., Suh, S. I., Min do, S., Chang, J. S., Lee, Y. H., Park, J. W., Kwon, T. K. (2004). Resveratrol inhibits phorbol myristate acetate-induced matrix metalloproteinase-9 expression by inhibiting JNK and PKC delta signal transduction. *Oncogene*, 23(10), 1845-1853.

Yang, C. S., Shin, D. M., JO, E. K. (2012). The role of NLR-related protein 3 inflammasome in host defense and inflammatory diseases. *International Neurourology Journal*, 16 (1), 2-12.

Yao, L., Wan, J., Li, H., Ding, J., Wang, Y., Wang, X., Li, M. (2015). Resveratrol relieves gestational diabetes mellitus in mice through activating AMPK. *Reproductive Biology and Endocrinology*, 13, 118.

Yu, C., Chen, Y., Cline, G. W., Zhang, D., Zong, H., Wang, Y., Bergeron, R., Kim, J. K., Cushman, S. W., Cooney, G. J., Atcheson, B., White, M. F., Kraegen, E. W., Shulman, G. I. (2002). Mechanism by which fatty acids inhibit insulin activation of insulin receptor substrate-1 (IRS-1) associated phosphatidylinositol 3-kinase activity in muscle. *Journal of Biological Chemistry*, 277(52), 50230-50236.

Yucel, C., Gokce¸ Karatoprak G. S., Aktas, Y. (2018). Nanoliposomal resveratrol as a novel approach to treatment of diabetes mellitus. *Journal of Nanoscience and Nanotechnology*, 18(6), 3856-3864.

Zaino, B., Goel, R., Devaragudi, S., Prakash, A., Vaghamashi, Y., Sethi, Y., Patel, N., Kaka, N. (2023). Diabetic neuropathy: Pathogenesis and evolving principles of management. *Disease-a-Month*, 69(9), 101582.

Zhang, J., Chen, L., Zheng, J., Zeng, T., Li, H., Xiao, H., Deng, X., Hu, X. (2012). The protective effect of resveratrol on islet insulin secretion and morphology in mice on a high-fat diet. *Diabetes Research and Clinical Practice*, 97(3), 474-482.

Zhang, J., Dong, X. J., Ding, M. R., You, C. Y., Lin, X., Wang, Y., Wu, M. J. Y., Xu, G. F., Wang, G. D. (2020). Resveratrol decreases high glucose-induced apoptosis in renal tubular cells via suppressing endoplasmic reticulum stress. *Molecular Medicine Reports*, 22(5), 4367-4375.

Zhang, L. X., Li, C. X., Kakar, M. U., Khan, M. S., Wu, P. F., Amir, R. M., Dai, D. F., Naveed, M., Li, Q. Y., Saeed, M., Shen, J. Q., Rajput, S. A., Li, J. H. (2021). Resveratrol (RV): A pharmacological review and call for further research. *Biomedicine & Pharmacotherapy*, 143, 112164.

Zhao, H., Zhang, Y., Shu, L., Song, G., Ma, H. (2022). Resveratrol reduces liver endoplasmic reticulum stress and improves insulin sensitivity in vivo and in vitro. *Drug Design, Development and Therapy*, 13, 1473-1485.

Zhao, W., Li, A., Feng, X., Hou, T., Liu, K., Liu, B., Zhang, N. (2016). Metformin and resveratrol ameliorate muscle insulin resistance through preventing lipolysis and inflammation in hypoxic adipose tissue. *Cellular Signalling*, 28(9), 1401-1411.

Zhou, Y., Lan, R., Xu, Y., Zhou, Y., Lin, X., Miao, J. (2020). Resveratrol alleviates oxidative stress caused by Streptococcus uberis infection via activating the Nrf2 signaling pathway. *International Immunopharmacology*, 89, 107076.

Chapter 26

Rutin in the Management of Diabetes Mellitus

Jyoti[1,*]
Meena Devi[1]
Nisham Rani[1]
Ritu Kataria[1]
Dev Raj Sharma[2]
Rinu Rana[2]
Mahendra Singh Ashawat[2]
Prabhat Singh[3]
Surbhi Gupta[4]
and Charu Bharti[4]
[1]G. V. M. College of Pharmacy, Sonepat, Haryana, India
[2]Laureate Institute of Pharmacy, Kathog, Jawalaji, Himachal Pradesh, India
[3]Faculty of Pharmacy, Swami Vivekanand Subharti University, Meerut, Uttar Pradesh, India
[4]Department of Pharmacology, School of Pharmacy, Bharat Institute of Technology, Meerut, Uttar Pradesh, India

Abstract

Diabetes has emerged as one of the most prevalent global health concerns, with its incidence steadily increasing. Current medications available for treating diabetes mellitus are often inconvenient and come with notable drawbacks. Numerous studies have highlighted the

[*] Corresponding Author's Email: jyotimalik127@gmail.com.

In: Naturally Occurring Chemicals …
Editors: A. Singh Grewal, G. Deswal, A. Kumar Dhingra et al.
ISBN: 979-8-89113-491-1

potential benefits of using medicinal plants with hypoglycemic properties for diabetes treatment. Flavonoids sourced from vegetables and medicinal plants have demonstrated positive effects on diabetes management by improving lipid profiles, antioxidant status, and glycemic control. Rutin, a widely found polyphenolic compound belonging to the flavonoid class, is present in various foods and plants. Rutin's capacity to lower blood sugar levels is attributed to several mechanisms, including the reduction of carbohydrate absorption in the small intestine, inhibition of tissue gluconeogenesis, promotion of glucose uptake by tissues, and stimulation of insulin production by beta cells. These multifaceted actions are believed to underlie rutin's potential to prevent complications such as nephropathy, neuropathy, liver damage, and cardiovascular issues that can arise from hyperglycemia and dyslipidemia. In conclusion, rutin shows promise as a candidate for the treatment of diabetes mellitus due to its substantial protective effects in managing this condition.

Keywords: diabetes, rutin, antioxidant, flavonoid, hyperglycemia, diabetes, antidiabetic activity

Introduction

Diabetes remains one of the most challenging global health issues. It is associated with an elevated risk of both macrovascular and microvascular complications in various organs, including the brain, kidneys, retina, and heart (Chandramohan et al., 2008). Diabetes, medically referred to as diabetes mellitus, encompasses a group of metabolic disorders marked by elevated levels of blood glucose resulting from deficiencies in insulin production, insulin action, or both. This condition is associated with chronic damage, dysfunction, and deterioration of numerous organs, including the heart, blood vessels, kidneys, nerves, eyes, and more. Diabetes stands as one of the most prevalent major metabolic conditions globally and ranks among the top five leading causes of mortality worldwide. Diabetes manifests in two primary forms: type 1 and type 2 diabetes. (Velingkar et al., 2009). While the underlying physiological processes of each type of diabetes vary, they both share the common feature of hyperglycemia, which is elevated blood glucose levels. Additionally, both types of diabetes are associated with a range of potentially life-threatening complications (Chen et al., 2008). Approved oral medications for diabetes come in various types. However, managing diabetes often requires a polypharmacy approach, where individuals need to take multiple medications. Unfortunately, many of these medications are associated with adverse side effects and potential interactions with other drugs. As a result, diabetes treatment can become costly, both in terms of expenses and potential health risks (Chitra et al., 2010). Long before the advent of modern treatments in the post-genomic era, plants and their derivatives served as valuable sources of bioactive compounds used in medications (Harvey et al., 2008). A diverse array of phytochemicals have demonstrated considerable benefits in both the prevention and management of various ailments. Over the past several years, numerous important medications derived from plants have significantly influenced and altered the landscape of current medical treatments (Dar et al., 2017). Flavonoids, primarily found in a wide range of commonly consumed fruits, have garnered extensive attention as one of the most extensively researched natural compounds (Benavente et al., 2008). Flavonoids obtained from vegetables, fruits, and medicinal plants have the potential to assist in diabetes management by improving glycemic control, lipid profiles, and antioxidant status.

Rutin

Rutin, also known as quercetin-3-rutinoside, rutoside, or sophorin, is a flavonoid glycoside found in citrus fruits. Its chemical structure is represented as 3,3,'4,'5,7-pentahydroxyflavone-3-rhamnoglucoside, as shown in Figure 1 (Kreft et al., 1997). Flavonols, including rutin, are abundantly found in various plants such as apples, buckwheat, tea, and passion flower. They contribute significantly to the nutritional content of foods (Harborne et al., 1986). Rutin (also known as vitamin P) is found in many plants, with three notable sources being *Fagopyrum esculentum* (buckwheat), *Sophora japonica* (Japanese pagoda tree), and *Ruta graveolens* (rue). This flavonoid exhibits a range of biological actions, including antioxidant and anti-inflammatory effects. Additionally, it demonstrates nephroprotective, neuroprotective, and hepatoprotective activities (Ghorbani et al., 2017). The term "rutin" is derived from the herb *Ruta graveolens*, commonly known as "common rue," which contains a significant amount of rutin in its aerial parts. Rutin is also referred to as purple quercitrin and vitamin P. This flavonoid glycoside is present in over 70 plant species and various plant-derived dietary items. Foods rich in rutin include buckwheat seeds, grapes, apricots, cherries, onions, grapefruits, oranges, and plums

(Kreft et al., 1997; Yang et al., 2008; Calzada et al., 2018). The isolation of rutin from various plants and their parts is described in Table 1.

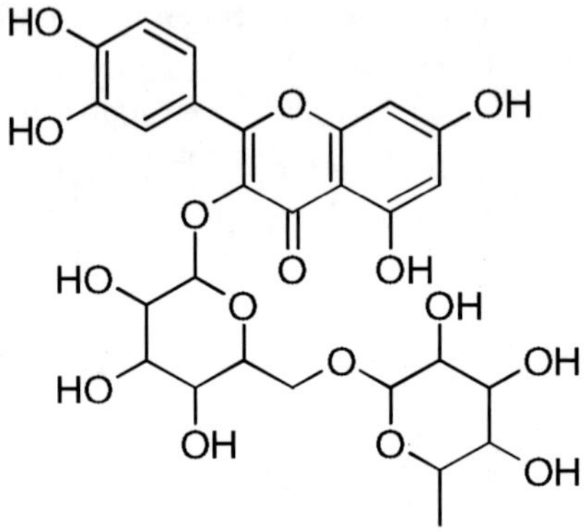

Figure 1. Chemical structure of rutin.

Table 1. Different plants species and their parts for rutin isolation

Plant species	Plant part used	Common name	References
Asparagus officinalis	Stem	Sparrow grass	Makris et al., 2001
Ribes nigrum	Fruits	Berry	Maatta et al., 2003
Capparis orientalis, C. spinosa and C. sicula	Flower bud	Capers	Inocencio et al., 2000
Fagopyrum esculentum Moench	Whole grain flour, groats (thermally treated), seeds	Buckwheat	Dietrych-Szostak et al., 1999, Kreft et al., 1999
Olea europaea	Fruits	Olive	Romani et al., 1999
Prunus domestica	Fruits	Plums	Kim et al., 2003
Rubus idaeus, R. occidentalis	Fruits	Red and black raspberry	Wada et al., 2002

Pharmacological Activity of Rutin

Numerous pharmacological features of rutin, such as its antioxidant activity used in people's nutrition as well as medicine. Traditionally, rutin has been employed as an antibacterial, antifungal and antiallergic agent. However, recent research has shown that it has broad-spectrum pharmacological benefits for the treatment of a variety of chronic conditions, such as diabetes, malignancies, high blood pressure, and high cholesterol level (Al- Dhabi et al., 2015). Rutin works against diabetes by increasing insulin sensitivity, and glucose storage and decreasing lipid accumulation in the liver.

Antidiabetic Property

Table 2. Recent advancement of rutin as antidiabetic drug

Drug/Combination	Formulation	Activity	Reference
Annona cherimola, rutin, and streptozocin	Ethanolic extract (50 mg/kg)	Reduce hyperglycemia, % HbA1c, and lipid profiles	Valdes et al., 2023
Rutin trihydrate loaded silica	Nanoparticles (100 μg/ml)	Hypoglycemia	Kerry et al., 2022
Rutin loaded chitosan-alginate	Nanoparticles	Increase in glucose uptake, reduce cell viability	Surendran et al., 2022
Combination of catechin, epicatechin, and rutin	Noval Formulation 10 mg/kg	Antihyperglycemic activity	Mechchate et al., 2021
Rutin trihydrate loaded formulation	Liposomal gel	Anti-inflammation activity stabilize cholesterol	Sharma et al., 2021
Rutin	Phospholipid (13.20 μg/mL)	Enhancing glycemic control mechanisms and increasing the secretion of insulin	Vankudri et al., 2016

Flavonoids offer positive effects on diabetes management. Rutin has the potential to lower blood sugar through mechanisms like reducing carbohydrate absorption in the small intestine, inhibiting tissue gluconeogenesis, increasing tissue glucose consumption, stimulating insulin secretion from pancreatic beta cells, and protecting Langerhans islets from degeneration (Sattanathan et al., 2011). Rutin therapy has shown to reverse hepatocyte hypertrophy, restore beta islet histo-architecture, and effectively decrease blood sugar levels. This is achieved by reducing cytokine-related inflammation, enhancing antioxidant levels, and improving plasma lipid profiles. Rutin's effects include lowering the production of inflammatory cytokines, reactive oxygen species, sorbitol, and advanced glycation end products (Niture et al., 2014). These effects are complemented by rutin's antihyperglycemic properties and its protective effects against the progression of diabetes-related complications (Jadhav et al., 2012). Rutin's antidiabetic effects are thought to stem from increased peripheral glucose uptake, either directly or by enhancing insulin secretion. Additionally, it may inhibit glucose transporter function. Rutin supplementation is also capable of reducing oxidative stress-related damage in the context of diabetic pathophysiology. This suggests that rutin has potential to both prevent and treat Type 2 diabetes (Dhanya et al., 2014). Flavonoids, specifically rutin, have been documented to possess antidiabetic properties. These include promoting beta-cell regeneration in the pancreas and improving insulin secretion. Rutin is also known to enhance insulin-mediated glucose absorption by targeting specific cells, increase calcium uptake, and inhibit the enzyme aldose reductase (Marella et al., 2017). There are some recent advancements in rutin for antidiabetic activity as given in Table 2.

Conclusion

Rutin, a flavonoid, holds promise as a potential aid in managing diabetes mellitus. Several studies have indicated that rutin could enhance insulin sensitivity, regulate blood sugar levels, and mitigate inflammation linked to diabetes. Beyond its influence on blood glucose management, rutin has also been explored for its potential anti-inflammatory properties. As chronic inflammation often accompanies diabetes and contributes to complications like cardiovascular disease, neuropathy, and nephropathy, rutin's effects on blood glucose, insulin sensitivity, and inflammation are of interest. However, these findings are in their early stages, and further research is required to confirm their validity, establish the optimal rutin supplementation dosage and duration, and ascertain any potential side effects. Extensive research is necessary to comprehensively determine its effectiveness and safety.

References

Al-Dhabi, N. A., Arasu, M. V., Park, C. H., Park, S. U. (2015). An up-to-date review of rutin and its biological and pharmacological activities. *EXCLI Journal*, 14, 59.

Benavente-Garcia, O., Castillo, J. (2008). Update on uses and properties of citrus flavonoids: new findings in anticancer, cardiovascular, and anti-inflammatory activity. *Journal of Agricultural and Food Chemistry*, 56(15), 6185-6205.

Calzada, F., Solares Pascasio, J. I., Valdes, M., Garcia Hernandez, N., Velázquez, C., Ordoñez-Razo, R. M., Barbosa, E. (2018). Antilymphoma potential of the ethanol extract and rutin obtained of the leaves from Schinus molle Linn. *Pharmacognosy Research*, 10(2), 119-123.

Chandramohan, G., Ignacimuthu, S., Pugalendi, K. V. (2008). A novel compound from Casearia esculenta (Roxb.) root and its effect on carbohydrate metabolism in streptozotocin-diabetic rats. *European Journal of Pharmacology*, 590(1-3), 437-443.

Chen, J., Li, W. L., Wu, J. L., Ren, B. R., Zhang, H. Q. (2008). Hypoglycemic effects of a sesquiterpene glycoside isolated from leaves of loquat (Eriobotrya japonica (Thunb.) Lindl.). *Phytomedicine*, 15(1-2), 98-102.

Chitra, V., Varma, P. V., Raju, M. V. R. K., Prakash, K. J. (2010). Study of antidiabetic and free radical scavenging activity of the seed extract of Strychnosnuxvomica. *International Journal of Pharmacy & Pharmaceutical Sciences*, 2, 106-110.

Dar, R. A., Shahnawaz, M., Rasool, S., Qazi, P. H. (2017). Natural product medicines: A literature update. *Journal of Phytopharmacology*, 6(6), 349-351.

Dhanya, R., Arun, K. B., Syama, H. P., Nisha, P., Sundaresan, A., Kumar, T. S., Jayamurthy, P. (2014). Rutin and quercetin enhance glucose uptake in L6 myotubes under oxidative stress induced by tertiary butyl hydrogen peroxide. *Food Chemistry*, 158, 546-554.

Dietrych-Szostak, D., Oleszek, W. (1999). Effect of Processing on the flavonoid content in Buckwheat (Fagopyrum e sculentum Möench) grain. *Journal of Agricultural and Food Chemistry*, 47(10), 4384-4387.

Ghorbani, A. (2017). Mechanisms of antidiabetic effects of flavonoid rutin. *Biomedicine & Pharmacotherapy*, 96, 305-312.

Harborne, J. B. (1986). Nature, distribution and function of plant flavonoids. In: *Plant Flavonoids in Biology and Medicine*, Buffalo, New York (USA), 22-26.

Harvey, A. L. (2008). Natural products in drug discovery. *Drug Discovery Today*, 13(19-20), 894-901.

Jadhav, R., Puchchakayala, G. (2012). Hypoglycemic and antidiabetic activity of flavonoids: boswellic acid, ellagic acid, quercetin, rutin on streptozotocin-nicotinamide induced type 2 diabetic rats. *International Journal of Pharmacy and Pharmaceutical Sciences*, 4, 251-256.

Kerry, R. G., Mohapatra, P., Jena, A. B., Panigrahi, B., Pradhan, K. C., Khatua, B. R., Mahari, S., Pal, S., Perikala, V., Kisan, B. and Lugos, M. D. (2022). Biosynthesis of rutin trihydrate loaded silica nanoparticles and investigation of its antioxidant, antidiabetic and cytotoxic potentials. *Journal of Inorganic and Organometallic Polymers and Materials*, 32(6), 2065-2081.

Kim, D. O., Chun, O. K., Kim, Y. J., Moon, H. Y., Lee, C. Y. (2003). Quantification of polyphenolics and their antioxidant capacity in fresh plums. *Journal of Agricultural and Food Chemistry*, 51(22), 6509-6515.

Kreft, S., Knapp, M., Kreft, I. (1999). Extraction of rutin from buckwheat (Fagopyrum esculentum Moench) seeds and determination by capillary electrophoresis. *Journal of Agricultural and Food Chemistry*, 47(11), 4649-4652.

Määttä, K. R., Kamal-Eldin, A., Törrönen, A. R. (2003). High-performance liquid chromatography (HPLC) analysis of phenolic compounds in berries with diode array and electrospray ionization mass spectrometric (MS) detection: Ribes species. *Journal of Agricultural and Food Chemistry*, 51(23), 6736-6744.

Makris, D. P., Rossiter, J. T. (2001). Domestic processing of onion bulbs (Allium cepa) and asparagus spears (Asparagus officinalis): effect on flavonol content and antioxidant status. *Journal of Agricultural and Food Chemistry*, 49(7), 3216-3222.

Marella, S. (2017). Flavonoids-the most potent poly-phenols as antidiabetic agents: an overview. *Modern Approaches in Drug Designing*, 1(3), 2-5.

Mechchate, H., Es-Safi, I., Haddad, H., Bekkari, H., Grafov, A., Bousta, D. (2021). Combination of Catechin, Epicatechin, and Rutin: Optimization of a novel complete antidiabetic formulation using a mixture design approach. *The Journal of Nutritional Biochemistry*, 88, 108520.

Niture, N. T., Ansari, A. A., Naik, S. R. (2014). Anti-hyperglycemic activity of rutin in streptozotocin-induced diabetic rats: an effect mediated through cytokines, antioxidants and lipid biomarkers. *Indian Journal of Experimental Biology*, 52(7), 720-727.

Romani, A., Mulinacci, N., Pinelli, P., Vincieri, F. F., Cimato, A. (1999). Polyphenolic content in five tuscany cultivars of Olea europaea L. *Journal of Agricultural and Food Chemistry*, 47(3), 964-967.

Sharma, D., Upadhyay, S., Upadhyay, P. (2021). Rutin trihydrate loaded liposomal gel formulation and characterization. *International Journal of Pharmaceutical Research*, 13(1), 2852-2862.

Surendran, V., Palei, N. N. (2022). Formulation and Characterization of Rutin Loaded Chitosan-alginate Nanoparticles: Antidiabetic and Cytotoxicity Studies. *Current Drug Delivery*, 19(3), 379-394.

Valdes, M., Calzada, F., Martínez-Solís, J., Martínez-Rodríguez, J. (2023). Antihyperglycemic Effects of Annona cherimola Miller and the Flavonoid Rutin in Combination with Oral Antidiabetic Drugs on Streptozocin-Induced Diabetic Mice. *Pharmaceuticals*, 16(1), 112.

Vankudri, R., Habbu, P., Hiremath, M., Patil, B. S., & Savant, C. (2016). Preparation and therapeutic evaluation of rutin-phospholipid complex for antidiabetic activity. *Journal of Applied Pharmaceutical Science*, 6(1), 090-101.

Velingkar, V. S., Dandekar, V. D., Murugananthan, K. (2009). Synthesis and pharmacological evaluation of some novel potent type II antidiabetic agents. *International Journal of Pharmacy and Pharmaceutical Sciences*, 1(1), 149-158.

Wada, L., Ou, B. (2002). Antioxidant activity and phenolic content of Oregon caneberries. *Journal of Agricultural and Food Chemistry*, 50(12), 3495-3500.

Yang, J., Guo, J., Yuan, J. (2008). In vitro antioxidant properties of rutin. *LWT-Food Science and Technology*, 41(6), 1060-1066.

Chapter 27

Silymarin in the Management of Diabetes Mellitus

Pravin Kumar[1]
Shiv Kumar Kushawaha[1,*]
Priyanka Chandolia[2]
and Mahendra Singh Ashawat[1]
[1]Laureate Institute of Pharmacy, Kathog, Jawalaji, Himachal Pradesh, India
[2]Department of Pharmacology, NIMS Institute of Pharmacy, Jaipur, Rajasthan, India

Abstract

The rapid advancement of modern society and significant shifts in individual dietary habits have emerged as increasingly prominent global health issues. Diabetes mellitus stands out as a chronic metabolic disorder characterized by elevated blood glucose levels. Silymarin, derived from Silybum marianum, holds promise for employment in both nutraceuticals and pharmaceuticals to manage this disease. It has garnered growing attention from researchers due to its multifaceted health benefits, resulting in a surge of scientific publications. Numerous studies have highlighted silymarin's potential therapeutic advantages in regulating carbohydrate metabolism in diabetes mellitus. This chapter provides an introductory overview of silymarin, delves into its physicochemical attributes, explores its pharmacokinetics, and examines its pharmacological effects in diabetes mellitus, with a focus on the underlying molecular mechanisms.

* Corresponding Author's Email: shiv.kushawaha@gmail.com.

In: Naturally Occurring Chemicals …
Editors: A. Singh Grewal, G. Deswal, A. Kumar Dhingra et al.
ISBN: 979-8-89113-491-1

Keywords: diabetes, silymarin, insulin resistance, hyperglycemia, phytoactive, antidiabetic activity

Introduction

Diabetes mellitus, a medical condition with potentially severe consequences, has exhibited a rising prevalence in recent decades, thereby presenting a substantial public health challenge in the twenty-first century (Zimmet et al., 2001). It is characterized by prolonged metabolic dysfunction, resulting in elevated blood glucose levels due to inadequate insulin release, action, or both. The ailment of diabetes has been acknowledged for millennia, with its earliest documented accounts tracing back to 1552 BCE in ancient Egypt. The medical scholars of ancient Egypt observed a condition that led patients to excrete urine with a sweet taste, a symptom that was later identified as diabetes. In the ensuing centuries, other civilizations, including the Greeks and Romans, also recognized and extensively studied this affliction. Aretaeus of Cappadocia, a Greek physician who lived in the 2nd century CE, detailed a condition he termed "diabetes," a Greek word meaning "siphon," alluding to the excessive urine output associated with the disease (Gemmill, 1972; Laios et al., 2012). Throughout the Middle Ages, diabetes remained inadequately comprehended, and effective treatments remained elusive. It wasn't until the 19th century that significant strides were taken in unraveling the intricacies of this ailment. In 1869, Paul Langerhans, a German medical student, uncovered pancreatic islets, which are clusters of cells responsible for producing insulin within the pancreas. The landscape of diabetes care underwent a profound transformation with the discovery of insulin in 1921, credited to Frederick Banting and Charles Best. By the 1930s, insulin had become widely accessible and continues to be a vital therapy for individuals with full insulin-dependent DM. In the subsequent decades, scientists continued to advance their comprehension of diabetes, including the identification of additional hormones influencing glucose regulation, such as glucagon and amylin. In recent times, research has honed in on devising novel approaches to treating diabetes, including medications targeting the root mechanisms of the condition. Today, diabetes stands as a formidable global health concern, impacting millions across the world. According to the International Diabetes Federation (IDF), the global diabetic population currently numbers 425 million, with an anticipated surge to 700 million cases by 2045 (Cho et al., 2018). The economic impact of diabetes is also considerable, with estimates indicating that diabetes constituted around 10% of the total global healthcare expenditures in 2019. Despite advancements in treatment and management, diabetes continues to stand as a noteworthy contributor to both illness and mortality, and the quest for a cure remains ongoing.

Silymarin

Table 1. Identification of important components of Silymarin

Identification process details	Identified components	Retention time (min)	References
• UHPLC –MS • Estimation by UV (288 nm) • Caffeine as internal standard	Taxifolin Isosilychristin Silychristin Silydianin Silybin A Silybin B Isosilybin A Isosilybin B	1.80 2.69 2.96 3.41 4.78 5.02 5.61 5.71	Graf et al., 2016
• Gradient elution column chromatography • Methanol: dichloromethanol as solvent • Reverse Phase Preparative HPLC	Silybin A Silybin B Isosilybin A Isosilybin B	8.03 9.01 11.98 13.12	Lee & Liu, 2003

'Milk Thistle' (Silybum marianum L. Gaertn), a member of the Composite/Asteraceae family, synthesizes silymarin within its seeds, leaves, and fruits. This medicinal plant, referred to as milk thistle, has the potential to reach a height of 2.0 meters and commonly exhibits an annual or biennial growth pattern (Zhu et al., 2012). The lipophilic extraction from the seeds, recognized as silymarin, constitutes the pivotal active component of milk thistle. Silymarin comprises an array of flavonoids, flavonolignans (which are isomeric forms of flavonolignans), and numerous other constituents (AbouZid et al., 2016). Structurally, flavonolignans exhibit a diverse array of configurations due to the linkage of the C6-C3 unit to the flavonoid core via C-O or C-C bonds in various positions. This linkage results in the creation of furan, dioxane, cyclohexane rings, or even straightforward side chains. As a whole, these molecules possess numerous chiral centers, rendering them commonly present as stereoisomers in nature. The formation of flavonolignans involves the oxidative pairing of taxifolin (a flavonoid) with a phenylpropanoid, typically coniferyl alcohol, followed by the coupling of these two radicals (Bijak, 2017). Table 1 encapsulates significant research particulars concerning the identification of key constituents within the silymarin extract.

Pharmacokinetics

Silymarin, classified within the second group of phytoactives according to the biopharmaceutical classification system, demonstrates limited systemic absorption through the oral route (23-47%) and possesses low polarity (Di Costanzo & Angelico, 2019). Upon oral ingestion, silymarin attains its peak systemic concentration within a span of 4-6 hours, and its elimination half-life is roughly 6 hours (Lorenz et al., 1993). Following absorption, silymarin undergoes metabolic transformation facilitated by the enzyme CYP450-2C8, leading to the creation of the major metabolite, ortho-demethylated silybin. A minor portion of silymarin is excreted through the renal pathway, whereas roughly twenty to forty percent is eliminated through the biliary route after undergoing conjugation with sulfate and glucuronide (Wu Lin & Tsai, 2009). In clinical trials, notable gastrointestinal (GIT) side effects associated with silymarin, such as irregular stools, nausea, diarrhea, and dyspepsia, were documented in 2-10% of patients (Saller et al., 2001). Silymarin has also been associated with minor adverse effects, including headache, itching, dizziness, skin papules, discomfort, and weakness, as reported in some instances.

Therapeutic Potentials of Silymarin

Silymarin offers a range of advantageous effects, including documented hepatoprotective, anti-Parkinson's, anti-Alzheimer's, antiviral, antibacterial, anticancer, and immunomodulatory benefits (Valková et al., 2021). Since ancient times, silymarin has been documented for its utilization in managing hepatic disorders and promoting lactation in women following childbirth (Salomone et al., 2017). Experimental studies have showcased the potential beneficial therapeutic effects of silymarin on conditions like non-alcoholic fatty liver disease, non-alcoholic steatohepatitis, and fibrosis within human hepatocytes. Additionally, silymarin has exhibited a favorable impact against certain viral infections (Lani et al., 2015), bacterial infections (Evren &

Yurtcu, 2015), and hepatoprotective activity. Silymarin clinically demonstrated therapeutic benefit against Parkinsonism and Alzheimer's (Ullah & Khan, 2018). Silymarin also exhibits anticancer activity by impeding tumor growth in animal models induced with breast cancer. Moreover, when applied topically, formulations containing phytoactives have shown a reduction in skin tumors and the inhibition of oxidative free radical reactions triggered by exposure to UV rays in mouse models. Additionally, for individuals with breast cancer, silymarin has demonstrated a soothing effect against radiation dermatitis (Karbasforooshan et al., 2019). Silymarin powdered extract exerts a regulatory influence on the immune system. Owing to its immunomodulatory effects, it has proven beneficial in managing the inflammatory cascade in patients undergoing abdominal dialysis (Sharma et al., 2023). Silymarin plays an active role in addressing metabolic disorders, and its combined use with berberine can augment this effect. Silymarin also demonstrates a beneficial regulatory impact on pre and post-meal blood glucose levels in individuals with diabetes mellitus (DM) (Voroneanu et al., 2016). Furthermore, it has also exhibited a potential preventive effect in mitigating the progression of diabetes mellitus (DM) complications (Stolf et al., 2017).

Silymarin in DM

A wide array of phytoconstituents are employed for diabetes mellitus (DM) management, though not all of them have undergone pharmacological testing (Baharvand et al., 2016). Numerous plants with antioxidant properties are being investigated for their potential in treating diabetes or mitigating its consequences. Silymarin, in particular, has garnered significant attention in recent times for its potential role in diabetes management. This chapter seeks to evaluate the available evidence regarding silymarin's capacity to address diabetes or preempt unfavorable DM-related manifestations such as neurological and nephrological complications, as well as its impact on signaling cascades. Silymarin has exhibited a range of mechanisms that might prove advantageous in DM treatment. One of its pivotal mechanisms is the enhancement of insulin sensitivity. Substantiating evidence has indicated its ability to augment the activity of AMP-activated protein kinase (AMPK), a regulator of glucose uptake and metabolism within cells (Choi et al., 2016). Through the activation of AMPK, silymarin has the potential to enhance insulin sensitivity and facilitate glucose uptake in cells, thus aiding in the regulation of blood glucose levels. Silymarin has also exhibited anti-inflammatory effects, which could prove beneficial in the management of diabetes (Karimi et al., 2011). Chronic inflammation is a prevalent hallmark of diabetes mellitus (DM), contributing to insulin resistance and disrupted glucose metabolism. Research has indicated that silymarin can impede the release of inflammatory mediators like chemokines, specifically TNF-α and IL-6, which are intricately linked to the genesis of insulin resistance (Shams et al., 2011). Furthermore, silymarin's antioxidant attributes have been established, potentially carrying substantial implications for diabetes management. Diabetic complications such as neuropathy and retinopathy often stem from oxidative stress, a prevalent feature in diabetes. (Pan et al., 2008). Research has indicated an augmented activity of superoxide dismutase (SOD) and catalase in response to silymarin treatment, which can contribute to the mitigation of oxidative stress.

Biological Role of Silymarin via Modulation of AMPK in DM

The activation of AMPK is considered one of the mechanisms through which silymarin is thought to exert its effects in diabetes management (Salomone et al., 2017). AMPK is a crucial enzyme responsible for regulating glucose and lipid metabolism within cells. Its activation fosters improved insulin sensitivity and heightened peripheral glucose utilization. Silymarin has exhibited the ability to activate AMPK across various cell types, including muscle, liver, and adipose cells. Moreover, silymarin's AMPK activation prompts the upregulation of glucose transporter 4 (GLUT4) expression on cell surfaces. This, in turn, facilitates the transport of glucose into cells, leading to elevated glucose uptake within these cells (Świderska et al., 2018). Furthermore, silymarin-triggered AMPK activation has been demonstrated to induce the breakdown of fatty acids within adipocytes. This action contributes to diminishing the presence of fatty acids in the bloodstream and enhancing insulin sensitivity. Silymarin has also exhibited the ability to activate AMPK by elevating intracellular cyclic AMP (cAMP) levels. Serving as a secondary messenger, cAMP regulates diverse metabolic functions, including glucose and lipid metabolism (Hussain et al., 2020). Furthermore, it diminishes the production of glucose by inhibiting the activity of hepatic glucose-6-phosphatase and phosphoenolpyruvate carboxykinase enzymes, owing to the activation of AMPK. Likewise, it could aid in reducing hepatic glucose synthesis and improving glucose homeostasis by downregulating the expression of these enzymes (Kheiripour et al., 2019).

Biological Role of Silymarin via Modulation of Proinflammatory Cytokines in DM

A potential mechanism through which silymarin might yield benefits in diabetes mellitus (DM) is by reducing the levels of chemokines like TNF-α and IL-6. The heightened insulin resistance, a pivotal feature of DM, is associated with the participation of TNF-α and IL-6. Notably, TNF-α has been documented to disrupt insulin activation, resulting in compromised glucose uptake within cells (Nieto-Vazquez et al., 2008). Additionally, IL-6 can augment glucose production in the liver, thereby contributing to the emergence of insulin resistance. Silymarin has been demonstrated to impede the generation of IL-6 and TNF-α across various cell types, encompassing liver cells and adipocytes (Ginwala et al., 2019). This could be attributed to its capacity to modulate various signaling pathways implicated in the generation of these cytokines, including the nuclear factor-kappaB (NF-kB). Silymarin could potentially contribute to the enhancement of insulin sensitivity and glucose uptake within cells by suppressing the production of TNF-alpha and IL-6. Consequently, this mechanism might aid in maintaining systemic glucose levels in diabetes mellitus (DM). Notably, diminishing the production of pro-inflammatory cytokines might not only regulate glucose levels in DM patients but also potentially thwart the progression of health issues correlated with DM, such as diabetic nephropathy, retinopathy, and neuropathy. These complications frequently stem from chronic inflammation (Halim & Halim, 2019).

Biological Role of Silymarin via Modulation of Oxidative Stress in DM

Silymarin has been shown to effectively scavenge reactive oxygen species (ROS) and thwart oxidative damage in both liver cells and pancreatic beta cells (Banjarnahor & Artanti, 2014). Research has shown that silymarin can heighten the activity of crucial antioxidant enzymes, including catalase and superoxide dismutase. These enzymes function to neutralize ROS and prevent oxidative stress. Furthermore, it has been demonstrated that silymarin can decrease the levels of advanced glycation end products (AGEs) in diabetic rats. AGEs are recognized contributors to the advancement of oxidative stress and complications associated with diabetes mellitus (DM) (Cao et al., 2019).

Silymarin in Major Complications of DM

Silymarin in Neuropathy

Neuropathy impacts around 50% of individuals with diabetes, presenting with diverse symptoms such as numbness, tingling, pain, allodynia, or even remaining asymptomatic. In severe instances, neuropathy can result in the amputation of toes, feet, or even entire legs (Roghani & Baluchnejadmojarad, 2010). Studies have suggested that silymarin holds promise as a potential therapeutic option for neuropathy, as evidenced by findings from in vitro and in vivo models. In particular, research has examined the effects of α-tocopherol and silybin therapy in cultures of rat cortical astrocytes and the SH-SY5Y cell line, both exposed to oxaliplatin (Mannelli et al., 2016). Such toxicity, leading to neuropathic pain, arises due to oxidative damage affecting nervous system tissues. The administered therapy safeguarded the cells against superoxide anions, malondialdehyde, carbonylated proteins, and DNA damage. Notably, when assessed in neoplastic cells, the therapy exhibited no impact on the apoptotic effects of oxaliplatin. In a parallel study conducted on rats, intraperitoneal oxaliplatin administration was followed by the administration of silybin and α-tocopherol, resulting in improved comfort levels for the rats and enhanced coordination among motor neurons. Moreover, rats with streptozotocin-induced diabetes mellitus displayed alleviated hyperalgesia and improved sciatic motor nerve transmission following a daily therapy of 100 mg/kg silymarin over two months. This regimen led to decreased malondialdehyde levels and restored superoxide dismutase (SOD) activity (Roghani & Baluchnejadmojarad, 2010). While clinical studies are necessary to corroborate these findings, the authors propose that silymarin shows potential for the prevention and treatment of diabetic neuropathy.

Silymarin in Nephropathy

The impairment of the glomerular filtration barrier, triggered by oxidative stress, inflammation, and elevated blood glucose levels, represents a characteristic feature of diabetic nephropathy (Conserva et al., 2016). Silymarin has demonstrated favorable outcomes in the context of renal disorders, as indicated by existing evidence. In an animal model of renal ischemia-reperfusion injury (mouse), the administration of silymarin resulted in decreased serum creatinine and urea levels. Beyond its impact on these biomarkers, silymarin therapy conveyed further advantages, including the attenuation of renal tubule cell damage and a reduction in apoptotic cells. Similar studies have observed that silymarin treatment contributes to diminishing oxidative stress in renal tissue by restoring antioxidant enzyme levels (Taleb et al., 2018). In laboratory experiments, silymarin showcased a reduction in oxidative stress markers, evident through lowered levels of malondialdehyde (MDA) and restoration of catalase enzyme activity in kidney tissue samples of streptozotocin-induced diabetes mellitus (DM) (Stolf et al., 2017).

Conclusion

DM stands as one of the most pervasive health burdens globally, impacting human populations at large. The emergence of silymarin as a novel phytoactive for the prolonged treatment of DM presents an avenue to overcome limitations associated with insulin and other oral hypoglycemic agents, including resistance development, injection site discomfort, and other adverse effects. The management of DM could potentially witness enhancement through the integration of silymarin, which exerts its effects by modulating AMP-activated protein kinase (AMPK), pro-inflammatory cytokines like TNF-α and IL-6, and activating antioxidant mechanisms. Silymarin's capacity to influence these pathways holds promise for DM management. Furthermore, silymarin also holds potential to mitigate significant long-term complications like neuropathy and nephropathy in DM. Moving forward, the impact of silymarin on DM management warrants exploration through clinical studies.

References

AbouZid, S. F., Ahmed, H. S., Moawad, A. S., Owis, A. I., Chen, S. -N., Nachtergael, A. (2017). Chemotaxonomic and biosynthetic relationships between flavonolignans produced by Silybum marianum populations. *Fitoterapia*, 119, 175-184.

AbouZid, S. F., Chen, S. -N., Pauli, G. F. (2016). Silymarin content in Silybum marianum populations growing in Egypt. *Industrial Crops and Products*, 83, 729-737.

Baharvand-Ahmadi, B., Bahmani, M., Tajeddini, P., Naghdi, N., Rafieian-Kopaei, M. (2016). An ethno-medicinal study of medicinal plants used for the treatment of diabetes. *Journal of Nephropathology*, 5(1), 44.

Banjarnahor, S. D., Artanti, N. (2014). Antioxidant properties of flavonoids. *Medical Journal of Indonesia*, 23(4), 239-244.

Bijak, M. (2017). Silybin, a major bioactive component of milk thistle (Silybum marianum L. Gaernt.). Chemistry, bioavailability, and metabolism. *Molecules*, 22(11), 1942.

Cao, X., Xia, Y., Zeng, M., Wang, W., He, Y., Liu, J. (2019). Caffeic acid inhibits the formation of advanced glycation end products (AGEs) and mitigates the AGEs-induced oxidative stress and inflammation reaction in human umbilical vein endothelial cells (HUVECs). *Chemistry & Biodiversity*, 16(10), e1900174.

Cho, N. H., Shaw, J., Karuranga, S., Huang, Y., da Rocha Fernandes, J., Ohlrogge, A., Malanda, B. (2018). IDF Diabetes Atlas: Global estimates of diabetes prevalence for 2017 and projections for 2045. *Diabetes Research and Clinical Practice*, 138, 271-281.

Choi, E. J., Kim, E. K., Jeoung, N. H., Kim, S. H. (2016). Effect of silymarin on gluconeogenesis and lactate production in exercising rats. *Food Science and Biotechnology*, 25, 119-124.

Conserva, F., Gesualdo, L., Papale, M. (2016). A systems biology overview on human diabetic nephropathy: from genetic susceptibility to post-transcriptional and post-translational modifications. *Journal of Diabetes Research*, 2016.

Di Costanzo, A., Angelico, R. (2019). Formulation strategies for enhancing the bioavailability of silymarin: the state of the art. *Molecules*, 24(11), 2155.

Evren, E., Yurtcu, E. (2015). In vitro effects on biofilm viability and antibacterial and antiadherent activities of silymarin. *Folia Microbiologica*, 60, 351-356.

Gemmill, C. L. (1972). The Greek concept of diabetes. *Bulletin of the New York Academy of Medicine*, 48(8), 1033.

Ginwala, R., Bhavsar, R., Chigbu, D. G. I., Jain, P., Khan, Z. K. (2019). Potential role of flavonoids in treating chronic inflammatory diseases with a special focus on the anti-inflammatory activity of apigenin. *Antioxidants*, 8(2), 35.

Halim, M., Halim, A. (2019). The effects of inflammation, aging and oxidative stress on the pathogenesis of diabetes mellitus (type 2 diabetes). *Diabetes & Metabolic Syndrome: Clinical Research & Reviews*, 13(2), 1165-1172.

Hussain, T., Tan, B., Murtaza, G., Liu, G., Rahu, N., Kalhoro, M. S. (2020). Flavonoids and type 2 diabetes: Evidence of efficacy in clinical and animal studies and delivery strategies to enhance their therapeutic efficacy. *Pharmacological Research*, 152, 104629.

Karbasforooshan, H., Hosseini, S., Elyasi, S., Fani Pakdel, A., & Karimi, G. (2019). Topical silymarin administration for prevention of acute radiodermatitis in breast cancer patients: A randomized, double-blind, placebo-controlled clinical trial. *Phytotherapy research*, 33(2), 379-386.

Karimi, G., Vahabzadeh, M., Lari, P., Rashedinia, M., Moshiri, M. (2011). "Silymarin," a promising pharmacological agent for treatment of diseases. *Iranian Journal of Basic Medical Sciences*, 14(4), 308.

Kheiripour, N., Karimi, J., Khodadadi, I., Tavilani, H., Goodarzi, M. T., Hashemnia, M. (2019). Hepatoprotective effects of silymarin on liver injury via irisin upregulation and oxidative stress reduction in rats with type 2 diabetes. *Iranian Journal of Medical Sciences*, 44(2), 108.

Laios, K., Karamanou, M., Saridaki, Z., Androutsos, G. (2012). Aretaeus of Cappadocia and the first description of diabetes. *Hormones*, 11, 109-113.

Lani, R., Hassandarvish, P., Chiam, C. W., Moghaddam, E., Chu, J. J. H., Rausalu, K. (2015). Antiviral activity of silymarin against chikungunya virus. *Scientific Reports*, 5(1), 11421.

Lorenz, D., Luker, P., Mennicke, W., & Wetzelsberger, N. (1984). Pharmacokinetic studies with silymarin in human serum and bile. *Methods and Findings in Experimental and Clinical Pharmacology*, 6(10), 655-661.

Mannelli, L. D. C., Zanardelli, M., Landini, I., Pacini, A., Ghelardini, C., Mini, E. (2016). Effect of the SOD mimetic MnL4 on in vitro and in vivo oxaliplatin toxicity: possible aid in chemotherapy induced neuropathy. *Free Radical Biology and Medicine*, 93, 67-76.

Morazzoni, P., Montalbetti, A., Malandrino, S., Pifferi, G. (1993). Comparative pharmacokinetics of silipide and silymarin in rats. *European Journal of Drug Metabolism and Pharmacokinetics*, 18, 289-297.

Nieto-Vazquez, I., Fernández-Veledo, S., Krämer, D. K., Vila-Bedmar, R., Garcia-Guerra, L., Lorenzo, M. (2008). Insulin resistance associated to obesity: the link TNF-alpha. *Archives of Physiology and Biochemistry*, 114(3), 183-194.

Pan, H. Z., Zhang, H., Chang, D., Li, H., Sui, H. (2008). The change of oxidative stress products in diabetes mellitus and diabetic retinopathy. *British Journal of Ophthalmology*, 92(4), 548-551.

Saller, R., Meier, R., Brignoli, R. (2001). The use of silymarin in the treatment of liver diseases. *Drugs*, 61, 2035-2063.

Salomone, F., Barbagallo, I., Godos, J., Lembo, V., Currenti, W., Cina, D. (2017). Silibinin restores NAD+ levels and induces the SIRT1/AMPK pathway in non-alcoholic fatty liver. *Nutrients*, 9(10), 1086.

Shams, M. E., Al-Gayyar, M. M., Barakat, E. A. (2011). Type 2 diabetes mellitus-induced hyperglycemia in patients with NAFLD and normal LFTs: relationship to lipid profile, oxidative stress and pro-inflammatory cytokines. *Scientia Pharmaceutical*, 79(3), 623-634.

Sharma, S., Kumar, P., Ashawat, M. S., Pandit, V., Verma, C. S., Sharma, D. K. (2023). Silymarin: A Phytoconstituent with Significant Therapeutic Potential-A Narrative Review. *Current Drug Therapy*, 18(2), 89-97.

Stolf, A. M., Cardoso, C. C., Acco, A. (2017). Effects of silymarin on diabetes mellitus complications: a review. *Phytotherapy Research*, 31(3), 366-374.

Swiderska, E., Strycharz, J., Wroiblewski, A., Szemraj, J., Drzewoski, J., Sliwinska, A. (2018). Role of PI3K/AKT pathway in insulin-mediated glucose uptake. *Blood Glucose Levels*, 1, 1-18.

Taleb, A., Ahmad, K. A., Ihsan, A. U., Qu, J., Lin, N., Hezam, K. (2018). Antioxidant effects and mechanism of silymarin in oxidative stress induced cardiovascular diseases. *Biomedicine & Pharmacotherapy*, 102, 689-698.

Ullah, H., Khan, H. (2018). Anti-Parkinson potential of silymarin: Mechanistic insight and therapeutic standing. *Frontiers in Pharmacology*, 9, 422.

Valkova, V., Duranova, H., Bilcikova, J., Haban, M. V. (2021). Milk thistle (Silybum marianum): a valuable medicinal plant with several therapeutic purposes. *Journal of Microbiology, Biotechnology and Food Sciences*, 2021, 836-843.

Voroneanu, L., Nistor, I., Dumea, R., Apetrii, M., Covic, A. (2016). Silymarin in type 2 diabetes mellitus: a systematic review and meta-analysis of randomized controlled trials. *Journal of Diabetes Research*, 2016, 5147468.

Wu, J. W., Lin, L. C., Tsai, T. H. (2009). Drug–drug interactions of silymarin on the perspective of pharmacokinetics. *Journal of Ethnopharmacology*, 121(2), 185-193.

Zhu, R., Wang, Y., Zhang, L., Guo, Q. (2012). Oxidative stress and liver disease. *Hepatology Research*, 42(8), 741-749.

Zimmet, P., Alberti, K., Shaw, J. (2001). Global and societal implications of the diabetes epidemic. *Nature*, 414(6865), 782-787.

Chapter 28

Curcumin in Diabetes Management: Nanotechnological Approaches for Bioavailability Improvement

Ashutosh Shukla[1,*]
Anupamaa Shukla[1]
Parjanya Kumar Shukla[1]
Sanjay Kumar[2]
Mahendra Singh Ashawat[2]
Tarun Kumar[2]
Shavinder Kumari[2]
Ajay Kumar[2]
C. P. S. Verma[2]
Rinu Rana[2]
and Keshav Dhiman[2]
[1]Krishnarpit Institute of Pharmacy, Prayagraj, Uttar Pradesh, India
[2]Laureate Institute of Pharmacy, Kathog, Jawalaji, Himachal Pradesh, India

Abstract

In recent times, diabetes has emerged as a significant global health concern, with a growing number of people suffering from this disease, and its prevalence is steadily increasing. Furthermore, diabetes can have

* Corresponding Author's Email: ashutosh.shukla96@gmail.com.

In: Naturally Occurring Chemicals …
Editors: A. Singh Grewal, G. Deswal, A. Kumar Dhingra et al.
ISBN: 979-8-89113-491-1

devastating consequences. Plant-based medicines have gained significant attention for their potential in preventing and managing Type 2 Diabetes Mellitus (T2DM), according to recent surveys. Within the scientific community, among the various herbal remedies, curcumin, an active component derived from turmeric, has shown substantial promise in the treatment of Type 2 DM. In both Ayurveda and traditional Chinese medicine systems, turmeric (Curcuma longa), obtained from the rhizomes of a biennial plant belonging to the ginger family, has been used for diabetes treatment for an extensive period. Curcumin, a bioactive compound found in turmeric, possesses numerous physiological and medicinal properties, including antioxidant capabilities, anti-inflammatory effects, and potential activity against cancer and diabetes. Due to its diverse physiological and pharmacological properties, including antimicrobial activity, antidiabetic properties, antiviral effects, and anticancer activities, curcumin exhibits significant potential in both preventing and managing various health disorders. The mechanisms through which curcumin exerts its effects on various molecular pathways are attributed to its unique chemical structure, enabling it to target a wide range of molecular sites. This chapter aims to comprehensively explore the physiological activities of curcumin and its modes of action in reducing the risks associated with T2DM and its complications.

Keywords: diabetes mellitus, curcumin, turmeric, *Curcuma longa*, antidiabetic activity

Abbreviations

CATA	Catalase
DM	Diabetes mellitus
FDA	Food and Drug Administration
GDM	Gestational diabetes mellitus
Gpx	Glutathione peroxidase
HbAlc	Hemoglobin A1C
HCV	Hepatitis C virus
HPV	Human papillomavirus
HSV-1	Herpes simplex virus
HuNoV	Human norovirus
IGT	Impaired Glucose Tolerance
IMPDH	Inosine-mono phosphate dehydrogenase

Ng	Nanogram
Nm	Nanometer
SODs	Superoxide dismutases
T2 DM	Type 2 diabetes mellitus.

Introduction

Diabetes is a complex and chronic condition characterized by the body's inability to produce or effectively utilize insulin, resulting in disturbances in the metabolism of various macromolecules, including carbohydrates, fats, and proteins (Mancia et al., 2018). It has become one of the most prevalent chronic diseases globally and is steadily increasing in both numbers and significance. This rise can be attributed to lifestyle changes that have led to reduced physical activity and an increase in obesity (Shaw et al., 2019). Diabetes is essentially a metabolic disorder that results from a defect in the secretion, action, or both of insulin, leading to persistent hyperglycemia. This hyperglycemia, in turn, triggers metabolic abnormalities in macromolecules due to insulin's crucial role as an anabolic hormone (Kharroubi et al., 2015). There are three major types of diabetes: type 1 diabetes (T1DM), type 2 diabetes (T2DM), and gestational diabetes (GDM) (Artasensi et al., 2020). According to the World Health Organization, approximately 311 million people worldwide are affected by T2DM, and this number continues to rise, especially in developing and low-income countries in Asia and elsewhere. It's important to note that as of now, T2DM is considered non-curable. However, it can be managed and prevented through various strategies, with a common approach involving the lifelong use of anti-diabetes medications (Chuengsmarn et al., 2012). Individuals with T2DM are at a heightened risk of various complications associated with the condition, and these complications can even lead to premature mortality (Olokaba et al., 2012).

Curcumin

This compound is chemically known as diferuloylmethane and is a primary constituent of the food flavoring agent turmeric. Turmeric is obtained from the rhizomes of the biennial East Indian plant Curcuma longa, which belongs to the ginger family, Zingiberaceae. It is a perennial plant native to Southeast Asia. Turmeric contains three major curcuminoids: curcumin, demethoxycurcumin, and bisdemethoxycurcumin (Figure 1), with curcumin being the primary ingredient. Curcumin makes up about 2-5% of the plant's overall constituents and is responsible for the yellow color as well as most of the medicinal properties of turmeric (Chattopadhyay et al., 2004). Turmeric has played important roles in traditional medicine systems such as Ayurveda. It has been used for various purposes, including as an antioxidant, disinfectant, pain reliever, treatment for malaria, and anti-inflammatory agent (Aggarwal et al., 2007). In dietary supplements, curcumin has been consumed for centuries and is considered pharmacologically safe (Ammon & Wahl, 1991). Turmeric, the food flavoring agent, has been employed in the management of diabetes mellitus (DM) in Ayurveda and the conventional Chinese healthcare system for a long time. Curcumin, the primary ingredient in this herb, has gained attention as a valuable therapeutic agent in experimental DM and in the management of patients with serious complications. This is mainly due to its hypoglycemic properties and its ability to reduce lipid levels in mammal models. Curcumin is also relatively affordable and considered safe (Zhang et al., 2013). The structure of curcumin consists of seven carbon linkages and three primary structural groups. Two carbonyl groups are connected by aromatic ring systems, which are phenols. Curcumin exists as a diketone tautomer, which can be found in both the enolic and keto forms. The specific form it takes depends on the pH conditions, with the bis-keto form predominating under acidic and neutral conditions, and the enol form being more prevalent at a pH above 8 (Urosevic et al., 2022).

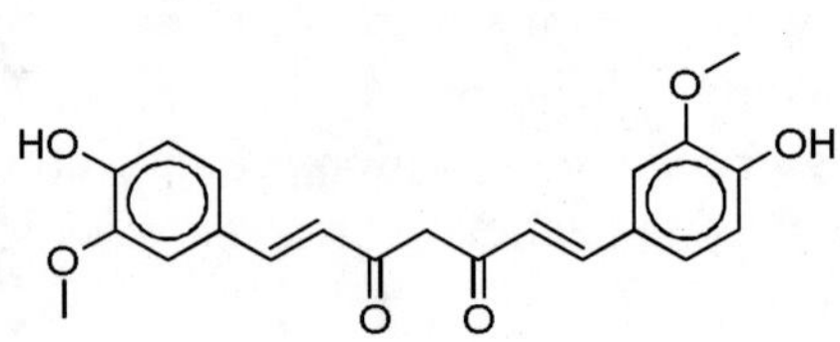

Curcumin

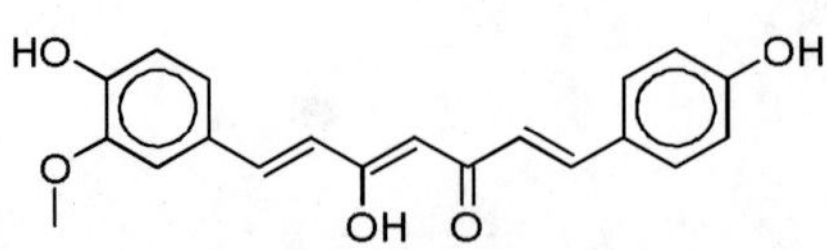

Demethoxycurcumin

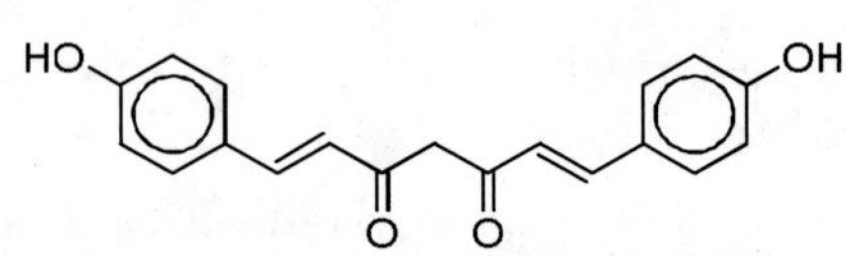

Bisdemethoxycurcumin

Figure 1. Structures of curcumin, demethoxycurcumin and bisdemethoxycurcumin.

Curcumin enjoys worldwide acceptance and is used globally in various forms for its medicinal properties. Turmeric, containing curcumin, is employed in a range of applications, including food preparation, cosmetics, coloring, antiseptic use, anti-inflammatory purposes, preservation, and as an anti-diabetic agent. It is available in different dosage forms such as solids, semi-solids, liquids, and in cosmetics preparations (Gupta et al., 2013). Turmeric-based formulations find utility in treating fresh injuries and wounds and act as counter-irritants for insect bites. Furthermore, it is used in the management of urological diseases, hepatic biliary diseases, and as an anthelminthic (Nelson et al., 2017). The United States Food and Drug Administration (USFDA) has authorized the use of curcumin and recognizes it as generally recognized as safe (GRAS). Clinical trials have demonstrated good acceptability of curcumin in patients, with safety established even at higher doses ranging from 4000 to 8000 mg/day (Basnet et al., 2011).

Use of Curcumin in T2DM

The use of curcumin, in conjunction with dietary supplements, has been shown to reduce oxidative stress in individuals with diabetes who have proteinuric CKD (chronic kidney disease), as well as in non-diabetic individuals, as demonstrated in a study conducted in Mexico. Another study has confirmed that curcumin, when administered at a considerably low dose, exhibits positive effects in Type 2 diabetes (T2DM) patients, with no reported adverse events. The study compared two groups and conducted various biological tests, including blood glucose, hemoglobin, body mass index (BMI), and a complete lipid profile test. The results of these tests showed improvements in the tested parameters in response to curcumin supplementation. Curcumin has also shown promising effects in reducing lipid levels in T2DM patients. In a study, individuals were divided into two groups and instructed to consume turmeric powder regularly for 56 days. The outcome of the study suggested that curcumin could serve as a supportive therapeutic agent to reduce the severity of diabetes, atherosclerosis, and obesity. Another report indicated that curcumin supplementation could reduce diabetes-related complications by decreasing markers of inflammation in T2DM patients. When patients were treated with 1,500 mg of curcumin daily for ten weeks, significant improvements were observed in various health parameters. A trial investigating the effects of curcumin on diabetes demonstrated that oral administration of curcumin had a beneficial impact on kidney function by significantly reducing albuminuria, making it a promising adjunctive treatment for T2DM patients, even with a modest decrease in glomerular filtration rate (GFR). The use of nano-curcumin capsules for managing T2DM patients showed potential benefits in alleviating depression and anxiety. Another clinical trial revealed that curcumin intake regulated glitazone-reverse insulin resistance receptors in peripheral blood mononuclear cells of individuals with T2DM and atherosclerotic heart disease (Marton et al., 2021).

Bioavailability of Curcumin

Curcumin is often referred to as a "wonder drug" due to its multiple identified effects, particularly its potential in managing various disorders such as diabetes. However, curcumin faces limitations in its medical application due to several factors, including its poor solubility (aqueous solubility of about 11 ng/ml), rapid metabolism, low bioavailability, and susceptibility to physiological degradation under different pH conditions. These limitations restrict its utilization in medical treatments, highlighting the need for advanced technologies to address these pharmaceutical challenges (Gupta et al., 2020). It exhibits minimal absorption in humans and is rapidly eliminated from the gastrointestinal tract when administered alone. To overcome this issue, numerous studies have explored methods to enhance the bioavailability of curcumin. One significant discovery is the use of piperine, derived from black pepper (Piper nigrum), which can increase the absorption of curcumin by up to 2000% (20 times). Piperine has been found to enhance the absorption of various substances by improving their bioavailability. Without such enhancements, even high doses of up to 4,000 mg of curcumin may be largely inactive. Scientific investigations have shown that curcumin, the active component of turmeric, is challenging to absorb and consequently has poor bioavailability. Studies have also suggested that piperine, the primary component of black pepper, enhances the absorption of poorly absorbed components. Combining both of these components with unsaturated fatty acids further enhances their absorption (Guneri, 2021).

Nanotechnology Approaches to Improve the Bioavailability of Curcumin

Nano-particles have emerged as a valuable tool in the field of nanotechnology, especially for addressing the challenges associated with the bioavailability and solubility of hydrophobic substances like curcumin. The use of nano-particles has gained significant attention in recent years due to their effectiveness in enhancing the therapeutic outcomes of encapsulated drugs. Nano-particles offer several advantages, including protection against enzymatic degradation, controlled release of drugs, prolonged circulation in the bloodstream, modification of pharmacokinetics, reduction of adverse effects, and prevention of nonspecific uptake. Numerous nano-technological approaches have been explored to improve the bioavailability of curcumin, as reported in studies (Ghalandarlaki et al., 2014). These approaches leverage nano-particles to encapsulate curcumin, thereby enhancing its solubility and bioavailability. This innovative use of nanotechnology holds great promise for improving the effectiveness of curcumin-based treatments and expanding its therapeutic applications.

Liposomes

Liposomal vesicles have wide-ranging applications, spanning from pharmaceuticals to cosmetics, and they play a significant role in facilitating the transfer of various nanomaterials. These vesicles typically exhibit a spherical shape and consist of phospholipids and steroids, with sizes ranging from 50 to 450 nanometers. Liposomal vesicles serve as excellent delivery systems, mimicking cellular structures and offering perishable yet precise compositions. In pharmaceuticals and cosmetics, liposomal vesicles find extensive use due to their ability to encapsulate and deliver substances effectively. Their round shape and composition make them versatile carriers for a variety of therapeutic and cosmetic compounds. Liposomal vesicles have a pivotal role in enhancing the bioavailability and targeted delivery of substances in these fields (Quispe et al., 2022).

Polymeric Micelles

These nanoformulations typically feature smaller sizes, often below 100 nm, and consist of amphiphilic co-polymers that form their essential outer structure. The chosen drug is typically enclosed within the hydrophobic core of these nanoformulations. This encapsulation serves the purpose of slowing down drug release and facilitating its delivery to the specific target site or tissue (Quispe et al., 2022).

Conjugate Structures

Conjugate structures involve the formation of a complex through covalent linkages between two or more substances. In the case of curcumin, conjugation to water-soluble polymers and tiny particles has been found to significantly improve its bioavailability and bioaccumulation when administered orally (Ghoran et al., 2022).

Nano Gels

Nano gels are a method in which substances are linked together using water-soluble polymer enzymes, resulting in structures with sizes typically ranging up to 200 nm. The unique feature of nano gels is their biological absorption through receptor-mediated endocytosis, making them effective for delivering active ingredients (Grimaudo et al., 2019; Idoudi et al., 2022).

Conclusion

T2DM is a complex health issue affecting a significant number of people worldwide. Its treatment involves lifestyle changes, a focus on a healthy diet, physical activity, and lifelong medical care with medications. Curcumin, as a natural anti-inflammatory and potential antidiabetic agent, presents a safe and cost-effective option for addressing this condition. However, more extensive and rigorously controlled clinical research is needed to establish the role of curcumin in the medical treatment of T2DM.

References

Aggarwal, B. B., Sundaram, C., Malani, N., Ichikawa, H. (2007). Curcumin: the Indian solid gold. *Advances in Experimental Medicine and Biology*, 595, 1–75.

Ammon, H. P., Wahl, M. A. (1991). Pharmacology of Curcuma longa. *Planta Medica*, 57(1), 1–7.

Araújo, C. C., Leon, L. L. (2001). Biological activities of Curcuma longa L. *Memorias do Instituto Oswaldo Cruz*, 96(5), 723–728.

Artasensi, A., Pedretti, A., Vistoli, G., Fumagalli, L. (2020). Type 2 diabetes mellitus: a review of multi-target drugs. *Molecules*, *25*(8), 1987.

Basnet, P., Basnet, S. N. (2011). Curcumin: An anti-inflammatory molecule from a curry spice on the path to cancer treatment. *Molecules*, 16, 4567–4598.

Chattopadhyay, I., Biswas, K., Bandyopadhyay, U., Banerjee, R. K. (2004). Turmeric and curcumin: biological actions and medicinal applications. *Current Science*, 87, 44–50.

Chuengsmarn, S., Rattanamongkolgul, S., Luenchapudiporn, R., Phisalaphong, C., Jirawatnotai, S. (2012). Curcumin extract for prevention of type 2 diabetes. *Diabetes Care*, 35, 2121–2127.

Ghalandarlaki, N., Alizadeh, A. M., Ashkani-Esfahani, S. (2014). Nanotechnology-applied curcumin for different diseases therapy. *BioMed Research International*, 2014, 394264.

Ghoran, S. H., Calcaterra, A., Abbasi, M., Taktaz, F., Nieselt, K., Babaei, E. (2022). Curcumin-based nanoformulations: a promising adjuvant towards cancer treatment. *Molecules*, *27*(16), 5236.

Grimaudo, M. A., Concheiro, A., Lorenzo, C. A. (2019). Nanogel for regenerative medicine. *Journal of Controlled Release*, 313, 148–160.

Guneri, N. (2021). A review on turmeric (Curcuma longa L.) and usage in seafood. *Marine Science and Technology Bulletin*, 10(1), 71–84.

Gupta, S. C., Patchva, S., Aggarwal, B. B. (2013). Therapeutic roles of curcumin: lessons learned from clinical trials. *AAPS Journal*, 15, 195–218.

Gupta, T., Singh, J., Kaur, S., Sandhu, S., Singh, G., Kaur, I. P. (2020). Enhancing bioavailiability and stability of curcumin using solid lipid nanoparticles (CLEN): a convenant for its effectiveness. *Frontiers in Bioengineering and Biotechnology*, 8, 879.

Hewlings, S. J., Kalman D. S. (2017). Curcumin: a review of its' effects on human health. *Foods*, 6(10), 92.

Idoudi, S., Bedhiaf, T., Hijji, Y. M., Billa N. (2022). Curcumin and Derivatives in Nanoformulations with Therapeutic Potential on Colorectal Cancer. *AAPS PharmSciTech*, 23, 115.

Jurenka J. S. (2009). Anti-inflammatory properties of curcumin, a major constituent of Curcuma longa: a review of preclinical and clinical research. *Alternative Medicine Review*, 14(2), 141–153.

Kharroubi, A. T., Darwish, H. M. (2015). Diabetes mellitus: The epidemic of the century. *World Journal of Diabetes*, 6(6), 850–867.

Lao, C. D., Ruffin, M. T., Normolle, D., Heath, D. D., Murray, S. I., Bailey, J. M., Boggs, M. E., Crowell, J., Rock, C., Brenner, D. (2006). Dose escalation of a curcuminoid formulation. *BMC Complementary and Alternative Medicine*, 6, 10.

Mancia, S. R., Trujillo, J., Chaverri, J. P. (2018). Utility of curcumin for the treatment of diabetes mellitus: Evidence from preclinical and clinical studies. *Journal of Nutrition & Intermediary Metabolism*, 9, 29–41.

Marton, L. S., Pescinini-e-Selzedas, L. L., Carnargo, M. E. S., Barbalho, S. M., Haber, J. F. S., Sinatora, R. V., Detregiachi, C. R. P., Girio, R. J. S., Buchaim, D. V., Bueno, P. C. S. (2021). The effects of curcumin on diabetes mellitus: a systematic review. *Frontiers in Endocrinology*, 12, 669448.

Nelson, K. M., Dahlin, J. L., Bisson, J., Graham, J., Pauli, G. F., Walters, M. A. (2017). The essential medicinal chemistry of curcumin. *Journal of Medicinal Chemistry*, 60, 1620-1637.

Olokaba, A. B., Obateru, O. A., Olokaba, L. B. (2012). Type 2 diabetes mellitus: a review of current trends. *Oman Medical Journal*, 27(4), 269–273.

Pandey, A., Tripathi, P., Pandey, R., Srivatava, R., Goswami, S. (2011). Alternative therapies useful in the management of diabetes: A systematic review. *Journal of Pharmacy & Bioallied Sciences*, 3(4), 504–512.

Quispe, C., Bravo, J. H., Javed, Z., Khan, K., Raza, S., Konuskan, Z. G., Daştan, S. D., Sytar, O., Martorell, M., Rad, S. J., Calina, D. (2022). Therapeutic Applications of Curcumin in Diabetes: A Review and Perspective. *BioMed Research International*, 2022, 1375892.

Shaw, J. E., Sicree, R. A., Zimmet, P. Z. (2010). Global estimates of the prevalence of diabetes for 2010 and 2030. *Diabetes Research and Clinical Practice*, 87(1), 4–14.

Urosevic M., Nikolic L., Gajic I., Nikolic V., Dinic A., Miljkovic V. (2022). Curcumin: Biological activities and modern pharmaceutical forms. *Antibiotics*, 11(2), 135.

Wilken, R., Veena, M. S., Wang, M. B., Srivatsan, E. S. (2011). Curcumin: A review of anti-cancer properties and therapeutic activity in head and neck squamous cell carcinoma. *Molecular Cancer*, 10(1), 12.

Zhang, D. W., Fu, M., Gao, S. H., Liu, J. L. (2013). Curcumin and diabetes: a systematic review. *Evidence-Based Complementary and Alternative Medicine*, 2013, 636053.

About the Editors

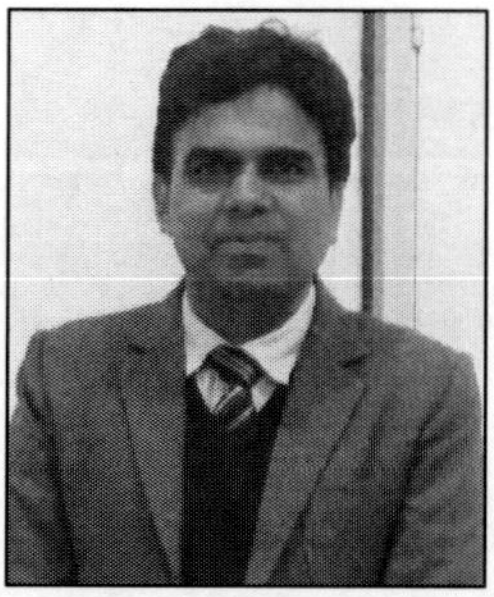

Dr. Ajmer Singh Grewal, Associate Professor, Department of Pharmaceutical Chemistry, Guru Gobind Singh College of Pharmacy, Yamuna Nagar, Haryana (India), has academic and research experience of over 11years in medicinal chemistry. His present areas of research include structure-based drug design and medicinal chemistry of MMP2 and MMP9 inhibitors as anticancer agents, antibacterial drug resistance (NDM-1), GK activators as anti-diabetic agents, AR inhibitors for diabetic complications, PPAR agonists for metabolic syndrome, multi-potent anti-Alzheimer's agents, selective PDE4 & 7 inhibitors as anti-inflammatory agents and environmental chemistry. He has written a total of 75 publications in national and international journals of repute, 9 book chapters, 4 books, and 4 design patents. He serves as a reviewer for reputed international journals published by Elsevier, Springer, Wiley, SAGE, and Frontiers. He had worked on various sophisticated analytical instruments including UV-Vis and FTIR spectrophotometer, Flash chromatography, and HPLC; and, on various chemistry softwares including ChemSketch, ChemDraw, and Marvin Sketch; Open Babel and Frog2 for structure optimization; PyMOL for molecular graphics, Glide (Schrodinger), AutoDock, AutoDock Vina, Discovery Studio (Dassault), Omega and Open Eye for in silico molecular docking studies.

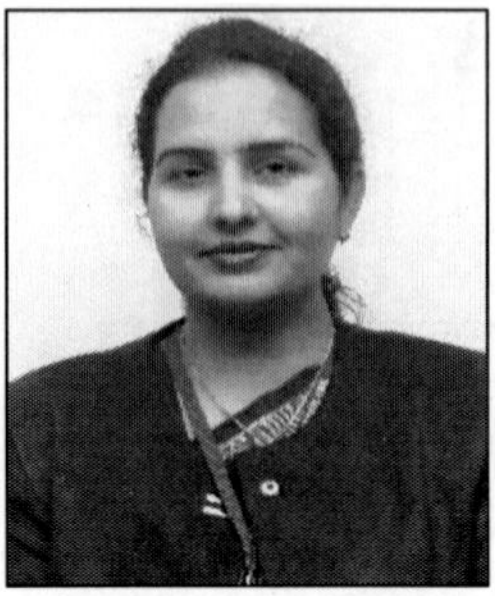

Dr. Geeta Deswal is presently working as Professor (Pharmacognosy) at Guru Gobind Singh College of Pharmacy, Yamuna Nagar, Haryana, India. She has obtained PhD from M.M. University, Mullana, Haryana (India) in Quality Audit of Herbal Formulations. She is an expert in bioactivity-guided extraction and isolation of phytoconstituents, standardization of drugs and herbal formulations, and phytochemical screening of medicinal plants and plant tissue culture. She is also working on the formulation and evaluation of herbal products as antimicrobial agents. She has worked on HPLC, UV spectrophotometer, Soxhlet Apparatus, Clevenger Apparatus, Sonicator, Rota evaporator, and Thin Layer and Column Chromatography. She has written 30 publications in national and international journals of repute and 2 book chapters. She received the Young Achiever Award on Occasion of Pharma Vision 2K25 by Shree Balaji Books and Innovational Ambassador by MHRD Innovational Cell, AICTE, New Delhi.

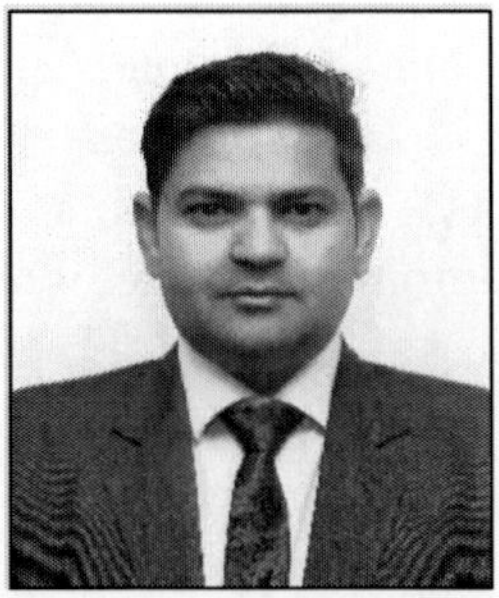

Dr. Ashwani K. Dhingra, Professor, Department of Pharmaceutical Chemistry, Guru Gobind Singh College of Pharmacy, Yamuna Nagar, Haryana (India), has academic and research experience of over 13 years in medicinal and pharmaceutical chemistry. He has completed his PhD in Pharmaceutical Sciences in the subject area of Pharmaceutical Chemistry from I.K. Gujral Punjab Technical University, Jalandhar, Punjab (India) in 2017. His present areas of research include the medicinal chemistry of antimicrobial and anti-inflammatory agents and drug discovery from natural products. He has written a total of 60 publications in national and international journals of repute, 7 book chapters, 6 books, 10 design patents, 8 copyrights and various poster presentations at several conferences (both national and international). He serves as a reviewer for reputed international journals published by Elsevier, Springer, Wiley, and SAGE with the status "Bentham Ambassador" from 2019 to 2022. He was awarded "Highly Cited Research" in Fitoterapia by Elsevier. He is a life member of APTI. He had worked on various sophisticated analytical instruments including UV-Visible spectrophotometer, and HPLC.

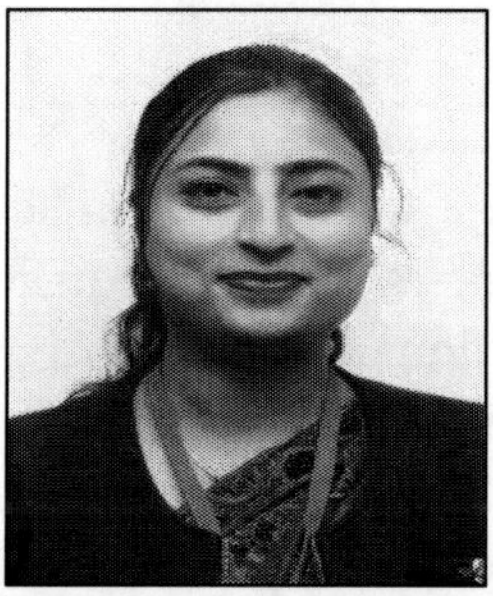

Dr. Priyanka Kriplani is presently working as a Professor at Guru Gobind Singh College of Pharmacy, Yamuna Nagar. Her field of specialization is Pharmaceutics. She received her PhD from I.K Gujral Punjab Technical University, Jalandhar in 2019 and has done her M. Pharmacy in Pharmaceutical Sciences from Rajiv Academy for Pharmacy, Mathura. Her research areas include the pulsatile drug delivery system, transdermal drug delivery system, and novel herbal drug delivery system. Before joining this institute, she worked as an Assistant Professor at Chaudhary Devi Lal College of Pharmacy, Yamunanagar. She has 30 research/review publications in journals, 3 design patents, 2 book chapters and 8 copyrights to her credit. She has guided 5 M. Pharmacy students and is currently guiding 3 M. Pharmacy students and 1 PhD student. She has completed 2 consultancy projects from Indswell Ayurveda. She is also a Fellow/Life member of APTI and the Indian Pharmacy Graduates Association, New Delhi.

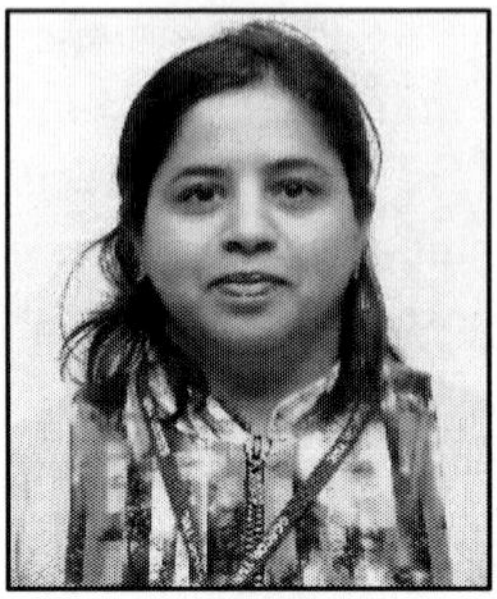

Dr. Bhawna Chopra, Professor, Department of Pharmaceutical Chemistry, Guru Gobind Singh College of Pharmacy, Yamuna Nagar, Haryana (India), has academic and research experience of 13+ years in medicinal and pharmaceutical chemistry. She completed her PhD in Pharmaceutical Sciences in the subject area of Pharmaceutical Chemistry from I.K. Gujral Punjab Technical University, Jalandhar, Punjab (India) in 2018. Her present areas of research include the medicinal chemistry of antimicrobial and anti-inflammatory agents and drug discovery from natural products. She has written a total of 55 publications in national and international journals of repute, 5 book chapters, 5 books, 8 design patents, 10 copyrights and various poster presentations at several conferences (both national and international). She serves as a reviewer for reputed international journals published by Elsevier, Springer, Wiley, and SAGE with the status "Bentham Ambassador" from 2019 to 2022. She was awarded "Highly Cited Research" in Fitoterapia by Elsevier. She is a life member of the Association of Pharmaceutical Teachers of India.

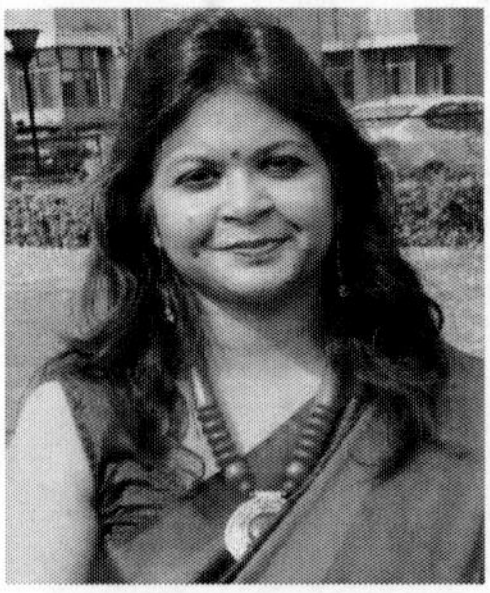

Dr. Shikha Baghel Chauhan is presently working as an Associate Professor (Pharmaceutics) at Amity Institute of Pharmacy, Amity University, Noida,

Uttar Pradesh (India). She is a self-motivated and passionate academic with more than 12 years of experience in teaching and 4 years of experience in the Pharmaceutical Industry. She has obtained her PhD from Amity University, Noida, Uttar Pradesh (India) in pharmaceutical sciences. She has extensive knowledge of functions related to regulatory affairs, product development, laboratory operations, and documentation. She took the academics profession due to her passion for teaching and her quest of learning. She likes to learn new technology and try to keep herself updated. Her areas of research are Novel Drug Delivery system, Transdermal Drug Delivery System, Floating Drug Delivery System, and In Situ Drug Delivery system. She has written a total of 35 publications in national and international journals of repute and 3 book chapters. She had been on the panel of reviewers for various prestigious journals (Elsevier, Springer, Taylor & Francis, etc.).

Index

A

B

N

O

P

Q

R

S

T